THE INFANT AND FAMILY
IN THE TWENTY-FIRST CENTURY

The Mentor Series

Consulting Editors:

J. Gerald Young and Pierre Ferrari

Book Series of the
International Association for Child and Adolescent Psychiatry
and Allied Professions
IACAPAP

Gomes-Pedro, Nugent, Young, and Brazelton
The Infant and Family in the Twenty-First Century

THE INFANT AND FAMILY IN THE TWENTY-FIRST CENTURY

edited by

João Gomes-Pedro
J. Kevin Nugent
J. Gerald Young
T. Berry Brazelton

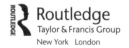

Routledge
Taylor & Francis Group
New York   London

Published in 2002 by
Routledge
Taylor & Francis Group
711 Third Avenue, New York,
NY 10017

Published in Great Britain by
Routledge
2 Park Square, Milton Park, Abingdon,
Oxfordshire OX14 4RN

First issued in paperback 2014

Routledge is an imprint of the Taylor and Francis Group, an informa business

Cover Design: Jen Crisp
Cover Image: Corbis

Library of Congress Cataloging-in-Publication Data
The infant and family in the 21st century / edited by João Gomes-Pedro . . . [et al.].
   p. cm.
   Includes bibliographical references and index.
   ISBN 978-0-415-93391-9 (hbk)
   ISBN 978-0-415-86092-5 (pbk)
   1. Infants—Congresses. 2. Parent and infant—Congresses. 3. Maternal and infant
welfare—Congresses. 4. Family—Congresses. I. Gomes-Pedro, João.

HQ774 .I5284 2002
305.232—dc21   2002018315

CONTENTS

INTRODUCTION AND DEDICATION FOR THE MENTOR SERIES

This is the first volume in a new series that will feature books by distinguished invited authors and editors in the fields of child and adolescent psychiatry and allied professions. It will also address topics of current interest, with a strong emphasis on education and dissemination of the most current knowledge for clinicians.

The breadth of media available for the communication of knowledge of all kinds is a gift to future generations, but it also carries with it the problem of selection. What is a busy clinician to read in order to bring the best of current professional knowledge to patients seeking help? The editors of the series and the Executive Committee of the International Association for Child and Adolescent Psychiatry and Allied Professions (IACAPAP) made the decision to use their combined wisdom periodically to select individuals and topics that might bring important new understanding of a topic, presented with clarity in an attractive and well-organized manner, to professionals caring for children and families across the world. With this first volume, and its many illustrious authors, we initiate this effort.

It is fitting that we dedicate The Mentor Series to a child and adolescent psychiatrist who was mentor and profound teacher to so many of his own and later generations, Donald J. Cohen, M.D. Dr. Cohen was Director of the Yale Child Study Center and Irving B. Harris Professor of Child Psychiatry, Pediatrics, and Psychology at the Yale University School of Medicine. He was also Chief of Child Psychiatry, Children's Hospital at Yale-New Haven. He was Past President of the International Association for Child and Adolescent Psychiatry and Allied Professions at the time of his death on October 2, 2001. His professional work encompassed multiple disciplines, and he was equally comfortable in his roles as psychoanalyst and neuroscientist. Professor Cohen brought to our professions the gift of an honest appraisal of the worth of data and concepts, notably free of the biased allegiance to a narrow perspective that too often afflicts us. Above all, he was a caring, insightful, and empathic clinician who had a flair for pragmatically matching pieces of his broad knowledge to a patient's needs at a given moment.

With all of these comments about his achievements, the dedication of The Mentor Series should not neglect a nodal point of Dr. Cohen's life work, his capacity for rapid, elegant, and unusually informative writing. Those of us who had the pleasure to work closely with him have embedded in our memories the picture of Donald typing as rapidly as possible, the ideas leaping over each other to the paper or computer screen—teaching us as he did so. Where did this passion to communicate so clearly and persuasively come from? I would suggest that Hemingway understood the roots of such writing very well: "Writers are forged in injustice as a sword is forged" (1935/1987, p. 71).

Dr. Cohen had a passion for caring for those whom misfortune had visited, and he knew how to do so with dignity and a wonderful humor, so that he did not slip into the righteousness that would make it easy to ignore him. His obituary in *The Economist* (October 20, 2001, p. 82) portrayed Donald well: "Curious, ebullient and ever the optimist, Dr. Cohen liked to reach out to damaged children and draw them back into the fold of normality." But, beneath these very adult qualities was something quite natural and basic, captured perhaps by the words of someone more likely to have been quoted by Donald than Hemingway—"the Rav," the distinguished rabbi known and admired by Donald and his wife, Phyllis, in their early days together:

> The great man whose intellect has been raised to a superior level through the study of Torah, gifted with well-developed, overflowing powers—depth, scope, sharpness—should not be viewed as totally adult . . . he remains the young and playful child, naive curiosity, natural enthusiasm, eagerness and spiritual restfulness have not abandoned him. Only the child with his simple faith and fiery enthusiasm can make the miraculous leap into the bosom of God. (Soloveitchik, 1974, cited in Sokol, 1997, p. 133)

J. Gerald Young, M.D.
Editor-in-Chief

Pierre Ferrari, M.D.
Editor

☐ References

Hemingway, E. (1987). *Green hills of Africa*. New York: Charles Scribner. (Original work published 1935)

Soloveitchik, J. B. (1974). "Ger ve-Toshav Anokhi": Modernity and traditionalism in the life and thought of Rabbi Joseph B. Soloveitchik. In M. D. Angel (Ed.), *Exploring the thought of Rabbi Joseph B. Soloveitchik* (p. 133). Hoboken, NJ: KTAV Publishing House.

PREFACE AND DEDICATION

Knowledge is power, but it is also true that knowledge is powerless if not applied. This book presents major themes developed by investigators regarding the optimal development of infants and families. These professionals from across the world met on several occasions during the 1990s to review and refine the most significant current knowledge concerning infants, and to identify significant themes emerging from this research. We now have well-substantiated data that can guide our efforts to aid infants and families, from the immediate caregiving of a mother to government policy decisions concerning children. Regrettably, the knowledge available about the specific conditions favoring the development of a child has been left substantially unapplied, so collecting this evidence, and presenting the resulting recommendations, is the purpose of this volume.

The book stands in recognition of, and in opposition to, the neglect of child care initiatives at every level, initiatives that could be undertaken if individuals and policy-making bodies had the courage and the will to do so. The book makes clear that there is both general knowledge and a plethora of data to guide our research and clinical efforts. The application of the well-documented knowledge presented here by clinicians, parents, and policymakers has begun, but the pace of these activities needs to be accelerated. This first volume of The Mentor Series, makes this knowledge available to child and adolescent psychiatrists and psychologists, pediatricians, nurses, social workers, teachers, and other clinical professionals concerned with the mental health and development of children. These professionals have contact with parents and other caregivers who create children's environments every day, so it is an essential first step toward the concrete application of this knowledge. It is our hope that the book will also be useful to day care administrators and agency administrators searching for policies that will enable children to develop in optimal ways.

For children, knowledge about their needs is not yet power, but we propose that the presentation of increasingly compelling data, in a form useful to clinicians and administrators, will help accelerate the transfer of power. As we do so, we recall with fondness and admiration a former President of the International Association for Child and Adolescent Psychiatry and Allied Professions, Professor Serge Lebovici. Professor Lebovici was Emeritus Professor of Child Psychiatry, University of Paris-Nord. There is a special pleasure in dedicating to Professor Lebovici this volume, which describes the care of infants and families, because it contains so many concepts and practices that were inherent in his every activity as a clinician. Serge did not wait for neuroscientists and geneticists to forge ahead with their elegant investigations. He anticipated many of their findings through his meticulous attention to every detail of the baby's behavior, and, especially, to each element of the interaction of the baby with its mother and father. All of us privileged to know and work with him professionally across the years vividly recall his early use of videotapes to capture what really happens when mother and infant dance their dance of love and fun—or of missed signals and confusion. The details of our neuroscience understanding of an infant's growing understanding of the world around him—how he or she learns to discriminate what is significant in the environment, with the vital help of his or her mother, and to store it in the early memory prototypes that will guide the infant through development—these are the microscopic details that Professor Lebovici focused our clinical attention on, so that we could understand how the mother was guiding the infant's emerging understanding of, and adaptation to, the enchanting world around him or her.

In order to conjure a vivid picture of Professor Lebovici for those who did not know him during his many years of superb contributions to children and their families, we might turn to another Preface to gather a sense of the purposefulness that characterized his many books, which were gifts to his colleagues from a man who was a leader in psychoanalysis, a model in clinical child and adolescent psychiatry, and a warmly remembered friend:

> So long as there shall exist, by reason of law and custom, a social condemnation, which, in the face of civilisation, artificially creates hells on earth, and complicates a destiny that is divine, with human fatality; so long as the three problems of the age—the degradation of man by poverty, the ruin of woman by starvation, and the dwarfing of childhood by physical and spiritual night—are not solved; so long as, in certain regions, social asphyxia shall be possible; in other words, and from a yet more extended point of view, so long as ignorance and misery remain on earth, books like this cannot be useless. (Hugo, 1909, p. 3)

João Gomes-Pedro
J. Kevin Nugent
J. Gerald Young
T. Berry Brazelton

☐ Reference

Hugo, V. (1909). Preface. In *Les Misérables* (p. 3). New York: Everyman's Library Alfred A. Knopf.

☐ Acknowledgments

The preparation of a book involves a cooperative spirit among many who contributed to its production, far beyond the editors whose names appear at the beginning. The pleasure of working with so many distinguished and patient colleagues, who gave their energy, time, and, most important, wisdom and vast knowledge, will not be forgotten. We are grateful to them for this joint effort to help the infants and families of the future. With a similar sense of gratitude, we thank the Executive Committee of the International Association for Child and Adolescent Psychiatry and Allied Professions (IACAPAP) for this opportunity to bring together the work of so many colleagues working in disparate fields, all of which bring aid to infants and mothers. The President of IACAPAP, Professor Helmut Remschmidt, the Treasurer, Professor Myron Belfer, and the Secretary-General, Professor Ian Goodyer, gave patient and consistent support to the production of this book, for which we are very grateful. Dr. Larry Maayan provided a generously meticulous reading of the manuscript, resulting in significant increase in its clarity. Ms. Patricia Torres was invaluable in her office management activities, making the steady and organized production of the manuscript at all stages an enjoyable task, even during some tense moments. George P. Zimmar, Ph.D., Executive Editor at Brunner-Routledge, gave us his wisdom and guidance, and his notable patience, as we proceeded through the various phases of manuscript review and book production. Kenneth J. Silver, Production Editor at Brunner-Routledge, has pushed ahead in all of our mutual efforts with similar good spirits, patience, and intelligent help as we put the book into print. Finally, we thank our families, who both encouraged us in our work and bore the brunt of our absence during its preparation.

INTRODUCTION
The Infant and Family
in the Twenty-First Century

This book examines the effects of experience for infants and children growing in their families and communities, and leads to recommendations for families based upon this knowledge. Genes and environment constitute the clay from which the lives of children are molded, and experience occurs in the warm—or sometimes hot—oven which hardens the clay into a durable vessel adapted to its functions.

There was a relative neglect of genetic influences among clinical theoreticians prior to the availability of current techniques for genetic research; accordingly, there was greater emphasis on clinical discoveries describing the impact of the environment on the growing child. This perspective subsequently stimulated caution among investigators who feared too much emphasis on environmental influences; the eruption of molecular biology was a final strong corrective to this emphasis, leading to extensive research on genetic influences, and a swing among some clinicians to a decided preference for genetic explanations of the behavior of children. However, the time is now ripe for a true reconciliation and merging of these perspectives, which, after all, describe the two interacting forces propelling development in a single organ, the brain-mind. This timeliness is the result of first, the collection of a rich array of diverse research describing the cognitive, emotional, and behavioral impact of varied environmental factors on the developing child, while the second is the emerging understanding of neural mechanisms underlying the development of cognition, emotion, and behavior, which has taken place through the blossoming of the developmental and cognitive neurosciences.

Thus, this book attempts to scrutinize the child's experiences and how they mold him or her, but the accent is on how environment sculpts these experiences. This strategy is not intended to neglect genetic contributions, but to better specify predictable and enduring effects of the environment on any child, making it increasingly possible to better recognize the effects of individual differences (with a strong genetic component) in the near future. The strategy has the favorable advantage of defining factors—the impact of varying environmental influences—that can be altered and improved as families agree upon the necessity of using better methods for nurturing the development of their children. Identifying factors favorable for development is not an academic exercise then, but is very practical. This is also a very difficult step, because the simple term *environment* encompasses multiple, interacting levels of influence on a child, from the effects of the feel and odor of a mother's skin on an infant, to government policies affecting the lives of millions of children. At each step of our journey we attempt to comment on an aspect of the dawning understanding of neural mechanisms in the developing brain that illuminates our examination of childhood experiences and suggests a neuroscience basis for how we can improve the lives of children.

Where do these chapters lead us? The book begins with the dream of a man who wishes to cultivate the flowering of the accumulated twentieth-century knowledge about young children. His dream contains the themes which follow in the book, approached from varied perspectives on the development of young children, and articulated by this group of acknowledged international experts at the turn of the century. We hope to take advantage of the proliferation of professional knowledge, in order to cull from it salient recommendations for the optimal care of these children, whether by a parent, professional, or policymaker.

João Gomes-Pedro
J. Kevin Nugent
J. Gerald Young
T. Berry Brazelton

PART

I

THE FAMILY
IN THE TWENTY-FIRST
CENTURY

João Gomes-Pedro

The Child in the Twenty-First Century

Baby XXI–Child and Family: Changing Patterns at the Turn of the Century, a conference held in Lisbon, was a great challenge because it inspired everyone present to reflect seriously on the baby. Living in a time of such rapid transition and evolution, it is imperative that we now act on the dream of our hopes for *Baby XXI.*

The sense of belonging, the belief in the continuity of the search, and the quest for adventure which any searching involves: These are, for me, the forces that, although impenetrably shrouded in the mystery of life, can balance destiny and coherence on one hand, with vulnerability and risk on the other. In pronouncing this faith, I nevertheless question whether my reflections are truly scientifically based. In fact, the proponents of the dominant genetic mode, deemphasizing the contributions of experience to the baby, argue systematically against the influence of the intangible human feelings that poets know so well. And if, by chance, there exist unequivocal signals of these feelings, they are explained as the result of outside influences on the individual, purely random and, therefore, not scientific. In the first half of the twentieth century, environmentalists' arguments predominated in the behavioral sciences. Technological progress and the avalanche of applications of the scientific method that provide a gauge of progress indubitably reinforced the proponents of the pathological model in medical science. Like the explorers' adventures with so many secrets to discover, we still have many mysteries present in our everyday scientific life.

In fact, how does one dispute statistical data with a clinical judgment? How does one argue against the significant results of a multivariate analysis of variance (MANOVA) utilized with data coming from a complex methodology, when we mainly count on parental feelings revealed through our conversations? How can we balance "parental science" with the accuracy of numbers? Keeping this all in mind, how can I validate my judgment on what I dream for my "Baby XXI"? I would like to do so by drawing a parallel between my dream and those that inspired the explorers of the past. However, as in the adventures of the caravels, inspiration was not enough. Along with the dream, scientific knowledge already existed in the use of the astrolabe. It was this combination that prompted explorers to raise masts and unfurl sails.

The pediatrician writing these lines is not merely a dreamer. He also wants to bring here his experience as a clinician and an educator, as well as the results of his research, in the hope that he can leave some messages to the future. More and more, when confronted with the challenge of reflection, I recall certain memories of the past. What moralists call values and researchers call data, I prefer to call the path of a continuum. In the wake of the sailing ship, sometimes the only thing that remains is the cawing of the sea gulls who inform one of the course of a journey where the continuity between the distance already covered and that which remains to be navigated is recognized, although not measured. More and more, I feel that it is in recognizing this continuity that we discover our competence, much like the navigator who finally sees land on the distant horizon.

The stories of my childhood are like the sea gulls who hover over the wake of the sailing ships. They come and go, come and go, as reminders of mysteries. I loved the stories my grandmother used to tell me about my great-grandparents, and my great-great-grandparents, about friends of my great-uncles, and about the vineyards and marshes where they worked, and which they loved. In all of them, Mr. Manuel is very often present in my memories. Mr. Manuel was a mason, working from dawn to dusk, who transformed rock into cut stone that could be used to make the little walls that sustained the grounds where my father planted grape vines. One day, during one of the many conversations that we had, Mr. Manuel sat on the step of the barn eating a slice of corn–wheat–rye bread, a type of rough peasant bread that today only a few shepherds are fortunate enough to taste. When I asked Mr. Manuel what that wheat–rye–corn bread tasted of—if it tasted of corn, of rye, or of wheat, or, by any chance, of the wine planted on the cold ground of the Dao—my friend Mr. Manuel answered with a phrase that reflected the philosophy of the pure: "Oh, little one, that depends on the soul of the moment."

If I were to express my fantasy for Baby XXI, I would need to be inspired in order to concentrate my mind on a happy baby, surrounded by a happy family. But what does happiness mean, especially happiness projected into the distant future? I feel my challenge here is to try to develop the techniques that enable this Baby XXI to have the happiness of prolonging his or her sense of identity and belonging, much like my own stories of youth. On my own journey, I rediscover what helped the explorers of the fifteenth century to build a dream and, later on, to transform it into reality. The course of this trip will be influenced by dreams, understood as a hope for certitude. I will embark upon a caravel that is laden with the proper instruments, which represent my knowledge. I will navigate on an ocean involving vulnerability and risk for those who sail on its waters. I will move ahead with the strength of the blowing wind, as a symbol of adaptation and change, and I will trim my sails to direct us to new discoveries. In this ambitious project, the route foretells adventure, with some of the risks already foreseen, some others unpredictable. In this adventure, I will add hope to the dream; it is through the uniting of hope with foresight that I envision a glimmer of certitude.

☐ Motivation: Building Our Dream with Creativity, Humility, and Knowledge

Along with Vasco da Gama, Columbus, Cabral, and Martin Luther King, Jr., I also have a dream. I would rather say that all of us have to have a dream. Without dreams, we do not fulfill our self-esteem, which is so crucial to our personal growth. Our dream is our strength, which must be built with creativity, humility, and knowledge.

Creativity is deeply linked to inspiration, but also to planning. Our explorers discovered new worlds five hundred years ago, inspired by dreams, a thirst for knowledge, and a hunger for discovery, all crucial elements that have forever driven people toward adventure and progress.

Together with that inspiration there also had to exist a project. The fact is that a strong political will, a desire for progress, as well as a desire for riches all enlightened and encouraged the spirit of the kings of the fifteenth century. The explorers' journeys of exploration were the keynote of a century of widening horizons, especially for Europeans. It would be Europe's particular combination of religious zeal, hard-headed acquisitiveness, and seafaring expertise that provided the necessary mixture of motivation and technical ability to accomplish this creativity and then to transform dream into reality. Although all those factors were common to several European nations, the additional factor of geographical and historical determinants explains how Portugal pioneered ocean routes. Furthermore, our heritage contains a deeply ingrained cultural script for novelty through invention and adventure.

The Muses, invented by the Greeks and sung by the poet Camões, are symbols of a past to be kept for the future. Creativity, the first component of the dream, can be seen as the Muse pushing toward the future, as in child development. In fact, creativity also has to be understood as the curiosity toward the external world that we may identify as the baby's main drive.

On the whole, if creativity is, in fact, the first drive for this progress, it has to be pursued with humility, which is, in a certain way, the motion for progress. When Vasco da Gama first arrived in India, one of his crew members was asked what on earth he was doing there. "We arrived, that's all," he said. This humility is, in my view, an essential component of a project. As a matter of unquestioned dogma, explorers of the past believed that their second duty was to dedicate their endeavors to the Creator. In the same manner, what immortalizes a scientist is his humility. So it was that Galileo, in his humility, accorded dignity to the most simple elements of nature. Discovering with a stone the notion of gravity, he established that force is not proportional to velocity, but to the change in that velocity. We revisit this concept of change later. All the formidable discoveries, identified as gifts of the Creator, are therefore embedded in attitudes of faith, which was later called basic trust by Erikson. Galileo, like the explorers, and like most of the researchers of our time, taught humanity intellectual humility as well as a basic trust in knowledge.

In our dream there is a tremendous amount of hope in human capacities and in our devotion to infancy. It is in this context that the third major element of our dream is knowledge. In fact, none of the discoveries would have been possible if only creativity and humility were involved. In terms of knowledge, what is critical is putting together in each period all the scientific data and using these in just the right proportion so that progress may be given a sense of coherence and evidence.

For the navigators of the fifteenth century, to lose sight of the coastline, particularly in the rough stormy waters of the Atlantic Ocean, was so dangerous that it was not merely a challenge that drove them. With all the familiar landmarks removed, navigation became largely a matter of guesswork. It was theoretically possible to get some idea of a vessel's north–south position by gauging the angle of the Pole Star or midday sun against the horizon. The problem was that the scholar's tool for making such a calculation, called the astrolabe, was in fact a fairly complex instrument that required tremendous expertise if it was to provide the navigator with adequate data. The angles changed slightly every day, making the use of charts indispensable, but an accurate measurement was hard to achieve when on board a pitching ship, even if the weather was favorable. In short, in the fifteenth century, navigation was a hard business in which expertise in using existing knowledge was clearly essential.

A parallel framework for this picture, in our times, lies in clinical knowledge. As a clinician, I have to use my scientific experience in order to make accurate decisions. As a clinician, too, I believe I should not be committed solely to any specific theoretical perspective, but rather should integrate perspectives from my experiences. For a clinician, however, knowledge is not only provided by clinical experience; personally, I find it very useful to add to that clinical experience my own research data and, in a very special way, the feedback from teaching.

Today we possess a tremendous amount of knowledge about the baby, especially compared to the knowledge we had little more than half a century ago. In the 1920s, behavioral research was directed at children below school age for the first time. This was done because so little was known about this group. In the 1930s, adolescence became another focus of concern for adults. This occurred after concerns arose about all the risks so prevalent during such a short period of a young person's life. It was not until the 1940s that infancy became the first pole of curiosity and investment. The great wish of professionals in different fields to have more scientific knowledge about babies and how they changed during the years made behavior and development a "must" in university curricula all over the world.

Mothers had long been recognized as an important influence on their child, and their behavior became a major subject of research. After the 1950s, the child-rearing practices of mothers started to be studied. Soon scholars "discovered" that there was also a father in the home who both directly and indirectly influenced the baby's behavior and development. The topic of parent–child interaction and the variables influencing parent behavior became priorities; in fact, the very first studies on baby behavior changed the direction and meaning of modern research in our field. The baby is, indeed, the major reality that changed the aims of professionals and researchers who dedicate their lives to the welfare of children and families in the world. The new view of the baby comes, very significantly, from the awareness of the baby's social and transactional role. Recent research about fetal behavior shows us that babies are social even before birth. In this context, they are no longer considered to be passive recipients of parental caregiving.

Human babies, genetically endowed with a capacity that ensures their survival by organizing their behavior, are able to respond adequately to sensory and social stimuli. They are capable of complex integrative behaviors and become progressively competent, interactive partners, influencing the effects of the environment on themselves. In order to be taken as a unique social partner, the human baby uses his behavior as a primary mode of communication, particularly with his parents (Nugent & Brazelton, 1989). In this context, reading and interpreting babies' signals is becoming a fundamental challenge for parents as well as for clinicians and educators, all of whom now recognize that to share these discoveries is a priority. Parents rely primarily on the intuition that we now call clinical intuition. Clinical scientists and professionals integrate that intuition with all the quantifiable data they receive before elaborating their decisions and interventions.

With this knowledge, we, like our explorers, are now able to sail far from the coast, giving Baby XXI new opportunities and showing the baby new horizons. One of these horizons is a new discovery of the sense of family, a knowledge that pushes us, in this millennial transition, toward more novelty and discovery. Taking stock of the situation, alongside the tiller of our caravel, I feel in my dream for Baby XXI the strong conviction that we must help today's parents and children (who will be parents tomorrow and grandparents in the next century) to believe in the future. This demands first and foremost that we believe in ourselves. We are aware of our risks and vulnerabilities, but we also have to believe that our difficulties are not calamities and that we may rely on hope.

In our society, children and adolescents still have few opportunities to test their caregiving skills before they have the responsibility for their first baby. Before they become parents, they certainly dream about their capacities and limitations in nurturing, but the immature and dependent human being is still an unknown for them. When the baby is finally born, parents need our support as they discover the magic of attunement or contingency already present in the baby's communicative system. Through this kind of discovery, parents begin to see that this system is infant centered, but that they, too, can learn more from their baby than they ever supposed possible. We know that the baby, in his or her own way, progressively consolidates his or her strength as a social partner by being a member of a very special group where common values are shared and respected.

There starts the dream. There starts the building of the sense of family, a process where all the members play an individual and unique role in transactions of discovery and enrichment. In the development of this system, each of the individual members influences the others and is consequently also changed. In interactive terms, partners in a dyad or in a triad are simultaneously both emitters and receivers, using turn-taking rules in the steps of their communicative game. In this way, every response represents a very significant stimulus for the partner: Doing this transforms a partnership into a communicative unit. The parent–infant dyad adds to that model a unique feature, which is that one of the members of that unit has not yet acquired spoken language. In this context, parent–infant communication includes strategies that are constantly changing according to the baby's progressive capacities, with every new emerging skill receiving more supportive feedback. Parental behavior is now acknowledged as anticipating the baby's competencies. One of the major responsibilities of clinicians and educators is to give support to these anticipatory behaviors, especially those related to the naturally evolving parent–baby intuition and those related to attentiveness in response to any unexpected or unusual behavior.

In my dream, and in my judgment, I believe we have to keep all these concepts in mind if we are to consider the newborn period a formative time that matures in parallel with the growth of the family system. In my dream for Baby XXI, I see a chance to use this period as a touch point in which parents can be assisted in their adjustment to the new member in their family system. It is part of the dream that baby and caregivers may become active participants in the two-way strategies that enable them to adapt to each other and, contingently, set the stimuli and motivation for further interaction (Brazelton, 1982). Throughout this process, each participant is also supposed to believe in the future, recognizing that it is worth trying. Nevertheless, there are risks and costs.

We face the future with knowledge, creativity, and humility. I referred to some elements of our knowledge that are supposed to transform hope into certitude. All of us, believers in the future, are the explorers of a new era. In each port, in each newly discovered land, we will represent the baby on the coat of arms of each landmark as a testimony of faith and progress.

☐ The Caravel and Identity: Social Inheritance and Cultural Identity

Several motivations were responsible for the Portuguese drive to achieve the great feats of global discovery. The Portuguese epic poem *Lusiadas*, written during the sixteenth century by Camões to honor the history of his country (especially that of the sailors), recalls the spirit that accompanied their feats—"they were men of no ordinary stature, equally at home in war and in dangers of every kind . . . achieving immortality through their illustrious exploits." There can be no doubt that the Portugal of the early fifteenth century provided a good foundation for those exploits, and that a sense of identity was a major component of that foundation.

By the term *identity,* I refer to the whole spectrum of the history of a people and its values. This identity is projected into each person through culture, carried by the social inheritance of cultural traditions. In each family, there are inherited stigmata and characteristics transmitted from generation to generation. In this transmission, the overall sense of power and pride that strengthens character and behavior is a major component of identity. In our everyday life, there are an almost infinite number of symbols that bring a plethora of characteristics to our identity. The family portrait we may have in our living room, the lullaby that we recall from our mothers and that we sing to our children or grandchildren, the way we celebrate our Christmas or Easter Sunday—each fulfills our destiny and forms our behavior.

Identity and Competence; Development and Self-Esteem

In my dream about the baby and the family living in the twenty-first century, keeping in mind the variables of vulnerability, my deepest concern is to find strategies that may strengthen individuals in terms of their cultural identity. In terms of child development, identity is deeply related to intimacy and trust, which are considered basic needs that are essential for the emergence of self-esteem and the establishment of structural relationships. Much of the research on identity development derives from Erikson's ideas. The model of stages utilized to characterize the developmental crises that emerge at different ages may be taken as one of his scientific testaments. Identity is a primary model and expression of social and affective support. The success of some guidelines for social support should be based on cultural and affective supports, conceived as organizers of a sense of belonging, which survive through beliefs and attitudes.

The clinical dimension that inspires our studies opens a new window into our spirit through which it is possible to recognize more general and eclectic perspectives. In this context, clinicians have come to recognize human development as a dynamic process influenced by determining factors both endogenous and exogenous, which, functioning together through the maturation of the central nervous system, contribute to the individual's processes of development. In this context, a goal of development is to reach a sense of competence identified as the total realization of humanness.

I see a parallel between identity and competence, as well as between development and self-esteem. Many of our strategies of intervention are based on the need to search for this sense of competence and self-esteem in the phenomenology of identity and development. In clinical terms it is relevant that the philosophy and strategies of intervention attempt to reestablish this flux of identity, which is particularly critical when specific touchpoints (as described by Brazelton) are guidelines for our intervention.

One of our intervention strategies to strengthen identity and to reduce risks in the critical perinatal period is the prenatal visit that occurs in a pediatric context. To be expecting a baby, especially the first one, is one of the most important events in a woman's life, and clearly represents a challenge to her maturity and to the structure of her personality. It is also an opportunity for new responsibilities concerning a new baby, in the face of which the woman feels, from the beginning, involved in a relationship of mutual dependence and progressive attunement. To be pregnant represents an enormous physical and psychological strain. In fact, the readjustment of various mechanisms that are responsible for the maintenance of global homeostasis in the pregnant woman consumes most of the energy during this period.

Cultural Traditions as Cultural Memories

The imaginary combines with the real to develop a new role for a woman, and this adaptation takes up most of the future mother's time. In this adaptation, cultural and family values are essential to conferring identity feelings on the mother-to-be. They also help her to guarantee her self-esteem, in terms of a continuity in her sense of competence. The most dramatic changes in the lifestyle of the woman who has become pregnant result from the awareness that she has stopped being a girl (who is basically responsible for herself) and begun assuming the responsibility for her baby. A sharing of responsibility is also progressively assumed by the couple, to the extent that both become aware of the division of their time and attention with another person—real, even if not yet present—in their world of verbal communication.

Prenatal interviews led us in the past to interpret a mother's anxiety, especially intense during the last month of pregnancy, as a pathological condition. However, this can now be understood in a different light. Indeed, these reactions of anxiety and fear may act as a sort of shock treatment that contributes positively to the reorganization of the woman in the face of her new role. This adaptation demands a quick adjustment to the baby, with whom the mother is not yet completely familiar. In this context, the roles of both the obstetrician and the pediatrician are fundamentally those of giving support during this adjustment, as well as during the development of the needed identity and trust. It is on this basis that the prenatal visit is confirmed by a large number of pediatricians as a priceless endeavor to capture all the potential of the process of "becoming a family," particularly in families at risk.

In very little time a pediatrician, or a family doctor, is able to start a significant relationship with parents-to-be. These opportunities reduce the stress of new parenthood, facilitate the development of more secure attachments, and confer identity. It should be emphasized, in this context, that in Portugal, as in many other countries, some patterns of child care face the risk of being discarded as cultural standards. One example of this is the failure to continue breast-feeding. In fact, after a full 100% at birth, we found the rate falling to 23% of mothers who were breast-feeding at 3 months. Another pattern related to identity is the fall in the continuity of the father's presence at the health visits. Using 15- to 20-minute interviews with both parents-to-be, we observed a significant change in two patterns of parental behavior in a middle-class Portuguese sample. Examining breast-feeding, 74% of the mothers who came to a prenatal visit were still breast-feeding their babies at 4 months. This compared to 18% of the control group (Gomes-Pedro et al., 1988). Similarly, 74% of the fathers who participated in a prenatal visit came in at least four times for their baby's routine visits during the first year of their infant's life. Only 23% of those fathers belonging to the control group did the same. Intervention through facilitation of identity formation may mean, in fact, the building of a new caravel able to cross new boundaries into the still unknown sea of a new century.

☐ The Sea and Vulnerability: Environment and Risk Factors

The sea at the time of the global discoveries represented not only the unknown, but also the fear of the infinite, the terror of depths, the imminent danger. In fact, in those times, there were few survivors, and there was a greater chance of drowning than of returning home. The great Portuguese poets sang dramatically about the sea, and even today, in the fishing ports along the coast, one breathes a sea-oriented culture. In my construction of the dream of Baby XXI, I consider vulnerability one of its fundamental components, and, metaphorically, I identify it with the sea. It is not the sea, however, that is vulnerable. Rather, the sea makes those who travel on it vulnerable beings, through the risks involved. In this perspective, risk is associated with vulnerability. In the case of the child, the characteristics of the sea are comparable to the environment (especially the family and other social environments). It is this identification of vulnerability that I will describe. This is necessary to conceptualize the interventions that are indispensable if we are to be able to support the child and the family of the twenty-first century. (By "support," I mean intervention so that they may feel happy and capable when they reflect on their future.)

Using a strict biomedical model, children are, at the end of this century, healthier than before. However, most scholars and clinicians consider this statement to be false in reality. Zuckerman, Weitzman, and Alpert (1988) wrote that American children are at risk "because of high rates of poverty, divorce, single parent households, chronic illness, school failure, teenage pregnancy, drug abuse, suicide, homicide, injuries and problems related to learning and behavior." Many other authors have written papers about the turmoil of children and families living under the stressful conditions that pervade the environment in our modern society (Arnold, 1990). Weak attachment processes, family discord, and violence are some of the other adverse conditions reported that support the argument that humans are increasingly vulnerable and at risk. The lives of our children, and I would say our own lives as well, are increasingly threatened by multiple menaces that undermine both general well-being and the family structure. Today, during the transition to a new millennium, and in spite of all the progress already made, a black cloud hovers over the lives of children throughout the world.

The Neglect of Children's Developmental Needs

Worthy of mention here is the fact that, despite the diminishing involvement of superpower military might, there are still too many bloody conflicts on our planet. The cost of the military equipment used in these conflicts is about $150 billion. This $150 billion would be more than sufficient to end poverty in the world. The last UNICEF Report, dedicated to the status of infancy in the world, estimated that an additional $25 billion per year is still necessary to guarantee protection for children around the world. In comparative terms, this sum is less than the cost of a Japanese motorway built to connect Tokyo to Kobe, is about equal to the price of the new airport in Hong Kong, and is much less than the amounts Europeans spend to drink wine and Americans spend to drink beer on an annual basis (UNICEF, 1996). A reversal of priorities may save the almost 50,000 children who die every day throughout the world, victims of dehydration and other easily preventable diseases. Each one of these deaths represents the physical death of a child. However, it is also the death of a future and the death of a hope for a family, as well as for a whole community.

The first right mentioned in the Convention on the Rights of Children (by which all countries must abide) is that "Men must assure, to the maximum possible, the survival as well as the development of children" (United Nations 1991 Convention on the Rights of the Child). There exists, however, a real ambiguity and inconsistency between what the United Nations signs and promises, and the reality of daily existence for the infant. One expression of this reality is apparent in the exploitation of the child. At different ages, the child appears in the media as an instrument of marketing, publicity, and political strategies. This contrasts with the infrequency with which the child is presented in true dimension as a child with developmental needs, evoking the respect and moral investment of all social partners. Child vulnerability sails with us in our caravel. All children are vulnerable. The problem of the balance of the child's developmental progress lies in the packaging, the structure of this vulnerability. Therefore, the evolving influences on each baby make all the difference. Of those factors, the family is the critical one.

Changing Family Structures Requires New Adaptive Patterns by Children: Attachment and Stress

In terms of structure, the family is changing very rapidly in Western cultures. The traditional family is disappearing, and this fact should be a concern for politicians as well as for professionals. Today there are many single-parent families. There are also couples who, while not divorcing, experience stress related to maladaptation. There are new families constituted by homosexuals, both male and female, who adopt babies and live according to a new model. Finally, accompanying these structural changes, and the decrease in the size of families, there are progressively fewer opportunities for children of both sexes to learn about parenting during their youth. In the same context, the emphasis on mothering as a primary role of females is reduced to a second priority. Every day new sources of interest rarely related to home and child care emerge for girls. It is hard for young mothers to combine mothering and working, causing a decrease in self-esteem. In addition to these patterns of change, the greater mobility of families means that relatives are less likely to be available as sources of parenting wisdom. Parents feel poorly prepared, and their behavior when responding to the needs of their sons and daughters reflects this. This behavior reflects the stress that society evokes in them in their parenting roles. Stress is, in fact, a major determinant of vulnerability.

Stress is exemplified by spending almost one quarter of a day in an overcrowded transportation system. It is manifested by parents and children who are faced with the abrupt separation that occurs when a baby is handed over to a day-care system where the baby will remain from morning to night. Regrettably, children often feel abandoned to their own still scarce and weak resources. Day-care centers are not always run by professionals, and even when they are, programs that are educationally adequate may not be linked with the family ecosystem. Furthermore, there are very often too many children in day-care groups. The turnover of teachers is sometimes very high also. In this kind of scenario, babies are subjected to multiple caregivers, which is a risk affecting the attachment process. Babies make successive adaptive adjustments and, in the process, may resist further deep relationships. In Portugal, just under a third (32%) of children aged 3–5 years attend publicly funded services, part of which are supported by education authorities. Part of these services are open only until 3 or 4 p.m., and include a 2-hour break at the noon hour. This means that they are not at all suitable for working mothers who very rarely finish their work activities before 5 p.m. Portugal's working index for women is about 80% in the reproductive age group. From this group, between 60 and 65% of women with a child under 10 are employed and nearly 10% of them have part-time jobs. This figure represents the second highest level in the European Union and should lead to a completely different policy concerning educational services in Portugal. The reconciliation of employment, continuing professional training, and family responsibilities is one of the most complex challenges facing Portugal and Europe at the turn of the century.

Humans are paradoxical beings, searching more and more for novelty, agitation, and change, while, above all, humans need stable symbols of peace and security. Humans reached a critical point of vulnerability at the turn of the century when we consider what is happening with the child and family. The family is the most significant ecosystem in which the child learns and gains identity. Within it, the child also learns to adjust and adapt to the vulnerable conditions that his social destiny brings. The genesis of the family from its primordial origins is one of the touchpoints proposed by Brazelton. It is perhaps the most important one because in the formation of the family the destinies of individuals confront potential identities, thus creating a new culture where transcendence and risk compete to survive. It is at this point that the vulnerability for Baby XXI is born.

Adolescents in our culture postpone that meeting, often because they only have access to conditions of denial. Difficulties getting a first job, difficulties finding a home for themselves, difficulties building self-esteem needed for a future parental role: All these circumstances act to prolong the time of adolescence in our society today. In the same context, the pregnancy of an adolescent girl is, most of the time, the tip of an iceberg, the base of which is found in a past that included persistent family stress. Joy Osofsky called attention to the importance of studying not only the conditions causing vulnerability, but also those conditions that exist in young mothers and babies that may lead to resilience and success (Osofsky, 1990).

Nevertheless, vulnerabilities exist in a continuum of change and success. When young couples finally gather the courage to marry or live together, and when they realize that they will have a baby, they discover that having a baby is something entirely different from taking care of it. This is one of the challenges that we face as educators and clinicians. In our diagnostic procedures, we are faced with multiple questions, one of which is mentioned by Thomas Boyce: "Is the source of vulnerability the individual child or the child's environment?" (Boyce, 1992). Each child has to be viewed as a self plus circumstances. Lewis Barness stressed the fact that "physicians need to learn and understand more about parents' perception of a child's vulnerability" (Barness, 1992). This represents one of the great challenges in medical education for the next century and is particularly critical when a family approach is taken into consideration.

Responding to the Vulnerability of Children

In summarizing, I would say that child vulnerability is a unique condition making the individual or group more susceptible to different kinds of stress; as a result, there is a greater probability of disease, deterioration, or other maladjustment.

Appraising this statement, at least four questions are relevant:

- Are we creating, in fact, a brighter, safer, and happier world for our babies?
- Are we eradicating risks and decreasing vulnerability, by promoting more adaptive skills and affectionate bonds, particularly when the birth of a family is possible?
- Are we helping parents to feel more competent, and to view themselves as more esteemed caregivers?
- Are we reinforcing the support that can help children to cope with too much stress as they near the threshold of deterioration?

Urie Bronfenbrenner responded to these questions brilliantly when he stated that discussion of our existence, our future, and our life cannot take place if we do not review our history and try to see how we fit into the social scheme of things. Bronfenbrenner and his colleagues wrote that what we need is a "humanism of science" (Bronfenbrenner, 1977).

In fact, vulnerability does not mean fatality. Rather, what we have to do is transform despair into hope: exactly what we did five centuries ago when we crossed the seas and transformed vulnerability into discovery.

In Portugal, we have been working on this transformation since the 1970s. We are aware of the vacuum that some societies have created by instituting new habits that, in anthropological terms, are destroying foundations that have existed for centuries. One of these foundations is the stable arrangement of the mother and baby together, without a break, following birth. We became convinced that the separation of mother and baby in our maternity wards after delivery was a determining factor in increasing vulnerability in the early postpartum period. Using the same rooming-in conditions, we studied the influence of extended early contact on both newborn infants' and their mothers' behavior. One of the main findings of our study was that interactive behavior—"interactive processes" as dimensions assessed in the infant through the Neonatal Behavioral Assessment Scale (NBAS)—was significantly better for the postpartum contact group. Some of these results continued through the 28th day (Gomes-Pedro, Bento de Almeida, Silveira da Costa, & Barbosa, 1984). As for the mothers' behavior, it was meaningful that the group with early contact got better results; the "affectionate behavior" dimension was more evident by the end of the first month of life.

Again, the sea represents vulnerability and uncertainty; yet symbols and events that cause anxiety are confronted in our dream by factors that represent hope and certainty.

☐ Wind and Sails, Change and Adaptation

One of the most influential elements in the voyages of the global discoveries was the wind. At a time when adventure materialized from dreams, it became necessary to confirm the image of the world that Ptolemy described in a map (probably the first geographic map in the history of the world). Much of the imagination and creativity of the navigators was humbly dependent on the wind. Therefore, an expedition of sailing vessels depended particularly on two factors: wind and sails. During the era of the global discoveries, the unpredictable and the unexpected dictated alterations of courses and destinies. In these cases, changes were a result of adaptations necessary when confronted with unpredictable natural and human elements. These symbolic reflections contain not only the components of the explorers' dreams, but also some fundamental mechanisms of human development. In relation to the child and family, we see the wind as a symbol of life and the changing environment that propels us in our need to adapt, while sails represent our adaptive capacities and behaviors, those vital and constant activities that determine homeostasis and are observable in day-to-day behavior. Ultimately, change encompasses everything related to alterations in the course of life, whether this course is calculated or not, and whether it is affected by adaptation or not.

Adaptation Across the Life Span

Clinical adaptation and change can be viewed as purveyors of concepts. The concept of adaptation that I would like to consider encompasses the life-span view of human development, attempting to explain interindividual differences emerging from change over a life span. The life-span concept is fundamental to the clinical notion that only a multidisciplinary approach may be meaningful and productive for nosology, diagnosis, and treatment. We learned from Ortega y Gasset that each person is himself and his own circumstance. The child's circumstance is first of all the family and, in its extension, the child's other relatives, friends, neighbors, teachers, and pets. The life-span approach allows us to think about change, taking into consideration the environment of each person and, consequently, the person's differences and adaptations. We must constantly be aware of not only the child, but also the meaningful others in each stage of change.

Doctors and, in a very special way, pediatricians of the twenty-first century will have to be more sensitive to the ideas and knowledge coming from other disciplines that attempt to explain the changes and events of life. Critical social changes, already referred to, involving marriage, breaking parental ties, violence, negligence, and many other developmental disruptions experienced by children and families, require the contribution of historians, economists, politicians, scientists, lawyers, urban planners, architects, sociologists, psychologists, psychoanalysts, educators, and many others.

Brazelton's view of child touchpoints is very much based on the constructs of circumstance and change, which make it much easier to develop comprehensive strategies of intervention. The notion of circumstance related to the child is often identified with environment. Furthermore, the meaning of *environment* has been conceived of mostly in a physical and social context. Nowadays, not only should we add new parameters to this meaning, including affective and moral factors, but we should also join the concept of change to the initial meaning. Environment is not a stable factor. It obviously changes both with time and with the evolving pattern of life related to the person living in that environment. This is particularly true where child development is concerned. Let us take as our example the meaning of growth. In the course of infant development, adaptation is a constant and a conditioning principle of the future. The phenomenon of adaptation explains the major part of the mechanism of survival and, also, of the child's successes. It is by observing adaptation that we begin to understand "why" we were born.

The Evolution of Human Adaptive Capacities

From the *Austra* to *Homo sapiens*, there were more than 65,000 generations. In the course of this whole evolutionary process, a progressively more differentiated brain emerged, becoming more and more complex. It gradually developed the capacity to integrate millions of sensations, including those affecting parental sensibilities, those capable of generating thought, and those capable of helping us resolve many of the delicate problems that progress implies. However, in terms of the adaptation of our species, the evolution of a large brain from a fetus whose mother is a biped created a complicated problem. How could a large head pass through a narrow cervix, in a species so well adapted for the long-distance traveling of the hunting–collecting ancient human? Our species was forced to adapt in a compensatory way through an evolution in human anatomy, one of the most significant examples of human adaptation in history. The pelvic ligaments of women became more flexible, compensating for the narrow pelvis of our erect bodies, and the head of the newborn became more elastic than that of other primates, so as to be able to be molded during labor. The price paid for this exceptional adaptation was, in terms of survival, the immaturity with which our babies are born. If our babies had a more prolonged maturation inside the womb, the increased size of their brains—their heads—would make vaginal birth impossible.

Thus, if the birth of a baby is no more than an ultimate separation, the baby should be fed, cleaned, warmed, protected, and cared for, both intimately and personally, by someone who loves this baby and wants to take care of him or her and make this baby happy. In terms of adaptation, the natural timing of birth represents the optimal balance between the increasing risks and the diminishing benefits of remaining in utero, and the dangers of birth and the demands of the extrauterine life. An adaptation, by its nature, raises the probabilities of one or two classes of events and therefore necessarily reduces or invalidates the probabilities of others. In our everyday clinical experience, we recognize multiple forms of adaptation, operating at various levels. Some of the most obvious examples are biological. When a newborn baby is in a cold environment that lowers the baby's body temperature, he or she metabolizes brown fat to generate heat. The cost of this physiological adaptation is an increased requirement for glycogen and calories, which can be easily met in normal conditions, but can represent a situation risky for low-weight or other vulnerable babies. Crying is another adaptive mechanism of the baby, who can manage a change of state in order to request an appropriate intervention by one of the parents, but at the cost of a lot of energy. The balance is achieved somewhere along the spectrum from a high degree of the baby's adaptability to a sensitive dependence on an adequate and supportive environment. In human infancy, Papoušek and Papoušek assign the fundamental role of adaptive behavioral regulation to "integrative nervous processes" active in the processing of perceived stimuli and in the organization of adaptive responses (Papoušek & Papoušek, 1979).

Cultural Threats to Human Adaptation

Recently published theories of socialization try to encompass new ways for humans to organize their adaptive processes. One of the most promising ones concerned with evolution and practicability derives from the field of behavioral ecology and distinguishes itself from others in that its proponents argue that prepubertal rearing experiences and behavioral development influence the timing of puberty. The authors argue that developmental events and processes affect adolescent sexual behavior and adult pair bonding (Belsky, Steinberg, & Draper, 1991). I believe that the threshold of child adaptability is at risk of being exceeded. This will be one of the major challenges for educators and health providers in the twenty-first century. Pediatricians, among others, need to recognize that the application of what researchers discover about early relationships may enable them to cope with the challenge of helping children and families evolve in the direction of adaptability and mastery, instead of psychopathology and despair. This represents another challenge for health and education planning in Portugal. Classic health indicators reveal that Portugal is in a period of transition. Infant mortality is now under 7 per 1,000, and perinatal mortality is approaching the psychological barrier of 8 per 1,000. All of these trends mean that health policies need to take into account indicators of well-being like birth rate, family dysfunction, adolescent pregnancy, reading abilities, and so on, so that rational interventions may begin helping parents and thus enhancing self-esteem in children. Portugal is a country with a population of about 10 million. The rate of population growth is 0%. The birth rate is 11.7 per 1,000 (the marriage rate is 7.1 per 1,000) and progressively decreasing. The divorce rate is going up (the official index of 1.3 per 1,000 does not cover the actual rate of family rupture). These indicators should guide us to culturally adapted, family-focused interventions.

The Advantages of Early Interventions

Over the last two decades, an increasing body of research emerged stressing early childhood as a privileged period for interventions. This research enlightens possible interventions contributing to significant improvements in both child and family development. In this context, the newborn period—being one of the fundamental steps in the growth of the family system—presents an excellent opportunity for enhancing parent–infant discoveries of one another and their potential for fulfillment as individuals. In research concerning another kind of early intervention, we studied the effects of a clinical intervention with mothers on the third day of their babies' lives. We examined whether a change in parents' attitudes would influence subsequent parent–infant interactions. Our results support the view that mothers become aware of their newborns' behavioral competencies when an appropriate intervention is designed with this purpose in mind (Gomes-Pedro et al., 1995). Using the NBAS as an intervention tool as well as an assessment instrument, we observed better performance on the "orientation cluster" in the experimental group. This group also had a more favorable interactive pattern, as measured through a specific interaction assessment repeated nine times during the first 2 years of the babies' lives. In order to develop strategies to help adaptation, we assume that a philosophy of early intervention should be based on a clinician sharing with parents emerging knowledge about their baby's behavior and temperament. Especially important is identifying what could eventually impede what may be called the "intuitive interaction." Other results appeared in the follow-up study, in which the babies were 6 years old. At this stage, no differences were evident between groups. This result suggested several hypotheses, among them that the follow-up itself may have acted as a significant intervention for both groups by unintentionally assembling them in a single, intervention sample. From research of this kind we are learning to better predict developmental outcomes, a responsibility that should become common for clinicians of the twenty-first century. One's capacity to predict some aspects of the developmental course of a child allows one to give anticipatory support to significant aspects of children's lives. This concept is intimately connected with the assessment of adaptability present within the caregiver–infant dyad.

Sailing makes use of the sails in order for the boat to remain on course. There are frequent changes in the wind and the need for adaptation to wind shifts. Responding to the capricious nature of the winds influencing development, we must organize our interventions adaptively as we attempt accurate predictions of developmental outcome. The result should be discovery of new knowledge, changing dream into reality.

☐ Sails, (Adaptation), Attachment, and Culture

The way the sails are set on the caravels, their shape, their size, and, most importantly, the functional relationship between them and their angles to the wind determine the performance of a sailing enterprise. In our dream, sails are a symbol of our systems of adaptation, and, as an example, a symbol of a specific model of those adaptive systems for the development of attachments. Sails function in relation to each other just as the threads of a spider web do. (What I call the "spider web" model is very similar to the model of the sail system of the caravel used in the global discoveries.) The spider builds its web in a progressive, consistent way. The central structure of the web is organized at the base of the principal threads, over which the spider interwines other secondary threads that provide elasticity, lightness, and resistance. In a corresponding manner, the mainsail, the lateen sail, the jib, and the mizzen of the caravel provided a harmonious structure in those ships used by the explorers. Consistency and flexibility are fundamental if spider webs, caravels, and human relationships are to function properly.

Attachment and Adaptation

Investigators of attachment processes suggest that the way love and caring are built and shared in the process of "becoming a family" influences the later experiences of the child. In this context, if the main threads or the mainsails are strong—that is, if the first experiences of the baby are ones of acceptance, nurturance, respect and empathy—then the baby views himself or herself as worthy of love as he or she becomes a child and later an adult. In contrast, babies who have experienced rejection, overstimulation, or unstable behavior from their parents will be more likely to view themselves as unworthy of love, and then it will be more difficult for them to become good caregivers themselves (Bretherton & Waters, 1985). The spider web and the sail system are metaphors for the working models of the attachment behaviors that Bowlby and his followers argued were fundamental frameworks to explain how interpersonal relationships are spawned from early experiences. I must stress that it is not only the early relationship between mother and child that will influence later development, but rather the initial special interactional experiences (especially with the mother). This is what conditions social development and later emotional states, both through the child's emerging expectations and through the mother's and father's feelings about themselves and others.

The critical nature of early experience lies at the interface between experience and the central nervous system. However, it should be stressed that experience is mediated by the individual nature of the organism on which it works. Through an explication of two essential concepts, experience-expectancy and experience-dependency, the formulations of Greenough, Black, and Wallace (1987) provide compelling evidence that the effects of experience during sensitive periods are specific and qualitatively different. On the other hand, following Bowlby, other studies revealed that mother–baby interactions are themselves regulators of diverse physiological and behavioral systems in the initial phases of life (Bowlby, 1958). For example, in various species the mother regulates basic functions of the baby, such as the baby's heart rate and respiration, while the baby's behavior induces maternal states whereby an outpouring of milk is provoked—a condition vital to survival. All these facts suggest that babies and their mothers are connected at the level of biological synchronies, leading to the notion that attachment itself has homeostatic functions throughout the life span. The human baby organizes biobehavioral responses in such a way as to regulate homeostasis and remain ready for and receptive to communication with the mother and father. Each time that the baby reaches this point of homeostasis the baby appears to achieve a feeling of competence, which makes the baby prepared for new interactions and consequently for new learning.

Attachment, Culture, and Individual Differences

Development is not, in fact, a continuous chain of events, but rather a journey of starts and stops. In this context, the major phases of acceleration contain, in general, periods of disorganization, while the periods of landing and apparent pause are fundamental phases of balance and reorganization. The whole structure of interpersonal relationships uses this model of stairs, facilitating the internalization of attitudes during each pause. Every adaptation in our life span is dependent on our relationships and on the way we regulate, through them, the interaction itself. We are continually involved in dialogue, either with our own intrinsic systems of regulation or with those of others. Thus we have an adaptive phenotype that is a consequence of the regulation of these various systems. In this context, the individual and unique expression of each person is a result of an apparently "mysterious," "unreachable" adaptation, at the base of which all relationships consist of numerous complex interactions that attain an aura of mystery. The mystery is greater when there is a disturbance, but this does not invalidate our persistent efforts to solve it.

In almost all of the studies of mother–infant separation, the babies appeared more disturbed when the mother–infant relationship was itself more disturbed. On the other hand, we already know that each individual is affected not only by the examples of others, but also (and mainly) by the way the person feels events or behaviors "ought to be." In the adult, this meaning develops to include the moral sense of a culture.

Robert Hinde proposed a comprehensive scheme encompassing the various didactic relationships between successive levels of social complexity, in which sociocultural structure and physical environments are simultaneously inspiring or influencing behavior and, in the same feedback system, are receivers from all the social variables, including individuals and their relationships (Hinde, 1991). The importance of this feedback inside the family system is now widely recognized. Pediatricians, family clinicians, psychotherapists, and many others already know that the great challenge both in prevention and in treatment is to maintain, as adequately as possible, the balance between persons, their relationships, and the group.

This adaptation is challenged every day by rapid transformations that make adaptation a "slower" process. In this adaptation, two of the major influences we have to keep in mind are individual differences on one hand, and culture on the other. In cultural terms, we can picture a macrocultural level that includes social expectations and a microcultural level that is more related to the family system. Cultures differ in the lifestyle they consider desirable; consequently, they differ in the way they treat maladaptation. That which is supposed to be "better" in one culture may not be in another. Therefore, when considering family educational strategies, we must be very careful not to consider as "optimal" any specific parent–infant relationship model. I believe that a great challenge for professionals in the next century will lie in helping each individual person adjust expectations and feelings to changing circumstances. Just as the knowledge of sailing techniques made the difference for the explorers, paying attention to expectations and emotions will make a difference for clinicians and educators in the future. The baby of the twenty-first century deserves and demands our respect within the matrix of the baby's culture. The promotion of attachment starts at this point, and research in this field is a strong starting point.

Other instructive data resulting from our research concerned mother–baby communication during the first weeks and months of life. We look at it today as a sailing expedition because it revealed so many discoveries. Using the data resulting from our analysis of interactions between mothers and babies during the first 2 years of life, and basing our methodology on the Greenspan and Lieberman Observation Scale (GLOS), we evaluated, among other things, the behavior resulting from those interactions (Greenspan & Lieberman, 1980). Although the analysis of maternal and infant behavior was done separately, a contingency emerged when the two statistical results were juxtaposed, appearing in the form of almost overlapping curves (Gomes-Pedro et al., 1995). This contingency is repeated in other ways in the most significant relationships of our lives. However, as with the spider web and the hoisting of the sails, it is the earlier events that set the tone for the outcome—an outcome that we clinicians must try to influence toward harmony and happiness through interventions respectful of the preferences of the family. Let us sail in search of opportunities to promote an understanding of the importance of attachments in each culture, in each child, in each dyad, in each family. All of this originates in our dream, but can be practiced every day.

☐ Epilogue and Conclusions

I am reaching the end of an expedition inspired by Baby XXI. Beginning with the creativity that dreams inspire, we move to a course that temperament and personal experience facilitate, and adapt to the changes that the shifting winds determine. I do not know if this voyage will end with land in sight or in a safe harbor. I hope that it will end in a dawn over the ocean, with a rising sun, a setting that a painter would be incapable of capturing. This dawn is the hope of a better world. When he tells us that "every living being searches for a better world and tries to remain or fluctuate in it," Popper (1972) challenges us to invent that world, each day and each instant.

As in a sailing voyage, we are recreating a journey. The dynamics of life are similar in that we reinvent our niches and our beliefs. It was at the crossroads of dream and sailing that the explorers made discoveries. In this epilogue, I call that crossroads of dream and journey "our project." All people of good faith have projects for a better world. That better world begins with a recognition of and respect for individual differences, and in the unique contributions of each individual toward a common aim. We intend that all the inhabitants of the world have the right and duty to leave to their descendants a planet in which it will be possible to drink pure water, breathe pure air, cultivate pure soil, enjoy a climate not spoiled by either the greenhouse effect or the ozone hole, use technology in order to progress more than to pollute, and to defend against disease, and accidents, and, above all, inhabit a planet in which a culture of love prevails over violence and lack of respect for others.

Aristotle, in his *Physics*, defined nature as something that means a "continuous movement originating from an internal principle and arriving at some completion." The impulse within nature in Aristotle has the same logic as the impulse that drove Vasco da Gama, Cabral, and Columbus to sail toward the horizon, beyond which no one had ever dared to venture. Throughout the evolution of that natural impulse we should distinguish between action and motion. Trying to understand development as an internal movement, we should have in mind that purposefulness of development may not be coincident with purposefulness of action, although they both could serve or fulfill the aim of nature. From Aristotle to Descartes, from Descartes to Claude Bernard, the discovery of nature involved constant action and intellectual movement.

Of all the forms of living matter, we are the only one to whom is granted the privilege of deciphering the logic of creation. I am not sure if dreaming helps to decipher that logic, but I feel that our coherence has to be inspired in a dream that, in fact, is a movement for progress. I have tried to revisit the mastery of discoveries to stimulate the mystery of foreseeing the future.

At the end of this expedition I feel that I have carried with me everyone and everything that conferred identity on my life and on my journey. It is very meaningful to me to share togetherness with friends who travel with me in this book.

The last reflection concerns the symbol of the transition from dream to reality, what I called hope and certitude. For those who interpret hope as still a dream, I would recall Fernando Pessoa, one of our great poets, who liked to sing of our sea: "Pode ser que para outro mundo eu possa levar o que sonhei, mas poderei eu levar para o outro mundo o que me esqueci de sonhar?" "Perhaps I will take to the other world that which I have dreamed, but will I be able to take to that world that which I forgot to dream?"

☐ References

Arnold, L. E. (1990). *Childhood stress*. New York: John Wiley and Sons.

Barness, L. (1992). Editor's introduction. *Advances in Pediatrics, 39*, 1.

Belsky, J., Steinberg, L., & Draper, P. (1991). Childhood experience, interpersonal development and reproductive strategy: An evolutionary theory of socialization. *Child Development, 62*, 647–670.

Bowlby, J. (1958). The nature of the child's tie to his mother. *International Journal of Psychoanalysis, 39*, 350–373.

Boyce, W. T. (1992). The vulnerable child: New evidence, new approaches. *Advances in Pediatrics,* *39,* 1–33.

Brazelton, T. B. (1982). Early intervention: What does it mean? In H. E. Fitzgerald, B. M. Lester, & M. W. Yogman (Eds.), *Theory and research in behavioral pediatrics* (Vol. 1, 1–34). New York: Plenum.

Bretherton, I., & Waters, E. (1985). Growing points of attachment theory and research. *Monographs of the Society for Research in Child Development, 50*(1–2).

Bronfenbrenner, U. (1977). Toward an experimental ecology of human development. *American Psychologist, 32,* 513–531

Gomes-Pedro, J., Bento de Almeida, J., Silveira da Costa, C., & Barbosa, A. (1984). Influence of early mother–infant contact on dyadic behavior during the first month of life. *Development Medicine & Child Neurology, 26,* 657–664.

Gomes-Pedro, J. C., Monteiro, M. B., Carvalho, A., Patricio, M., Torgal-Garcia, F., Fiadeiro, I., & Levy, M. L. (1988). Early interventions and pediatric practice. In S. Doxiadis (Ed.), *Early influences shaping the individual* (pp. 299–317). NATO ASI Series 160. New York: Plenum.

Gomes-Pedro, J., Patricio, M., Carvalho, A., Goldschmidt, T., Torgal-Garcia, F., & Monteiro, M. B. (1995). Early intervention with Portuguese mothers: A two-year follow-up. *Journal of Developmental and Behavioral Pediatrics, 16,* 21–28.

Greenough, W. T., Black, J. E., & Wallace, C. S. (1987). Experience and brain development. *Child Development, 58,* 519–559.

Greenspan, S. T., & Lieberman, A. F. (1980). Infants, mothers and their interaction: a quantitative clinical approach to development assessment. In S. I. Greenspan & G. Pollack (Eds.), *The course of life. Psychoanalytic contributions toward understanding personality development. Infancy and early childhood* (pp. 271–312). Washington, DC: Government Printing Office.

Hinde, R. A. (1991). Relationships, attachment and culture: A tribute to John Bowlby. *Infant Mental Health Journal, 12,* 154–163.

Nugent, J. K., & Brazelton, T. B. (1989). Preventive intervention with infants and families: The NBAS Model. *Infant Mental Health Journal, 12,* 154–163.

Osofsky, J. D. (1990). Risk and protective factors for teenage mothers and their infants. *Society for Research in Child Development Newsletter,* winter.

Papoušek, H., & Papoušek, M. (1979). The infant's fundamental adaptive response system on social interaction. In E. B. Thoman (Ed.), *Origin of the infant's social responses* (pp. 175–208). Hillsdale, NJ: Lawrence Erlbaum.

Popper, K. R. (1972). *Objective knowledge: An evolutionary approach.* Oxford: Clarendon Press.

UNICEF. (1996). *State of the world children.* New York: Author.

United Nations. (1991). *Convention on the rights of the child.* New York: Author.

Zuckerman, B., Weitzman, M., & Alpert, J. J. (1988). Preface. Children at risk: Current social and medical challenges. *Pediatric Clinics of North America, 35*(6), 1169–1452.

T. Berry Brazelton

Strengths and Stresses in Today's Families: Looking Toward the Future

The United States is one of the richest countries in the world. And yet, the indications for breakdown in families are higher here than in any other civilized nation. Twenty-five percent of children are living in poverty (Zill, 1993). Fifty percent of children will spend a significant part of their lives in a single-parent family, largely because of divorce. One in every two marriages ends in divorce (Zill, 1993). Twenty-seven percent of children are in single-parent families. These children are being raised primarily by women—either because of divorce or because of the influence of our welfare system, which prejudices against marriage and families (National Commission for Children, 1991; Zill, 1993). The poverty rate of children in these single-parent families is four times higher than that of children with both parents present (U.S. Select Committee on Children, Youth and Families, 1990).

Having just been to Denmark, my dream is for a socialist democracy with the support systems for families that have been instituted in that country. Most of these are present in other European nations. Japan, China, and many of the Eastern countries seem to support children and families far more than we do in the United States. Their farsightedness contrasts dramatically with our lack of interest in the stresses that overwhelm our young families. What is the likelihood for change in policy in this country? The future of our society resides in our children. The stresses of poverty and of growing up in the war zones of our inner cities surely predict violence in the future lives of these children (Garbarino, 1991).

I would like to see a new American agenda for children. We do know what to do, and if we don't do it, we can anticipate more and more problems, more and more violence from the breakdown of our families. A child who is raised in a chaotic, violent environment with sexual and physical abuse is predicted to repeat this (Greenspan, 1993). We do know what to do. We know a great deal about children's development and about stabilizing families (Brazelton, 1969, 1981, 1992; Brazelton & Cramer, 1990).

As a member of the National Commission for Children, 1988–1991, I witnessed the breakdown of stable communities and nurturing families for our children. But we have set out a four-part agenda for stabilizing our family life. The four parts are:

1. Ensuring income security for all members of society. The problems of being poor and depressed in our inner cities affect children in several ways. Before they are born, they may be exposed to drugs and they may be malnourished, which produces an at-risk and disorganized baby. This baby can face a chaotic environment—low parent educational level, family disorganization, limited opportunities, run-down housing, poor schools, and hazardous neighborhoods (Zill, 1993). Furthermore, the labels of being poor or ethnically different set up a cycle of disadvantage.
2. Ensuring that all members of our society have health care and that preventive and early intervention services are paid for.
3. Changing our education system to reach out for parents, and to start in the 0–3 years to strengthen families to provide a decent self-image for children so they can be educable.
4. Creating a moral climate for children and families with family life as a priority—in the workplace, in community life respecting ethnic and religious diversity, and counteracting and controlling the influences of television, addiction, and sexual irresponsibility.

This program is outlined in the document *Beyond Rhetoric* (National Commission for Children, 1991), and we have formed a grass-roots organization, called Parent Action (Baltimore, MD), to advocate for these changes.

Stable families and stable communities are the keystone of any success for our children's future (Zill, 1993). How do we create or re-create them? There are programs that do work (Schorr, 1989, 1993). The four attributes that seem to be important and are characteristic of successful programs are that they are:

1. Comprehensive, intensive, flexible, and responsive. For example, a worker will help a new mother cook, clean house, and diaper her baby while offering her the advice or support for intervention from the worker's program.
2. Able to deal with children as part of families, and families as part of neighborhoods and families. Head Start has worked because it got families involved in their children's education (U.S. Select Committee on Children, Youth and Families, 1990). Communities must be involved and families need to feel a part of those communities.
3. Staffed with workers who have the time and skills to build relationships of trust and respect with children and families. They must establish a continuing warm welcome and supportive relationship based on shared belief systems that are sensitive to ethnic, religious, and socioeconomic values. This is not an easy challenge, but it can be done and has been by successful programs. The melting pot has not worked; respect and attention to diversity will.
4. A long-term orientation, with prevention and the development of children and families, as a prerequisite (Schorr, 1993).

With these goals in mind, we have developed a system for reaching out to new parents called "touchpoints" (Brazelton, 1992). Touchpoints are predictable periods in a child's development that can disrupt family relations, but can also provide an opportunity for practitioners to connect with parents. The use of each touchpoint to bring parents together in peer groups could be used to create a sense of community (Stadtler, O'Brien, & Hornstein, 1995). Each touchpoint can be shared with other parents who are struggling with the same ethnic and religious values that are the underpinning of parenting. Valuing this diversity is at the base of success in this model. If we could use diversity in a positive way, stressed parents would feel backed up at many different levels. For example, treating adolescent, unwed mothers-to-be in a positive way could turn around their future. We have already lost the opportunity for preventing the pregnancy. We know that the most successful programs for preventing repeated pregnancies enhance the teenager's success with her first baby. By valuing her and her baby, we can optimize her chance of success with her baby. Getting teenagers together to share touchpoints with each other and to feel a sense of community with peers could be a step toward continuing success.

☐ Bringing About a Sense of Community

In order to bring about a sense of community, I would start with the new family. In pregnancy, bring expecting parents together in a community center of their own choice—a school, a church, a community meeting place. Give the parents-to-be a chance to be together in groups with common values and common expectations. The groups would form around ethnic value systems, or because of mutual values. For example, a group of teenage parents could become the center of one, whereas Spanish Americans and African Americans could form other groups. Because their focus would be on the future newborn, they should be treated with respect and for a positive future. Each group would be given the chance to know each other and to share common concerns. Their prenatal medical care as well as the childbirth information they would need could be provided in this center of their choice. Any benefits, such as WIC (Women, Infants, and Children program) or Food Stamps, could be provided in this one-stop center. At each visit, the emphasis would be on the sense of shared community.

After the delivery of the newborn, a representative from the community center would visit the newborn nursery, to share the newborn's behavior with the new parents. Using the Neonatal Behavioral Assessment Scale (NBAS; Brazelton & Nugent, 1995), the new parents would have the chance to understand the individuality of their baby. Our research has demonstrated a significant increase in the sensitivity to the newborn's behavioral cues as well as to the individual temperament of the baby after the NBAS has been demonstrated to new parents in the neonatal period. The health visitor from the community center would concentrate on recruiting the parents to return at 3 weeks to the center. The sense of community would be emphasized: "Remember that all your peers have had their babies. They want to compare theirs with yours. If you return at 3 weeks, the baby and you can have your checkups. All of you can compare your babies, can be prepared for the 'colicky crying' that will be coming soon afterward. You will get your WIC supplement and food stamps." Combining health in preventive checkups, the education for the child and family's development, the food supplements, and a sense of community becomes a powerful way of maintaining the group's peer relationships.

Each subsequent visit and health checkup can be geared to the times in the infant's development when parents will need the preventive advice necessary to help them understand and optimize the baby's future (Brazelton, 1983). We have a map of such times in the first year that can serve to prevent sleep and feeding problems, and that will prepare new parents for each spurt in the child's development. I am sure that if the groups can share their ideas and their issues at each of these times, they will feel a sense of shared success as their babies make progress. At each spurt in development, the parents will feel the success that the baby will demonstrate. By the end of the first year, they will be ready to continue in the peer group, three or four times in the second year, and twice a year thereafter. Immunizations and health checkups for the baby and family can be administered at the center. Child care and then Head Start education can proceed with these groups participating actively (Zigler & Muenchow, 1992). Parents will feel empowered and will remain in their children's educational process.

With this preventive model of health, education, and shared development, we can return a sense of empowerment to all new families in our country.

☐ Touchpoints for Anticipatory Guidance

If we can begin to reach out for families and to re-create communities for them, we can begin to provide the layers of an envelope in which families can begin to feel secure and empowered. They will pass this on to their children. Their ability to take an active, understanding role in their child's development can enhance the self-image of each child. That is my dream for the future—that each child feels he or she is important and is loved.

The opportunity for supportive workers to play a role as they work with families in the prevention of failures in child development is enormous. The importance of their role in optimizing each stage of a child's developmental progress—motor, cognitive, and emotional—is equal to the pediatrician's role in prevention of disease and physical disorders (Brazelton, 1983). We have found that when we emphasize the individuality of the infant, it enhances the capacity of the family to offer him or her an optimally nurturing environment (Brazelton, 1974). This becomes critical if one assumes that the outcome of a developing child is dependent on the interaction between genetic endowment and environmental influences that are appropriate to the child's temperament.

Systems theory presents an optimistic approach for all of us who are interested in prevention. First, each member of the system must react to every stress incurred by that system—such as to the birth and the adjustment to the new baby, as well as to each developmental step in the baby's development. Because each member shares the reactions, our presence as a member of the system could soften the stress. Second, at each stress point, there is an opportunity for learning—learning to succeed or learning to fail. If we, as supportive physicians, can offer the necessary information and modeling for the parents to understand the baby's development and to enhance it, we can play a crucial role toward the success of the family system. With parents at risk for stress and/ or failure in our complex societies, this can be a critical balance. Since all new parents are likely to be stressed parents, our role can be a critical one in the development of most of the families in our clinical practices.

For this role, I devised the map of "touchpoints," the points at which a change in the system is brought about by the baby's spurt in development. No developmental line in the baby makes steady upward progress. Each line of development progresses in spurts, leveling off to consolidate all that has just been learned (Piaget, 1972). The spurts are expensive, costing the baby and parents sleep, anxiety, and energy. Parents are unable to enlist help. They're too exhausted. The times of leveling off are easy, and parents don't need help at those times.

Just before each spurt in any line of development (motor, cognitive, or emotional), there is a short but predictable period of disorganization in the baby. The parents are likely to feel disorganized themselves and to fear that the baby is regressing to problem behavior. This period of disorganized, regressive behavior represents a period of reorganization before the next spurt in development. Because these are predictable (one in pregnancy, seven in the first year, three in the second, and two in each subsequent year), they can be mapped out to fit the ends of each family with a developing infant. I have found in my own practice, and in outreach programs for families at risk, that I can predict and participate with them in these times. By scheduling the routine pediatric visits for immunizations and checkups to coincide with these points of reorganization, I can offer parents the information necessary to understand these periods (Brazelton, 1992) and predict the subsequent spurt in the child's development. Because these are the times when parents are likely to put more pressure on the infant or child, and they occur at a time when the child needs less pressure, I can help them make the choices they need to make them feel successful when the child reorganizes for the next developmental spurt. The child's success in development becomes experienced as their own success as parents. The family as a system feels fueled toward success.

Touchpoint 1

The first touchpoint is an important one for forming a relationship with parents-to-be. If I can meet and share concerns with parents in the seventh month of pregnancy, we will have created a trusting relationship between us before the new baby arrives (Brazelton, 1981; Brazelton & Cramer, 1990). This visit need not demand more than 10 to 15 minutes, but because it occurs at a time when parents' concerns about the new baby are at a peak, I can share these concerns. All parents worry about whether they'll be able to nurture the new baby. They dream of two babies—a perfect one, with the behavior and appearance of a 3-month-old, and an impaired one, which is damaged and dissimilar compared to any baby from the parents' past experience. The dread of this baby, matched with the parents' concern about how they would ever nurture such a baby, raises a kind of alarm reaction or energy in the parents to face whatever baby they get. But their real concentration is on the fetus. The fetus's behavior is already a burning concern. They wonder whether he is "too active" or "too quiet." Can we tell by ultrasound whether he is well formed or not? We can share their dreams and fantasies with them. I can assure them that I will support them and participate with them toward optimizing the baby's development, whatever baby they get. We have established our relationship in this first touchpoint, and we are ready to work as a system.

Touchpoint 2

The second touchpoint is in the hospital or at home, soon after the baby is born. I can demonstrate the new baby's remarkable repertoire to the parents in the immediate period after birth. Using the NBAS (Brazelton & Nugent, 1995), we have shown in numerous research studies that both mother and father can be captured to become significantly more sensitive to their new baby's behavior by sharing an assessment in the immediate neonatal period. Both parents can profit by such an observation if they participate in this 10- to 20-minute assessment. During the examination, they become aware of my interest in their baby, and of the fact that I am seeing and understanding the new baby as an individual. They begin to see the baby's individuality and remarkable capacity to respond to his or her world. If there are problems to be faced, we can begin to share them as well. In this shared interval, I can not only enhance their understanding of the new baby, but I can capture them to return for the subsequent touchpoints. Using the baby as our language, we can now return to their questions about breast or formula feeding, and about their prospective handling of the baby's rhythms and responses. We are already speaking a shared language that includes the baby's temperament and style of responses to the new world. I remind them at this time that I would like to see the three of them at each subsequent touchpoint.

Touchpoint 3

The third touchpoint occurs optimally at 2–3 weeks. Before the regular fussing that occurs in most infants (85% in the United States; Brazelton, 1962) at the end of each day between 3 and 12 weeks of age, I like to evaluate the new baby with the parents. I need to predict this fussy period and to share ideas about why it occurs and what they can and can't do about it. At this time, I can see whether the mother is beginning to recover from the common postpartum exhaustion and depression. The checkup of mother and baby will be a major goal for the visit. In addition, I can help the parents toward organizing the baby for a predictable feeding and sleeping schedule. But the most important subject for the visit will be the touchpoint—that of predicting the fussy period at the end of the day. For most babies there is a period of irritable crying, which occurs after the immature nervous system has handled environmental stimuli all day, and I can help the parents to plan for it in advance. This fussy period seems to be an organizer for the 24-hour cycle. By predicting it and explaining its positive value to parents at this touchpoint, I have seen that the 2- to 3-hour period can be reduced significantly. The parents do not have to handle the baby and overload an already overloaded, immature nervous system. The baby is less frantic, and the parents feel successful in dealing with this period calmly each day.

Touchpoint 4

The next touchpoint, at 2 months, is a time for the first inoculations, a time for reevaluation of the feeding, sleep, and fussing cycles. But it is also a time to share a new and exciting development in the baby's awareness of the parents. By this age, a baby demonstrates by his or her behavior that the baby can match the parents' behavior (Brazelton, 1975; Brazelton & Cramer, 1990; Brazelton, Koslowski, & Main, 1974) in a face-to-face situation. In addition, the baby behaves differently with each parent. He or she has slow cycling of arms, legs, toes, fingers, eyes, and face with the mother. It looks as if the baby anticipates a feeding or other caretaking. For the father, the baby has a "pounce look," an anticipation of being played with. The baby's eyes, face, shoulders go up into a wide-eyed anticipatory look. His or her extremities reach out for the father jerkily, as if expecting him to poke them and play. If one comments on the patterns to hungry parents, they can see the learning that has already gone on in their new baby. This enhances their feelings of responsibility and success. And it enhances their feeling of having a meaningful relationship with such an observant caregiver.

Touchpoint 5

The next touchpoints become the focus for each subsequent visit. For example, at the 4-month visit, one can predict that there will soon be a burst in cognitive awareness of the environment. The baby will be difficult to feed. He or she will stop eating to look around and to listen to every stimulus in the environment. The baby will begin to awaken again at night, even though he or she may have been sleeping through it before. Both feeding and sleeping patterns will be disrupted for a short period in this next few weeks. This is coincident with the rapid burst in the baby's development. New awareness of the environment, of strangers, will be accompanied by a burst in motor development. The baby starts to try to sit, loves to be stood up, reaches successfully with each hand and plays with objects more effectively. This period of disorganization will have served its purpose in driving the baby on to develop—cognitively and motorically. When parents understand this period as a natural precursor to the rapid development that will follow, they will not need to feel as if it represents failure. They will not need to press the baby to eat at each feeding. A short feeding followed by his looking around will serve the purpose during the day. Two feedings in a dark, quiet room will be sufficient to stimulate the breasts to produce milk and to preserve breast-feeding. A formula-fed baby will take a formula well in a nonstimulating environment. Pressure to feed is not necessary for this brief period (Brazelton, 1969).

Sleep issues can be predicted at this same time. This visit at 4 months can be a time to discuss a preventive approach to sleeping problems. At this time, I ascertain whether the baby knows how to get to sleep when he or she is put in bed at night. If the baby is put to sleep in the parents' arms, he or she has not had the chance to learn to get to sleep. Then, when the baby comes up to light sleep every 3 to 4 hours during the night, he or she will fuss, cry out, and will need parents to intervene—to feed him or her, to pick him or her up, to try to get the baby back to sleep. If the baby has learned to find comfort with an independent pattern of getting to sleep, such as thumb sucking or clinging to a blanket, the baby can get back down to sleep at each 4-hour rousing. At this time, I can help the parents to make decisions about cosleeping, about whether to go to the baby at each rousing. I can help them understand the baby's sleeping behavior to make appropriate decisions about their responses. This is the first touchpoint to help to prevent sleep problems. This visit and the discussion of feeding disruptions can give parents insight into their feelings about feeding refusals. This visit, which may last 20 to 30 minutes, becomes a productive opportunity for parents to understand these issues from the standpoint of the baby's development, and it offers me important insights into their issues. I can rely on this information to help them in the future, no matter what their decisions will be about handling these issues.

Touchpoints 6, 7, and 8

At 6, 10, and 12 months, there are three more touchpoints in the first year—each of which presents opportunities for discussing parenting issues that will arise, and for preventing the tensions between them, which could lead to failure. Each touchpoint precedes a developmental spurt in one or more areas.

These are examples of the kinds of issues that can be addressed at each checkup. The parents will feel that the health caregiver is concerned about the baby's psychological development as well as his physical progress. They will feel more confident in themselves and in their baby, as a result of the support and interest of the caregiver.

These touchpoints can be useful and can be predicted as opportunities to support parents in understanding their child's development throughout childhood. The timing for them may be somewhat delayed for a premature or fragile infant, but they will be even more important as opportunities for supporting their anxious parents. Pediatricians and parents can join in optimizing the child's developmental progress.

☐ References

Brazelton, T. B. (1962). Crying in infancy. *Pediatrics, 29,* 579–588.

Brazelton, T. B. (1969). *Infants and mothers.* New York: Delacorte.

Brazelton, T. B. (1981). *On becoming a family: The growth of attachment.* New York: Delacorte.

Brazelton, T. B. (1983). Developmental framework of infants and children: A future for pediatric responsibility. *Journal of Pediatrics, 102,* 967–972.

Brazelton, T. B. (1992). *Touchpoints: Your child's emotional and psychological development.* Reading, MA: Addison-Wesley.

Brazelton, T. B., & Cramer, B. (1990). *The earliest relationships.* Reading, MA: Addison-Wesley.

Brazelton, T. B., Koslowski, B., & Main, M. (1974). The origins of reciprocity: The early mother infant interaction. In M. Lewis & L. Rosenblum (Eds.), *The effect of the infant on its caregiver.* New York: Wiley.

Brazelton, T. B., & Nugent J. K. (1995). *Neonatal behavioral assessment scale* (3rd ed.). London: MacKeith Press.

Garbarino, J. (1991). *No place to be a child: Growing up in a war zone.* New York: Lexington Books.

Greenspan, S. I. (1993). *Playground politics: Understanding the emotional life of your school aged child.* Reading, MA: Addison-Wesley.

National Commission for Children. (1991). *Beyond rhetoric: A new American agenda for children and families.* Washington, DC: Library of Congress.

Piaget, J. (1972). Intellectual evolution from adolescence to adulthood. *Human Development, 15,* 1–12.

Schorr, L. D. (1989). *Within our reach: Breaking the cycle of disadvantage.* New York: Anchor Press/ Doubleday.

Schorr, L. (1993, winter). Daring to learn from our successes. *Aspen Institute Quarterly,* pp. 78–107.

Stadtler, A. C., O'Brien, M. A., & Hornstein, J. (1995). The Touchpoints model: Building supportive alliances between parents and professionals. *Zero to Three, 16*(1), 24–28.

U.S. Select Committee on Children, Youth and Families. (1990). Federal program affecting children and their families. U.S. House of Representatives, 101st Congress, 2nd Session. Washington, DC: U.S. Government Printing Office.

Zigler, E., & Muenchow, S. (1992). *Story of America's most successful educational experiment.* New York: Basic Books.

Zill, N. (1993, winter). The changing realities of family life. *Aspen Institute Quarterly, 5*(1), 27–51.

3
CHAPTER

John H. Kennell

On Becoming a Family:
Bonding and the Changing Patterns
in Baby and Family Behavior

In 1973 Professor John Lind of Sweden wrote *Birth of the Family in the Obstetrical Hospital*, in which he emphasized the importance of keeping couples together during labor and delivery. "The family is born in the delivery room," he wrote (Klaus, Kennell, & Klaus, 1993).

Clinical experience and research have made it increasingly clear that events and perceptions during the perinatal period have a powerful influence, favorable or unfavorable, on the relationship between the members of this new family—the mother's bond to the infant, the father's and the siblings' bonds to the infant, and the father–mother tie. We now know that what happens during pregnancy, labor, and delivery affects how the mother and father feel about the child—feelings that may endure throughout their lifetime with that youngster. With such an overwhelming number of problems of child abuse and neglect, conduct disorders, behavioral difficulties, delinquency, alcohol and drug abuse, and marital strife and divorce, it is important for us to do everything we can to make events during the perinatal period a positive experience to improve the lives of both the parents and the child.

In the last two decades, a number of studies have investigated the effects of restoring one or more aspects of the centuries-old practices that were lost with the move of childbirth into the hospital. Examples include the studies by Dr. Gomes-Pedro (Gomes-Pedro, Bento de Almeida, Silveira da Costa, & Barbosa, 1984) and colleagues in Lisbon, Dr. Brazelton (Brazelton, 1973), and many of the other symposium speakers. Benefits were found in almost every one of these investigations for the group of mothers and babies who received a component lost in the move to the hospital and restored in the research, for example, the studies in which mothers were allowed early contact with their newborn infants (DeChateau, 1977; Kennell, 1974; Klaus and Kennell, 1982; Klaus et al., 1972).

Recent reports of tragic outcomes for infants and children have been shocking reminders of the importance of applying our research findings to all parents and babies in the perinatal period, and of intensifying or extending our studies with particular emphasis on factors that prepare and support prospective parents.

☐ Medicalization of Childbirth and Its Effects on Bonding

In the first half of this century, increasing numbers of women came into the hospital for delivery because of concern about high maternal and infant mortality rates. With this movement, two major issues drastically changed long-standing birthing practices. The first factor was concern about infection. As more deliveries took place in the hospital, maternal and infant mortality began to decrease. However, there were alarming outbreaks of infection that resulted in the death of many mothers and infants. In an attempt to protect mothers and babies and to control infection, visiting by family members was strictly limited. The babies were put in central nurseries where they received care only from "clean" doctors and nurses in white uniforms (Klaus & Kennell, 1982). As a consequence of these changes, the mother was cut off from most of her family and their support, and the mother and baby were separated for extended periods. More and more of the care of the baby was taken over by the nurses.

The second influence was the use of heavy sedation and analgesia, so-called "twilight sleep," for the mother during her labor, which produced amnesia for the pain and experience of labor and delivery. The confused and disorderly behavior of mothers who received this medication made it necessary to eliminate all family members from the labor and delivery division. Support for mothers was provided only by nurses. After delivery the mother was extremely sleepy and confused, in no shape to hold or become acquainted with her baby. As a consequence, the analgesia resulted in mother–infant separation for a number of hours.

To gain a long-term perspective on birth practices, an anthropologic sample of 186 representative nonindustrial societies was reviewed. Strikingly, 183 societies, or all but 3, expected mothers and babies to nest together for days or weeks after delivery, a rooming-in equivalent, and virtually none permitted the degree of separation that has been routine in many maternity hospitals in this century. In most societies the mother and baby are placed together with support, protection, and isolation for at least 7 days after birth. The provision of food, heat, and water and a private time for the mother and infant to get to know each other is common in most cultures. On the basis of our observations and the reports of parents, we believe that every mother has a task to perform during the postpartum period. She must look at and "take in" her real, live baby and reconcile the fantasized image of the infant she anticipated with the one she actually delivered.

Immediately after the birth, parents enter a unique period during which events may have many effects on the family. During this period, which lasts a short time, the parents' attachment to their infant sometimes begins to blossom. The first feelings of love for the infant are not necessarily instantaneous with the initial contact. The relation between the time when a mother falls in love with her baby and the sensitive period is not clear at present. Several mothers have shared with us their distress and disappointment when they did not experience feelings of love for their baby in the first minutes or hours after birth. It should be reassuring for them and similar mothers to learn about two studies of normal, healthy mothers in England.

Macfarlane and associates (Macfarlane, Smith, & Garrow, 1978) asked 97 Oxford mothers, "When did you first feel love for your baby?" The replies were as follows: during pregnancy, 41%; at birth, 24%; first week, 27%; and after the first week, 8%.

In a study of two groups of primiparous mothers, 40% recalled that their predominant emotional reaction when holding their babies for the first time was one of indifference. The same response was reported by 25% of 40 multiparous mothers. Forty percent of both groups felt immediate affection. Most mothers in both groups had developed affection for their babies within the first week. The onset of this maternal affection after childbirth was more likely to be delayed if the membranes were ruptured artificially, if the labor was painful, or if the mothers had been given meperidine (Demerol).

Donald Winnicott (1971), who started as a pediatrician and became a distinguished psychoanalyst, has made remarkably perceptive observations that suggest he was describing this period, which we have called the maternal sensitive period. From these observations, Winnicott proposed that a healthy mother goes through a period of primary maternal preoccupation. He found that the mother who developed this state provided a milieu for the infant's personality to begin to make itself evident. He believed that it was necessary for a mother to reach this state of heightened sensitivity so that she could sense her infant's feelings and so meet the infant's needs.

This special state increases during pregnancy, is maintained at a heightened level right after delivery, and then decreases in the early weeks following birth. It is interesting that the timing and course of primary maternal preoccupation are similar to those described for the maternal sensitive period. We suspect that endocrine changes play a significant role in starting and enhancing both these processes. Are they initiated by the rise in estradiol and drop in progesterone in the weeks before delivery? Are they due to the cerebral effects of oxytocin, which has been associated with maternal attachment in animals? Interestingly, the heightened sensitivity of primary maternal preoccupation is sometimes misinterpreted by physicians and nurses as excessive anxiety.

The clinical observations of Rose (Boggs & Alderstein, 1960) and our own (Kennell & Rolnick, 1960) suggested that affectional ties can be easily disturbed and may be permanently altered during the immediate postpartum period. Relatively mild illness in the newborn, such as slight elevations of bilirubin levels, slow feeding, additional oxygen for 1 to 2 hours, and the need for incubator care in the first 24 hours for mild respiratory distress, appear to affect the relationship between mother and infant. The mother's behavior is often disturbed during the first year or more of the infant's life, even though the infant's problems are completely resolved before discharge and often within a few hours. This raises a question about the impact of high-technology procedures in the neonatal period on the mother–infant relationship. Recently Kemper and colleagues (Kemper, Forsyth, & McCarthy, 1989) reported a comparison of healthy jaundiced and nonjaundiced newborns. By 1 month of age more mothers of jaundiced infants (bilirubin greater than 12 mg%) had stopped breast-feeding, and had never left the baby with anyone else or for less than 1 hour one time only. They had taken the baby for more than two well-child visits, more than one sick visit, and more emergency room visits. This emphasizes again that identification of a condition such as jaundice in a newborn may lead to continued concern and the vulnerable child syndrome. That early events have long-lasting effects is a principle of the attachment process. A mother's anxieties about her baby in the first few days after birth, even about a problem that is easily resolved, may affect her relationship with the child long afterward.

In the past 20 years, studies have focused on whether additional time for close contact of the mother and infant in the first minutes, hours, and days of life alters the quality of the attachment. In three studies the extra time was added not only during the first 3 hours but also during the next 3 days of life (Klaus et al., 1972; Kennell et al., 1974; Siegel et al., 1980). At 1 month the mothers in the group who had extra contact showed significantly more affectionate behavior toward their infants. They stood closer and watched over them more during physical examination, soothed them more when they cried, engaged in more eye-to-eye contact and fondling during feeding, and were more reluctant to leave them with someone else.

In six out of nine randomized trials of only early mother–infant contact during the first hour of life with suckling, the length of breast-feeding was significantly increased (DeChateau & Wiberg, 1977a, 1977b; Klaus & Kennell, 1982). In these studies the women who benefitted the most from early contact were poor, inner-city mothers with low levels of social support.

Extended contact for the mother and infant during the first days of life may be a more potent intervention than early contact (for 1 hour or less) in altering maternal behavior. Supporting this view are the observations that in nonindustrialized societies early contact for mother and infant is routine in only 50% of the cultures, while extended contact for a week or more following birth for mother and infant is observed in the great majority of societies.

When additional time is given for close mother–infant contact following the first 8 hours after delivery, differences in later mothering behavior also occur. In a study of 301 primiparous patients, O'Connor and others noted that increasing the time by 12 hours (6 hours on days 1 and 2) significantly decreased the number of mothering disorders, with 10 such occurrences in the control group but only 2 in the group of mothers who received extra time with their infants (O'Connor, Vietze, Sherrod, Sandler, & Altmeier, 1980). Siegel and associates, looking at a group composed of new and multiparous mothers, did find differences in parenting at 4 and 12 months, but no difference in mothering disorders (Siegel et al., 1980). A woman was defined as having a mothering disorder if her infant was battered, had nonorganic failure to thrive, was abandoned, or was given up for an unplanned adoption.

Several questions come to mind. Is the time a mother spends with her newborn in the first hour as significant as a longer period together on the second or third day of life? Is the effect in the first hour due to the quiet, alert state of the infant, to the state of the mother, or to a combination of the two? In the first hour after birth the newborn infant is in a heightened state of alertness and responsivity. Interestingly, no matter when increased amounts of contact between mother and infant are added in the first 3 postpartum days, there appears to be improved mothering behavior. It is not known why significant alterations in caretaking have been noted when mother–infant contact is increased for a short time in the first hours of life. When we make it possible for parents to be together with their baby, in privacy, for the first hour and throughout the hospital stay, we establish the most beneficial and supportive environment for the beginning of the bonding process.

Detailed studies of the amazing behavioral capacities of normal neonates in the quiet alert state have shown that the infant sees, hears, imitates facial gestures, and moves in rhythm to his mother's voice in the first minutes and hours of life, resulting in a beautiful linking of the reactions of the two and a synchronized "dance" between the mother and infant (Brazelton, Koslowski, & Main, 1974; Condon & Sander, 1974; Gomes-Pedro et al., 1984; Robson, 1967; Stern, 1971). The infant's appearance coupled with this broad array of sensory and motor abilities evokes responses from the mother and father and provides several channels of communication that are most helpful in the initiation of a series of reciprocal interactions and the process of attachment (DeChateau & Wiberg, 1977a, 1977b; Klaus & Kennell, 1982; Klaus, Kennell, & Klaus, 1995; Parke, 1979; Rödholm & Larsson, 1979; Trevarthen, 1977).

Lang noted that immediately after a home delivery most mothers suckle their infants (Lang, 1972). She observed that the neonates do not suck but lick the area around the nipple. The licking of the nipple induces a marked increase in prolactin secretion in the mother, and, at the same time, an increase in oxytocin, to contract the uterus, decrease bleeding, and, on the basis of recent animal research, increase social and emotional bonds. Macfarlane has shown that 6 days after birth infants can distinguish reliably by scent their mother's breast pad from the breast pads of other women (Macfarlane, 1975). The mother has an intense interest in looking at her newborn baby's open eyes (Klaus & Kennell, 1982; Robson, 1967). In the first 45 minutes of life the infant is awake and alert and will visually follow the mother for 180 degrees. With the mother's strong desire to touch and see her child, nature has provided for the immediate and essential union of the two. The alert newborn rewards the mother for her efforts by following her with his or her eyes, thus maintaining their interaction and kindling the tired mother's fascination with her baby.

Lind and associates in Stockholm have shown that a surprising increase in blood flow to the breast occurs when a mother hears her infant (Lind, Vuorenkoski, & Wasz-Hoeckert, 1973). These intricate interactions have focused attention on the cascade of interlocking sensory patterns that quickly develop between mother and infant in the first hours of life.

Evidence suggests that many of these early interactions also take place between the father and his newborn child. In an interesting observation of fathers, Rödholm and Larsson noted that paternal caregiving greatly increased when the father was allowed to interact and establish eye-to-eye contact with his infant for 1 hour during the first hours of life (Rödholm & Larsson, 1979). Keller and others reported that the group of fathers who received extended postpartum hospital contact with their infants, compared to a traditional contact group, engaged in more "en face" behavior and vocalization with their infants and were more involved in infant caretaking responsibilities 6 weeks after the baby's birth (Keller, Hildebrandt, & Richards, 1985). They also had higher self-esteem scores than the other group of fathers.

In his work with a mother and her 3-month-old twins, Stern observed that the pattern of interaction between a mother and her child has a characteristic rhythm (Stern, 1971). Intricate interchanges occur within a few seconds. When these interactions are repeatedly out of phase—for example, if one partner looks away just as the other looks at him—many aspects of the relationship between the two individuals are disturbed. Our observations suggest that this dance of mother and infant, which may or may not be in rhythm, is initiated in the immediate postpartum period. Brazelton and his colleagues (Brazelton et al., 1974) have stated, "This interdependency of rhythms seems to be at the root of their attachment' as well as communication." Thus it seems important that the family have privacy in the first hours of life, in which the new and older members may become attuned to each other.

☐ Loss of Traditional Perinatal Practices and Support

In the movement of families across the Atlantic to settle in the United States, important ties to extended families, as well as a number of traditions and practices, were lost. Life in the United States emphasized mobility and change. Frequently, newcomers to the United States wanted to cast off old practices and adopt new American ideas, which often meant rearing children differently than had been the practice in their family for hundreds of years. At the beginning of the twentieth century, birth occurred in the home, usually with family members present. The baby remained with the mother from birth on and the baby was breast-fed. Traditions and practices affecting the mother, the infant, and the mother–infant pair that had developed over centuries, particularly social support, were lost as birth shifted from the home to the hospital. The research that my colleague Marshall Klaus and I have conducted suggests that this loss has exceeded the limits of adaptability of some mothers and infants (Kennell, DeChateau, & Wasz-Hoeckert, 1987; Klaus & Kennell, 1982). Let us consider the following situations based on our field research.

In a typical home in the Mayan Indian village of Santa María Cauqué in the Guatemalan Highlands there is no VCR, no color TV, no compact disc player, no stereo, no central air conditioning, no refrigerator, no Sealy Posturepedic mattress, no wall-to-wall carpeting, no indoor plumbing, and no running water. It is hard for us in Western, industrialized societies to believe that life can go on without these objects. But in fact, traditional practices that have been passed down for thousands of years give a new mother access to many important things: She is allowed to stay together with her baby from the moment of birth on, and she has support from close friends and family members during the pregnancy, labor, delivery, and the first months of the baby's life. By tradition, the mother is encouraged to keep busy working in early labor, to move about until the time of delivery, and to deliver in a vertical squatting position. These practices have continued from generation to generation for thousands of years because they work. These ways of doing things have developed through the rigorous process of evolution, and they have been crucial for the survival of these people. Even in recent history, the people living in these Mayan Indian villages have been exposed repeatedly to devastating earthquakes, wars, forced conscription of the young men into the armed forces, and extreme poverty.

Some of the Mayan Indian women who have left this village because of economic pressures have delivered their babies in the urban teaching hospital, where they receive the benefits of technology with sterile equipment, running water, expert medical care, the availability of newborn resuscitation techniques, and a neonatal intensive care unit. But the hospital routine requires these women to labor alone. They have lost the warmth, encouragement, and guidance that their family could provide.

These women provide examples of different levels of support from family, community, and culture during pregnancy, labor, delivery, and the first months of the infant's life. Cross-cultural observations such as these have stimulated productive research by Dr. Brazelton and others speaking at this symposium. When we were carrying out research on breast-feeding in a large maternity hospital in Guatemala, we were distressed to hear the plaintive, childlike cries of mothers who were laboring in a room alone. When we asked one of our Guatemalan research workers to stay by the side of a crying mother, we were impressed that she would stop crying and become relaxed even though the uterine contractions continued. We had the impression that labor progressed more rapidly as well as more peacefully with a companion present. This stimulated us to learn more about labor support in the United States and in other cultures and to plan a research study (Klaus, Kennell, & Klaus, 1993; Sosa, Kennell, Robertson, & Urrutia, 1980).

We have discovered that in all but 1 of 128 cultures studied by anthropologists, a family member or friend, usually a woman, remained with the mother during labor and delivery. Although more fathers, relatives, and friends have been allowed into labor and delivery rooms in the past 10 years, a significant number of mothers still labor and deliver in some hospitals without the presence of family members or close friends. There had been little systematic study of this issue since the Newtons reported in 1962 that mothers who were quiet and relaxed and had better emotional relationships with their attendants during labor and delivery were more pleased at the first sight of their babies (Newton & Newton, 1962).

The clinical importance of emotional support during labor is strongly supported by three randomized trials of continuous support during labor, provided by a woman we call a *doula*, involving nearly 1,200 women. Two studies in Guatemala showed significant effects on the course of the mother during labor (Klaus, 1986; Sosa, 1980). In a study in Houston, Texas (Kennell, McGrath, Klaus, Robertson, & Hinckley, 1991) primiparous mothers, supported continuously by a woman companion, had a smaller number of cesarean sections (18% vs. 8%), a shorter length of labor, requested fewer epidurals (11% vs. 64%), and required less frequent use of oxytocin compared to mothers who did not have continuous support. In spite of the measures used in modern obstetric care to shorten the length of labor, such as artificial rupture of membranes, pitocin, forceps, and cesarean sections, none of these interventions matched the shorter labor lengths of the women who had a doula in this study. Continuous social support appears to be an essential ingredient of childbirth that was lost when birthing moved from home to hospital.

What does a doula do that is associated with such powerful effects? A time-sampling study was carried out by Terri DeLay as part of the study of the effects of the doula in the United States. When the mothers were uncomfortable or in contraction, doulas touched the mothers significantly more. Doulas spent the majority of the time within 1 foot of the mother, possibly indicating that close proximity is a key factor in the behavior of a doula. Doulas spent almost half of their time talking with the mothers, suggesting that comforting, encouraging or didactic phrases are considered supportive, either directly by reducing the mother's anxiety, or indirectly by distracting her from the pain. Further, over half of the time, doulas used various styles of touching the mother, indicating that physical contact may be an important element of doula behavior. Finally, although caretaking behaviors generally occurred less frequently than other behaviors, those geared toward the physical comfort of the mother occurred most frequently.

The direct effects of the continuous support of a doula on the health of the mother and infant in our three studies are dramatic. However, there appear to be indirect effects that influence early mother–infant communication and make a mother's early attachment to her baby in the neonatal and puerperal period progress more easily.

In the first 25 minutes after they left the delivery room, the mothers who had a doula present during labor were awake more of the time when they were with their newborns (Sosa et al., 1980). They stroked their babies, and smiled at and talked to their infants significantly more than the control mothers when controlling for length of labor and the time the mothers were awake. We do not have evidence to indicate whether this has long-term implications. However, in the original study that we conducted on the effects of early and extended mother–infant contact, there are clues suggesting that the level of affectionate interaction between mothers and infants during the early postpartum period might significantly affect later behavior.

Fathers are now expected to be present at the birth of their infants by virtue of their biological relationship to those infants, but fathers may not be best suited to fulfill the role of sole labor support person. Currently in the United States, there is no long-standing tradition that defines the father's role during labor and delivery.

A male partner may be a poor source of support for the laboring woman because of his unsureness about his role, his anxiety about the alien hospital environment, and his worries about his partner and their baby, but his personal involvement with the woman makes his presence in labor and delivery of primary importance. In a study by Bertsch et al. (Bertsch, Nagashima-Whalen, Dykeman, Kennell, & McGrath, 1990), virtually all mothers stated that the father's presence during labor was terrifically helpful. In reality these fathers touched and spoke to their laboring partners significantly less often than a comparison group of doulas. Thus, women and their partners want the male partner to be present at labor and delivery, but behaviorally the father may provide very little of the type of active support given by doulas.

This leads to the important question: Can similar perinatal effects be achieved by doulas supporting both women and their male partners? We are attempting to find the answer in a randomized controlled study of labor support to couples at our hospital in Cleveland. Preliminary results show a significant decrease in cesarean sections when the mother is supported by her husband and doula. Hofmeyr, Nikodem, Wolman, Chalmers, and Kramer (1991) in South Africa in a randomized study of doula support found that labor support by a doula decreased anxiety and depression and improved maternal self-concept, mother–infant relationships, infant health, breast-feeding, and perceptions of the marital relationship.

If the effects of support supplied just during labor and delivery are so great, cannot similar benefits be expected from positive social support during pregnancy and the first weeks after the birth of the baby? Results from our Houston study introduce some interesting connections between social support during pregnancy and perinatal outcome. While examining the data about all the mothers and infants in that study in an effort to understand the continued high U.S. cesarean section rates, White, Black and Hispanic subgroups were found to have a significantly different incidence of cesarean sections (White = 5.6%, Black = 20.1%, Hispanic = 11.5%, $p < .004$). We wondered whether this finding is somehow related to the continued Black/White discrepancy in infant mortality in the United States. Infant mortality is usually twice as high in Blacks as in Whites.

In an effort to answer this question, the factors believed to be associated with differences in infant mortality rates were examined for their relationship with the cesarean rate discrepancy, even though the study was not designed for this purpose. By including only low-risk patients at full term, the study design excluded women with medical conditions often thought to account for Black/White differences in infant mortality. Physiological differences across the three groups that could increase the need for cesarean delivery were eliminated by preenrollment screening for diabetes, hypertension, obesity, and premature labor. In addition, the three groups did not differ on mean measures of prenatal factors such as income, maternal education level, maternal age,

age at first prenatal visit, and number of prenatal visits. Women with any evidence of drug or alcohol abuse were excluded from the study.

Differences in care and the course of labor and delivery were also considered as potential sources of the variation in cesarean rates. However, labor length, anesthesia use, medical and nursing staff time with the patient, and obstetric and neonatal complications (e.g., meconium staining, maternal fever, need for infant resuscitation) did not differ across the three groups. Mean postdelivery ratings of the labor and delivery experience by mothers did not differ across the three groups, whether or not they received continuous labor support.

Studies have suggested lack of social support during pregnancy as a cause of high infant mortality rates. In the current study, there were no group differences in social support as measured by income and education levels, but the pattern of family living arrangements differed strikingly across the three groups. Specifically, the majority of White and Hispanic mothers lived with their male partner (either independently or in the parental household), whereas most of the Black mothers resided only with their parent(s) or other family members. The presence or absence of a male partner in the home may not be a causative factor, but rather an indicator of the general attitudes about pregnancy, childbirth, and family, which determine the quality or quantity of support provided to the expectant mother. Although the information obtained in this study examined only family constellation, the intriguing results suggest that all aspects of social support in the perinatal period should be investigated as potential determinants of perinatal outcome.

☐ Substance Abuse and the Importance of the Family

A third occurrence that affects the perinatal period is the abandonment of motherhood due to alcohol, cocaine, and other substance abuse. There is probably no city and no premature or intensive care nursery in the United States that has not experienced cocaine-abusing parents who do not visit their infant, fail to take the baby home and abandon the baby or, after discharge, neglect the baby. I use the term *parent*, but the majority of these are single mothers.

Substance abuse may be a symptom of the crumbling of the family. It is one of many problems threatening the health and development of children that will continue until we reestablish the importance of the family. The early discharge of mothers and babies from the maternity hospital, the lack of a national parental leave policy (until 1993), and the pressures on mothers to return to work soon after delivery deprive most mothers and fathers in the United States of the opportunity to really "take in" and get in rhythm with their baby in the first hours, days, and weeks so that they develop a sturdy attachment. With less opportunity for support from the extended family and almost no available home help to assist the mother (in contrast to most European countries), we in the United States are clearly neglecting the admonitions of Donald Winnicott: "The mother's bond with the baby is very powerful at the beginning and we must do all we can to enable her to be preoccupied with her baby at this time—the natural time."

When a mother's early contact and interaction with her baby are abbreviated, rushed, or distracted by the demands of discharge, care of the household and husband, plus early return to work, is it possible for her to achieve the type of bond that will enable her to manage the child through the challenges and vicissitudes of the next 21 years?

Some mothers can, but many demonstrate that present priorities are exceeding their limits of adaptability. We need a national family policy to restore families to good health. These policies should support Winnicott-like concepts by establishing optimal perinatal practices, parental leave, home help, available and affordable quality day care, flexible working hours, and arrangements for mothers and fathers.

In 1959, Greta Bibring wrote about childbirth, "What was once a crisis with carefully worked-out traditional customs of giving support to the woman passing through this crisis period has become at this time a crisis with no mechanisms within the society for helping the woman involved in this profound change of conflict-solutions and adjustive tasks" (p. 113). In the three decades since then, many support systems have been developed. The widely assorted childbirth classes continue some of the traditional customs. However, more extensive support systems for all parents during pregnancy and after delivery are needed due to the loss of the extended family and due to the pressures on mothers and fathers that have increased greatly during this period.

Our research indicates the need for a supportive woman companion (a doula) continuously present with every woman and almost all couples during labor and delivery. Her supportive role would start in the third trimester so she could become well acquainted and help with questions, uncertainties, options, and explanations. She would make certain that the mother and father could interact with their undressed baby after delivery in privacy for the first hour. She would be certain to emphasize the amazing abilities of their infant by showing Brazelton Scale items, and she would keep the baby with the mother and father every possible minute in the hospital. The doula would assist with breast-feeding. She would arrange for support for the mother and baby in the first weeks so that the mother is protected, nurtured, and mothered, so that the mother could "take in" her baby, establish her breast-feeding, and progressively develop a robust attachment. The doula would also support the father and encourage his involvement in the care of the baby.

☐ Implications

The studies reported here on bonding, on the remarkable abilities of the newborn baby and the newly delivered mother, and on the benefits of relationships and support during pregnancy, labor, and delivery (doula) and in the weeks and months following delivery present a compelling argument for a change from the management of each mother and baby as a medical problem. In most medical centers, the increasing emphasis on the use of epidural analgesia and interventions to speed the progress of labor ("the medicalization of childbirth") have removed control and decision making from the parents and have greatly emphasized the medical management of the mother and the baby, often to the detriment of the early social, emotional, and humanistic experiences of the parents with their newborn infant.

The studies of infant abilities and of parent–infant attachment two decades ago resulted in changes in most maternity units, giving more attention to the needs and wishes of parents, infants, and families. At the present time, in many maternity hospitals these practices have become so modified that they are slapdash in nature and often violate components of the initial research. The practice of keeping parents and their newborn together in a private setting immediately after birth has been eliminated in other hospitals.

In addition, with the present emphasis on obstetric interventions, there has been a profound change in the role of the childbirth educator in many communities. For many years the childbirth educator described a variety of options for parents and explained advantages and disadvantages so that parents could make their own decisions. In recent years, the role of the childbirth educator has changed. Increasingly, the educator has had her role restricted to telling the parents what the course of care will be in the hospital where they plan to deliver or with the obstetricians who will be managing the delivery.

The positive physical and psychological results of continuous emotional support during labor by an experienced woman deliver new hope for parents and children, but also many challenges. The doula does not fit the medical view of obstetrics. Effects of the magnitude that have been reported almost certainly reflect psychoneuroendocrine changes. If studies can demonstrate these changes, bonding and the doula may fit better into the medical model and be more readily accepted.

Few doulas are currently available, but it is heartening to note the large number of women who wish to become doulas because of their desire to help other mothers through the crisis of childbirth. New information on the positive effects of doula support for different groups of mothers (e.g., women whose partners are present at the birth) may increase parents' interest in having a doula and may result in obstetric accommodations for the doula throughout the country.

The findings from the bonding and doula studies fit in well with the current emphasis on alternative methods of health care that focus on mind–body influences. Disease-oriented programs emphasizing supportive relationships show benefits in a variety of medical problems such as heart disease, cancer, and conditions unresponsive to traditional medical care. The doula studies provide a unique model for those interested in understanding how mind–body influences operate. The period of labor is relatively short and there are undoubtedly hormonal changes associated with the doula's effectiveness. When these have been elucidated, the doula may provide a model for testing in which individual components of alternative medical programs are particularly effective. The emphasis on the treatment of medical diseases should not distract attention from the needs of individuals and families facing the life stresses that are characteristic of our society, such as divorce, single parenthood, unemployment, aging, and retirement.

Studies on the doula and bonding are of obvious importance not only for the benefit of families during the perinatal period, but also for what they offer to families and individuals through the life span. Hopefully, the frightening evidence of the dissolution of the American family and the multiple disturbances of interpersonal relationships will lead to other studies on the needs of individuals and families. It is difficult to believe that it is necessary to have a further increase in family and individual dysfunction before close attention is paid to the benefits of supportive relationships throughout life.

For the many professionals concerned with psychological and social problems of children and families, the doula and bonding studies should point the way to various changes that enhance and provide supportive relationships throughout life: for individuals facing the problems of declining abilities and worsening health in old age, and for families and children from the perinatal period through early adulthood.

Finally, the results from studies on bonding and doula support should lead to an enhanced national appreciation of the necessity of giving every child the best start possible by providing optimal support and enhancement of the early relationships in the perinatal period to every new family.

The family is indeed born in the delivery room, but now we see that in its early infancy it requires careful feeding and nurturing.

☐ References

Bertsch, T. D., Nagashima-Whalen, L., Dykeman, S., Kennell, J. H., & McGrath, S. (1990). Labor support by first-time fathers: Direct observations. *Journal of Psychosomatic Obstetrics and Gynecology, 11*, 251–260.

Bibring, G. (1959). Some considerations of the psychological processes in pregnancy. *Psychoanalytic Study of the Child, 14*, 113.

Brazelton, T. B. (1973). Effect of maternal expectations on early infant behavior. *Early Child Development and Care, 2*, 259.

Brazelton, T. B., Koslowski, B., & Main, M. (1974). Origins of reciprocity: The early mother–infant interaction. In M. Lewis & L. A. Rosenblum (Eds.), *The effect of the infant on its caregiver* (pp. 49–76). New York: Wiley.

Condon, W. S., & Sander, L. W. (1974). Neonate movement is synchronized with adult speech: Interactional participation and language acquisition. *Science, 183*, 99.

Engel., G. L., Reichsman, F., Harway, V. T., & Hess, D. W. (1985). Monica: Infant-feeding behavior of a mother gastric fistula-fed as an infant: A 30-year longitudinal study of enduring effects. In E. J. Anthony & G. H. Pollock (Eds.), *Parental influences in health and disease* (pp. 29–90). Boston: Little, Brown & Co.

Gomes-Pedro, J., Bento de Almeida, J., Silveira da Costa, C., & Barbosa, A. (1984). Influence of early mother–infant contact on dyadic behavior during the first month of life. *Developmental Medicine & Child Neurology, 26*(5), 657–664.

Hofmeyr, G. J., Nikodem, V. C., Wolman, W. L., Chalmers, B. E., & Kramer, T. (1991). Companionship to modify the clinical birth environment: Effects on progress and perceptions of labour, and breastfeeding. *British Journal of Obstetrics and Gynaecology, 98*(8), 756–764.

Keller, W. D., Hildebrandt, K. A., & Richards, M. (1985). Effects of extended father–infant contact during the newborn period. *Infant Behavior and Development, 8*, 337.

Kemper, K., Forsyth, B., & McCarthy, P. (1989). Jaundice, terminating breast-feeding, and the vulnerable child. *Pediatrics, 84*, 773–778.

Kennell, J. H., DeChateau, P., & Wasz-Hoeckert, O. (1987). John Lind memorial symposium. *Infant Mental Health Journal, 8*, 190–209.

Kennell, J. H., McGrath, S., Klaus, M. H., Robertson, S., & Hinkley, S. (1991). Continuous emotional support during labor in a U.S. hospital. *JAMA, 256*, 2197–2201.

Kennell, J. H., & Rolnick, A. (1960). Discussing problems in newborn babies with their parents. *Pediatrics, 27*, 832.

Kennell, J. H., Jerauld, R., Wolfe, H., Chesler, D., Kreger, N. C., McAlpine, W., Steffa, M., & Klaus, M. H. (1974). Maternal behavior one year after early and extended post-partum contact. *Developmental Medicine and Child Neurology, 16*, 172.

Klaus, M. H., & Kennell, J. H. (1982). *Parent-infant bonding* (2nd ed.). St. Louis, MO: C. V. Mosby.

Klaus, M. H., Kennell, J. H., & Klaus, P. H. (1995). *Bonding: Building the foundations of secure attachment and independence.* Reading, MA: Addison-Wesley.

Klaus, M. H., Kennell, J. H., & Klaus, P. H. (1993). *Mothering the mother: How a doula can help you have a shorter, easier and healthier birth.* Reading, MA: Addison-Wesley.

Klaus, M. H., Jerauld, R., Kreger, N. C., McAlpine, W., Steffa, M., & Kennell, J. H. (1972). Maternal attachment: Importance of the post-partum days. *New England Journal of Medicine, 286*, 460.

Klaus, M. H., Kennel, J. L., Robertson, S. S., & Sosa, R. (1986). Effects of social support during parturition on maternal and infant morbidity. *British Medical Journal, 293*, 585–587.

Lang, R. (1972). *Birth book*. Ben Lomond, CA: Genesis Press.

Lind, J., Vuorenkoski, V., & Wasz-Hoeckert, O. (1973). The effect of cry stimulus on the temperature of the lactating breast primipara: A thermographic study. In N. Morris (Ed.), *Psychosomatic medicine in obstetrics and gynaecology*. Basel, Switzerland: S. Karger.

Macfarlane, J. A. (1975). Olfaction in the development of social preferences in the human neonate. In *The parent–infant interaction* (pp. 103–117). Amsterdam: Elsevier.

Macfarlane, J. A., Smith, D. M., & Garrow, D. H. (1978). The relationship between mother and neonate. In S. Kitzinger & J. A. Davis (Eds.), *The place of birth*. New York: Oxford University Press.

Newton, N., & Newton, M. (1962). Mother's reactions to their newborn babies. *JAMA, 181*, 206.

O'Connor, S., Vietze, P. M., Sherrod, K. B., Sandler, H. M., & Altemeier, W. A. (1980). Reduced incidence of parenting inadequacy following rooming-in. *Pediatrics, 66*, 183–190.

Parke, R. D. (1979). Perspectives on father-infant interaction. In J. D. Osofsky (Ed.), *The handbook of infant development* (pp. 549–590). New York: Wiley.

Parke, R. D., Hymel, S., Power, T., & Tinsley, B. (1979). Fathers and risk: A hospital based model of intervention. In D. B. Sawin, R. C. Hawkins, L. O. Walker, & J. H. Penticuff (Eds.), *Psychosocial risks in infant-environment transactions* (pp. 35–70). New York: Brunner/Mazel.

Rose, J., Boggs, T., Jr., & Alderstein, A. (1960). The evidence for a syndrome of "mothering disability" consequent to threats to the survival of neonates: A design for hypothesis testing including prevention in a prospective study. *American Journal of Diseases of Children, 100*, 776.

Siegel, E., et al. (1980). Hospital and home support during infancy: Impact on maternal attachment, child abuse and neglect, and health care utilization. *Pediatrics, 66*, 183.

Sosa, R., Kennell, J. H., Robertson, S., & Urrutia, J. (1980). The effect of a supportive companion on perinatal problems, length of labor, and mother–infant interaction. *New England Journal of Medicine, 303*, 597.

Stern, D. (1971). A micro-analysis of mother-infant interaction. *Journal of the American Academy of Child Psychiatry, 10*, 510.

Trevarthen, C. (1977). Descriptive analysis of infant communicative behavior. In H. R. Schaffer (Ed.), *Studies in mother-infant interaction* (pp. 227–270). New York: Academic Press.

Winnicott, D. W. (1971). *Playing and reality*. London: Tavistock.

CHAPTER 4

Urie Bronfenbrenner

Preparing a World for the Infant in the Twenty-First Century: The Research Challenge

As the twenty-first century dawns, we have several wishes for the babies of the new century, each one invoking and ensuring for each baby the blessing of a developmental principle that science reveals as furthering the realization of the newborn baby's unquestionably rich genetic potential for competence and character.

☐ Developmental Principle 1

In order to develop intellectually, emotionally, socially, and morally, Baby XXI requires the same thing: progressively more complex, reciprocally contingent interaction with one or more older people with whom he or she develops a strong, mutual, and irrational emotional attachment, and who are committed to her well-being and development, preferably for life (Bronfenbrenner, 1989; Bronfenbrenner & Morris, 1997).

What is meant by "progressively more complex reciprocally contingent interaction"? Perhaps an analogy will help. It's what happens in a ping-pong game once the play gets going. As the partners become familiar with each other, they adapt to each other's style. The game begins to go faster, and the shots in both directions tend to become more complicated as each player, in effect, challenges the other (Bronfenbrenner, 1979, 1993, 1995).

Thus far, it might appear that any person who repeatedly engages in progressively more complex reciprocal activity with a child will be equally effective in furthering the child's physical and psychological development. At its close, however, the invocation imposes some conditions in that regard; specifically, the person must be someone with whom the child develops a strong, mutual, irrational emotional attachment, and who is committed to the child's well-being and development, preferably for life.

If I were now speaking not here but in my own country, the United States, at this point there would be several hands raised in the air, people wishing to raise a question. With us, it is not always a friendly question: "What do you mean by 'an irrational emotional attachment'?"

In reply, I say: "Somebody's got to be crazy about that kid!"

And once again, in my own country, that response usually provokes a second question, hardly more friendly that the first: "Why does it have to be 'irrational'?"

By now, a short answer will no longer do; you have to give an explanation. So, I explain along the following lines. Any parent of course knows that his or her child is not the most intelligent, the most beautiful, the most wonderful in the world. Nevertheless, at some level deep inside, that is what most of us feel—that our own children are more magical and special than any other children we know. And what research shows is that this makes a critical difference for the following reason. Progressively more complex, reciprocally contingent interaction is hard work. It takes strong motivation and all your attention. As we Americans say, you have to hang in there. And "irrational emotional attachment"—what in plain language is called "love"—makes that possible.

But it is not that simple. Three points need to be emphasized:

1. Love is not enough. There must also be activity.
2. The activity cannot go just in one direction. It has to go in both directions—back and forth.
3. It cannot be the same back and forth. Sooner or later it has to become "more complex." But you can't rush it; the complexity has to come about gradually, not all at once.

By the way, in the beginning, which party should be the first to make it more complex—the infant, or the caregiver? Research indicates that the process works better if the infant is the one to introduce something new. In our case, it's Baby XXI, who starts his or her own birthday celebration. But then we have to respond, and continue to do so. And that has to happen just about every day from now on, not just on special days. Otherwise, he or she won't realize his or her unusual potential.

Another question: Who is better at this emotionally charged ping-pong game—mothers or fathers, women or men? The available evidence indicates that once they get into the game, either sex can play equally well, although they have somewhat different styles. However, such gender differences do not appear to be very important. Far more critical for Baby XXI's future is to grant the baby my second birthday wish, as follows.

☐ Developmental Principle 2

The establishment and maintenance of patterns of progressively more complex reciprocal interaction and emotional attachment between caregiver and child depend in substantial degree on the availability and involvement of another adult, a third party who assists, encourages, spells off, gives status to, and expresses admiration and affection for the person caring for and engaging in joint activity with the young child (Bronfenbrenner, 1989).

It also helps, but is not absolutely necessary, if the "third party" is of the opposite sex from that of the person dealing with the child.

Isn't science wonderful? We've reinvented the wheel!

Who is the third party—mother or father? It doesn't matter. The second blessing works both ways. Each partner enables the other to be a more loving and effective parent. In short, in the dance of development, ideally, it takes three to tango!

The third developmental principle tells us that you can't just dance anywhere. There has to be a time and a place.

☐ Developmental Principle 3

The process of gradually escalating, reciprocally contingent joint activity between a child and an adult who care about each other fosters the child's development only to the extent that it takes place on a regular basis over extended periods in the child's life under conditions that are generally free from frequent interruption and acute environmental or emotional stress. Why so? Because, otherwise, neither the child nor the adult can keep attending to and responding to the other. And if they don't, joint activities cannot really get going, and hence don't get a chance to become increasingly more complex. This means, in turn, that development proceeds at a slower pace so that the child may not get very far in reaching his or her potential for competence and character. Unless, of course, the necessary conditions for restarting, sustaining, and expanding the ping-pong game are reestablished.

It's never too late to do that. Indeed, it appears that we are the only species for whom there are no fixed, critical periods. Some recovery is always possible. But there are some qualifications. First, there must be a change in the child's immediate environment; it must become more responsive to the child's needs. Second, the longer one waits, the more difficult the task and the longer it takes for the child to recover lost ground.

Fortunately, there are other positive forces that help to foster and sustain psychological growth. The next developmental principle tells us that interaction with people is not the whole story.

☐ Developmental Principle 4

The establishment of patterns of progressive interpersonal interaction under conditions of strong, mutual attachment enhances the young child's responsiveness to other features of the immediate physical, social, and—in due course—symbolic environment that invite exploration, manipulation, elaboration and imagination. Such activities, in turn, also advance and support the child's psychological development (Bronfenbrenner & Morris, 1997).

Once again, a question arises. For young children today, how available are objects and settings that meet the developmental criteria set forth in the foregoing principle? Consider, from this perspective, the wide array of automated toys—animals, humans, space creatures, and monsters, all programmed to repeat the same series of actions over and over again. And even those that are not battery powered share with their activated counterparts the common suggested features of overwhelming physical prowess, violence, and sadistic cruelty. Today, in both stores and homes, such items far outnumber representations of more human figures and familiar objects that invite imaginative play about activities and relationships in everyday life (Bronfenbrenner, 1989).

For older ages, many of these same elements are incorporated in the rapidly proliferating series of board games, construction sets, and puzzles—nowadays specially diversified for successive age levels—and they are increasingly incorporated into preprogrammed audiovisual devices and computer games that need to be periodically updated. All of these items become the focus of high-pressure television advertising campaigns, often aimed directly at the children themselves. As a result, many homes are filled with so many gadgets and games that none of them gets played for any length of time.

In sum, in today's highly technological, hectic world, most of the toys and activities provided to children hardly fulfill the requirements stipulated in the fourth principle: Specifically, they do not invite exploration, manipulation, elaboration, or imaginative activity on the part of the child. They fail primarily because they are so rigidly structured as to allow little opportunity for introducing any spontaneous variation. To be sure, many products of modern technology do meet the stipulated criteria, but activities of this kind are by no means limited to the technological realm. Indeed, they are perhaps even more readily found in traditional cultures than in so-called "postmodern societies" (surely an oxymoron!). To cite a few examples: objects in nature—both animate and inanimate, large and small—like domestic animals, stones and shells, trees and caves; objects that can be put inside one another, or used to build things (and tear them down again); anything that can make rhythmic and musical sounds, such as pots, pans, and soup spoons; and materials that can be used to draw, paint, or mold shapes and forms. More broadly, whatever induces sustained attention and evolving activity of body and mind, such as songs, dances, stories, dolls, stuffed animals, picture books, and, of course, real books that can be read and then newly reimagined, and retold on one's own. (You will not be surprised that all these are well represented among the gifts I have brought for Baby XXI.)

But some children may not respond, even when provided with a wide range of objects and opportunities for activity. One obvious prerequisite is that the environment must include materials that are appropriate to the child's developing physical and psychological capacities. In addition, we have also seen that the youngster's active orientation toward the physical and symbolic environment is powerfully mediated by prior, persistent patterns of interpersonal interaction in the context of a strong, enduring emotional relationship with one or more adults, almost always including the child's parents. These ongoing experiences remain a potent liberating and energizing force in relation not only to the physical environment but to the social world as well. Thus, they enable the child to relate to other people beyond the immediate family—including peers as well as other adults—and to involve them effectively in meeting the child's own developmental needs. At a broader level, the child's newly acquired abilities make it possible for the child to benefit from experiences in other settings, most notably to learn in school.

In short, the informal education that takes place in the family is not merely a pleasant prelude but a powerful prerequisite for success in formal education from the primary grades onward. This empowering effect reaches further still, for, as evidenced in longitudinal studies, it appears to provide a basis—but offers no guarantee—for the subsequent development of the capacity to function responsively and creatively as an adult in the realms of work, family life, and citizenship (Bronfenbrenner, 1996b, 1996c).

This does not mean, however, that the absence of early opportunities for interactive experiences in the context of a mutual emotional attachment precludes the possibility of later achieving adult effectiveness. As indicated earlier, there are several other routes to the acquisition of competence and character. The problem is that they are much less efficient, and much more expensive in both time and money.

Taken as a whole, the research evidence indicates that when the elements stipulated in the first three principles are provided on a continuing basis, the positive effects on children's development are indeed substantial. Accordingly, a society that seeks the well-being and development of its children is well advised to provide them with the kinds of environments and experiences specified in the first three propositions.

But there is a catch. The research findings also reveal that the developmentally fostering processes of interaction between child and environment presented thus far operate efficiently only under certain environmental conditions. One of these conditions we have already mentioned—the active involvement of a "third party." What happens if there is no third party? The question is, of course, far from academic, for it speaks to one of the major changes now taking place in postindustrial societies, namely, the rapid rise in the proportion of single-parent households in both the developed and developing world. The overwhelming majority of such homes are those in which the father is absent and the mother bears full responsibility for the upbringing of the child. Many investigations of developmental processes and outcomes in families of this kind have now been conducted across a range of cultural and social class groups, including socialist countries and some developing nations as well (Bronfenbrenner, McClelland, Wethington, Moen, & Ceci, 1996).

In general, the findings lead to two complementary conclusions. First, the results indicate that children growing up in such households are at greater risk for experiencing a variety of behavioral and educational problems, including extremes of hyperactivity or withdrawal, lack of attentiveness in the classroom, difficulty in deferring gratification, impaired academic achievement, school misbehavior, absenteeism, dropping out, involvement in socially alienated peer groups, and, especially, the so-called "teenage syndrome" of behaviors that tend to hang together—smoking, drinking, early and frequent sexual experience, a cynical attitude toward work, adolescent pregnancy, and, in the more extreme cases, drugs, suicide, vandalism, violence, and criminal acts (Bronfenbrenner et al., 1996). Most of these effects are much more pronounced for boys than for girls. More intensive investigations of these phenomena have identified a common predisposing factor for the emergence of such problem behavior: namely, a history of impaired parent–child interaction and relationships beginning in early childhood.

Not all single-parent families, however, exhibit these disturbed relationships and their disruptive effects on development. Systematic studies of the exceptions have identified what may be described as a general "immunizing" factor: Children of single-parent mothers are less likely to experience developmental problems in those families in which the mother experiences strong support from other adults living in the home, or from nearby relatives, friends, or neighbors, members of religious groups, and, when available, staff members of family support and child care programs. Interestingly enough, the most effective agent of "third-party" support (in the minority of instances in which such assistance is provided) appears to be the child's father. And what counted most was not the attention given to the child, important as this was, but the assistance provided to the mother herself by serving as a backup in times of crisis, doing errands, spelling her off, sharing responsibility for discipline, and providing needed advice and encouragement. Once again, in the family dance, "it takes three to tango."

The developmental risks associated with a one-parent family structure are relatively small, however, in comparison with those involved in two other types of environmental context. The first and most destructive of these is poverty. Because many single-parent families are also poor, this places them and their children in double jeopardy. Even when two parents are present, research in both developed and developing countries reveals that in households living under stressful economic and social conditions, processes of parent–child interaction and environmentally oriented child activity are more difficult to initiate and to sustain. Much more effort and perseverance on the part of parents is required to achieve the same effect than in families living under more favorable circumstances, particularly when, as is often the case, the mother is the only parent or even the only adult in the home.

To be sure, research also indicates that when the mother, or some other adult committed to the child's well-being, does manage to establish and maintain a pattern of progressive reciprocal interaction, the typically disruptive impact of poverty on development is significantly reduced. But the proportion of parents who, despite their stressful life circumstances, are able to provide quality care is, under present conditions, not very large. And even for this minority the parents' buffering power begins to decline sharply by the time children are 5 or 6 years old and are being exposed to other impoverished and disruptive settings outside the home.

What is the effect of poverty on children's development? The answer to this question has already been given, for the consequences are similar to those for single parenthood in the absence of a third party, but the risks are substantially higher and the effects more pronounced, typically persisting well into adulthood (except in those as-yet-infrequent instances in which opportunities for continuing rehabilitative experiences become available).

It is not only the poor, however, for whom developmental processes are now at risk. In today's world, the well-educated and the well-to-do are no longer protected; over the past two decades other highly vulnerable contexts have evolved that cut across the domains of class and culture. Recent studies reveal that a major disruptive factor in the lives of families and their children is the increasing instability, inconsistency, and hecticness of daily family life (Bronfenbrenner & Morris, 1997). This growing trend is found in both developed and developing countries, but has somewhat different origins in these two worlds. Yet the debilitating effect on child-rearing processes and outcomes is much the same. I begin with examples from the so-called postindustrial world, because they may be more familiar.

In a world in which both parents usually have to work, often at a considerable distance from home, every family member, through the waking hours from morning until night, is "on the run." The need to coordinate conflicting demands of job and child care, often involving varied arrangements that shift from day to day, can produce a situation in which everyone has to be transported several times a day in different directions, usually at the same time—a state of affairs that prompted a foreign colleague to comment, "It seems to me that in your country, most children are being brought up in moving vehicles."

Other factors contributing to the disruption of daily family life include long commutes to and back from work; jobs that require one or the other parent to be away for extended periods of time; frequent changes in employment; associated moves for the whole family or those that leave the rest of the family behind waiting until the school term ends or adequate housing can be found; and, last but far from least, the increasing number of divorces, remarriages, and redivorces. (Incidentally, the most recent evidence suggests that the disruptive effects of remarriage on children may be even greater than those of divorce.)

What are the outcomes of "family hecticness"? Once again, the observed consequences are behavior problems and educational problems, including longer term effects that now also encompass children of the well-educated and the well-to-do.

It is obvious that to deal with such deeply rooted societal phenomena as poverty and the hectic pace of daily life will require nothing short of a restructuring of the social order. Nevertheless, the destructive impact of both these forces on the competence and character of future generations is so enormous that their elimination must be given the highest priority at the national and international level.

But such an undertaking is a long-term endeavor, and children can't wait. There are some immediate and practicable short-term strategies that can reduce the social disarray and human damage produced by both destructive forces. The general nature of these strategies is indicated in the next principle.

☐ Developmental Principle 5

The effective functioning of child-rearing processes in the family and other child settings requires establishing ongoing patterns of exchange of information, two-way communication, mutual accommodation, and mutual trust between the principal settings in which children and their parents live their lives. In contemporary societies, these settings are the home, child-care programs, the school, and the parents' place of work (Bronfenbrenner & Morris, 1997).

Why, you may ask, the parents' workplace? The answer from research is that today one of the principal sources of stress and disarray in the lives of families and their children lies in the conflict between the needs of the family and the demands of the job.

There is an interesting observation in this regard. In whose job does stress have the greater disruptive effect on the child, the mother's or the father's? The answer may appear counterintuitive—the available evidence points to the father. Why? The most apt response to this question was given by the distinguished American sociologist Robin M. Williams. Commenting on this differential effect of stress on the job, he pointed out, "It's because the mothers absorb it all, and the fathers don't even know that there's anything to be absorbed."

The sixth and last principle lays out the chief directions to be pursued in policies and practices aimed at enhancing child development and family life in contemporary societies.

☐ Developmental Principle 6

The effective functioning of child-rearing processes in the family and other child settings requires public policies and practices that provide place, time, stability, status, recognition, belief systems, customs, and actions in support of child-rearing activities, not only on the part of parents, caregivers, teachers, and other professional personnel, but also from relatives, friends, neighbors, coworkers, communities, and the major economic, social, and political institutions of the entire society (Bronfenbrenner, 1989).

However, the invocation of Principle 6 does not complete this summary of general findings of recent research on the forces now affecting the development of young children. Unfortunately, I am forced to bring with me yet another gift—one that is to be opened only if my birthday wishes for Baby XXI should not be granted. This last and I hope ungiven gift has a long history. It is called "Pandora's Box," and it contains all of Baby XXI's less welcome potentials—what all the babies of the twenty-first century can become if we do not heed the latest lessons of research in our field. What will then be released are powerful and persistent potentials for anger, hate, destruction of others and of self, and, perhaps the most dangerous of all, apathy and impotence—the inability to act and the inability to love.

Yes, from the findings and trends I have been monitoring now for half a century, such possibilities are not ruled out. Pandora's Box is real, and its contents are escaping. But we still command some forces that can seal it up again. They are the constructive forces embodied in the six principles that emerge from contemporary research on human development. Thus, examples of policies and practices of this kind appear in publications listed in the references at the end of this article. It becomes our responsibility as scientists and citizens to do our part in transforming the lessons of developmental research into developmental reality. That is the gift that Baby XXI, and all the children of the coming twenty-first century, deservedly ask of us today.

☐ References

Bronfenbrenner, U. (1979). *The ecology of human development: Experiments by nature and design.* Cambridge, MA: Harvard University Press.

Bronfenbrenner, U. (1989). Invited address to UNESCO. Bilingual publication No. 188. Paris: Unit for Co-operation with UNICEF and WFP. Reprinted in *Research and clinical center for child development, Annual report*, 1988–1989, No. 12 (pp. 27–40). Sapporo, Japan, Hokkaido University. Also reprinted in H. Nuba, M. Searson, & D. L. Sheiman (Eds.). (1994). *Resources for early childhood* (pp. 113–130). New York: Garland.

Bronfenbrenner, U. (1993). The ecology of cognitive development: Research models and fugitive findings. In R. H. Wozniak & K. Fischer (Eds.), *Scientific environments* (pp. 3–44). Hillsdale, NJ: Lawrence Erlbaum Associates.

Bronfenbrenner, U. (1995). Developmental ecology through space and time: A future perspective. In P. Moen, G. H. Elder, Jr., & K. Luscher (Eds.), *Examining lives in context: Perspectives on the ecology of human development* (pp. 619–647). Washington, DC: APA Books.

Bronfenbrenner, U. (1996a). *A ecologia do desenvolvimento humano* [Portuguese]. Porto Alegre, Brazil: Artes Medicas.

Bronfenbrenner, U. (1996b). Japanische Kindheit als Grundlage einer Lernkultur: Folgerungen für Forschung und Praxis [Japanese childhood as a foundation for learning. Lessons for reality and research]. In D. Elschenbroich (Ed.), *Anleitung zue Neugier, Grundlagen Japanischer Erziehung* (pp. 329–354). Frankfurt, Germany: Suhrkamp Verlag.

Bronfenbrenner, U. (1996c). Le modèle écologique dans l'étude du developpement de l'enfant [The process-person-context model in developmental research] [Principles, applications, and implications]. In R. Tessier, C. Bouchard, G. M. Tarabulsy, & C. Piche (Eds.), *Enfance et famille: Contextes de developpement [Child and family: Contexts for development]* (pp. 9–59). Quebec, Canada: Les Presses de l'Université Laval.

Bronfenbrenner, U., McClelland, P., Wethington, E., Moen, P., & Ceci, S. J. (1996). *The state of Americans. This generation and the next.* New York: The Free Press.

Bronfenbrenner, U., & Morris, P. A. (1997). The ecology of developmental processes. In R. M. Lerner (Ed.), *Handbook of child psychology, Vol. 1, Theory* (5th ed., pp. 993–1028). New York: Wiley.

NEW DIRECTIONS
IN INFANCY RESEARCH

5

CHAPTER

Lewis P. Lipsitt

Early Experience and Behavior in the Baby of the Twenty-First Century*

The life of the baby of the twenty-first century will be greatly enhanced by recent re-search advances in the field of infant behavior and development. As a result of the extensive scholarly attention paid the infant in the present century, we know a great deal now about (a) the sensory and learning capabilities of the very young child, (b) the role of stress or perinatal risk factors in compromising the brain function and cognitive capacities of babies, and (c) the importance of experiential or psychological and other environmental events as these affect the subsequent development of the baby.

Until recently, the psychophysiological and behavioral characteristics and the learn-ing potential of young infants had not been extensively explored, nor well used for diagnostic and intervention purposes. There were perhaps three or four major works until two decades ago on the behavioral development of infants, and these generally covered the entire age range of infancy. One of these was the classic volume of the German pediatrician Albrecht Peiper (1963), still used as an historic compendium of valuable information, summarizing virtually all of the world's literature on behavioral and neurological development available at that time. Perhaps the major review and critical synthesis of research relating to the sensory and behavioral functioning of new-borns was K. C. Pratt's chapter, "The Neonate," published in Murchison's (1933) sec-ond edition of *A Handbook of Child Psychology* (no chapter on the neonate and infancy appeared in the first, 1931 edition), which was then carried forward and revised for Carmichael's first edition of the *Manual of Child Psychology* (Pratt, 1946). None of these works used the word *cognition* in their descriptions of the capacities, traits, or behavior outputs of the infant. Cognitive psychology is a relatively recent specialty field, involv-ing the study of information-processing strategies and of memorial processes.

The term *cognition* relates to the act, capacity, faculty, or process of knowing. Some-what loosely, cognition refers to "mental processes" or operations by which organisms

---

*This article was presented at the *Bebe XXI* conference that took place at Aula Magna of the University of Lisboon from September 30–October 4, 1990.

become aware of objects of thought or perception. That the term is even used today implies acknowledgment that the newborn has a mind. That assumption has not been long in vogue. Of course, the assertion that the newborn is capable of mental operations ideally requires considerable clarification and qualification. Suffice it to say here that with the recent advent of a wealth of information indicating that at birth all sensory systems are functioning with a modicum of maturity, and with our new understanding that experiential inputs can produce perseverative or lasting changes in the behavior of the baby, it is reasonable to speak of the neonate as a cognitive being.

Because much of our information about the baby's cognitive capacities is derived from the documentation of behavioral changes in the presence of diverse sensory inputs, the examination of cognition inevitably entails study of behavioral development. By the same token, much of the behavior observed in infants is mediated by psychobiological responses of the baby to the pleasures and annoyances of various sensory experiences. Thus our review here necessitates discussion of hedonic aspects of infantile reactivity as well.

☐ The Neonatal Nervous System and the Effects of Experience

All human behavioral processes are mediated by the nervous system, and the nervous system changes with maturation. A very pronounced brain growth spurt occurs just before term birth and shortly afterward (Dobbing, 1975), and within 2 months or so brain cell division, or formation of new cells, diminishes and probably ceases by about 2 years of age (Winick & Rosso, 1975). Brain growth continues after such cell division ceases, however, due to cellular growth, the branching of dendrites, and the proliferation of dendritic spines (Pribram, 1971; Purpura, 1975).

The typical child developmentalist of the early twentieth century believed that the relationship between maturation and environment was a one-way street, with all experiential effects waiting on maturational changes that would permit the experience to have an effect or the behavior to occur. It is now well accepted on the basis of early-experience studies, some of which have shown profound neural tissue changes as a function of early experience, that the maturation–environment relationship is a two-way street (Jacobson, 1978; Jeffrey, 1980). Environmental enrichment, or the imposition of special experiences, can alter maturation rates in certain spheres, such as visual cortex development, which in turn can alter the readiness of the organism to appreciate or assimilate further stimulation in that sphere. Visual deficits of children, due to early strabismus and the consequent amblyopia usually accompanying this, apparently can never be properly compensated, regardless of anatomical correction.

Concerning the growth of dendrites and their spines up to the age of 2 years, there is considerable evidence in the recent literature to support the proposition that experience itself increases dendritic proliferation. In a study, for example, involving restriction of rabbits' vision, Globus and Scheibel (1967) showed that the apical dendritic spines became deformed. By the same token, Schapiro and Vukovich (1970) enhanced the formation of cortical spines and neurons by administering newborn rats about 30 minutes of handling, noise, and visual stimuli for 8 days. Now-classic experiments by Hubel and Wiesel (e.g., 1970) showed that a visual deprivation experience in cats, imposed by suturing one eyelid, would, especially if carried on in the 4th to 8th week "critical period," diminish the number of visual cortical neurons that would react to stimulation later in the previously occluded eye.

Although it is not a foregone conclusion that impairment effects imposed by experiential constraints will be matched eventually by similarly convincing data showing brain growth enhancement effects from experiential enrichment procedures, it is an exciting prospect that such effects are possible. As suggested by Wittrock (1980), the bold implication that experience can contribute through neural growth to increased ability to learn and remember is worth testing, because an "increase in brain size and weight, the increased density of arborization of dendritic spines, the profusion of intercellular connections, and changes in neurotransmitters might indicate a greater store of information in the brain, an increased ability to learn, or an increase in the neural substrates of the ability to learn and to remember" (p. 378).

☐ Sensory Processes

The normal newborn enters the world with all sensory systems functioning. Although there are individual differences in thresholds of response to stimulation in every modality, each one of the senses can be tested for the presence of response and documentation made of the stimulus intensity required to elicit the indicator response, such as leg withdrawal, head turn, startle behavior, or eye blink (Kessen, Haith, & Salapatek, 1970).

Vision

Sudden onset of light produces the eye-blink reflex and sometimes the eye–neck reflex, involving a backward thrust of the head. Illumination changes also result in diminution of the pupil size and changes in cardiac and respiratory activity. Cortically evoked potentials in response to illumination changes have also been produced. Preferences for intermediate brightness levels have been demonstrated in a study of twenty 3-day-old babies who were presented with paired combinations of three uniform gray panels differing in brightness (Hershenson, 1964).

Newborns respond to color. It has been shown in a study of 24 infants aged 15 to 70 days that from a very early age infants visually pursue moving objects (Chase, 1937). A spot of colored light was moved across a colorless background, with brightness controlled, and the baby followed the target lights. Numerous successful studies have been made of hue discrimination in older infants, such as from about 60 days onward, and these successes have prompted attempts to explore color perception at earlier and earlier ages. Studies by Peiper (1961) and Trincker and Trincker (1955) suggested that color perception is essentially the same for the very young infant as it is for the adult.

However, many of the infant studies unavoidably confounded brightness with the color dimension. Dobson (1976) has explored the spectral sensitivity of 2-month-old infants using visually evoked cortical potential. Spectral sensitivity was determined through measurement of implicit time of the visually evoked potential. It was concluded that the macular pigment in the young infant is probably less dense than that of the adult and therefore more shortwave radiation reaches the infant's photoreceptors.

The ability to discriminate details, such as line separation, has been explored by infant researchers. The optokinetic nystagmus response, which occurs when the eyes fixate on moving striped patterns, provides one procedure for assessing visual acuity. The infant is presented with a series of patterns differing in width, and the point is noted at which nystagmus fails to occur. Using this procedure it has been demonstrated that the newborn has at least 20/150 vision (Dayton et al., 1964). The response to a moving pattern may, of course, be unlike the "voluntary" responses that one assumes are involved in visual gaze and preference behavior, even of the newborn.

As part of an innovative and informative research program involving the ontogeny of visual perception, Fantz (1961) presented striped patterns in pairs with gray stimuli in order to assess comparative fixation times in infants under 1 month of age and up to 6 months. Presenting the stimuli 10 inches from the infants' eyes, the line width varied from $1/_8$ inch to narrower stripes. Under one month of age, the $1/_8$ inch stripe and none other was preferred over the gray field. Assessed in this way, acuity increased over age, and 6-month-old infants were able to discriminate stripes of $1/_{64}$ inch. Using these general procedures, infants as young as 2 months have been shown to discriminate regular from irregular stimulus patterns, and to prefer curved over straight contours (Fantz & Miranda, 1975).

A major determinant of visual preference in infants is amount of contour in the stimulus (Karmel & Maisel, 1975). Preference responses of infants as young as 13 weeks old have been demonstrated to be an inverted U-shaped function of amount of contour, with older infants preferring more contour than do younger infants (Karmel, 1969). The corneal reflection technique (Haith, 1969; Salapatek, 1975) also has shown contour to be important in infant visual preference. Eye movements tend to hover around stimulus contours or contrast borders; newborns tend to fixate on the vertices of triangles.

Depth perception has been studied in older infants using the now well-known "visual cliff" (Walk, 1966), a large table covered with heavy plate glass, with a runway down the middle, a "shallow" side, and a "deep" side. The depth cues are implemented by having the visual pattern some distance below the plate glass, in contrast to the shallow side on which the pattern is flush against the glass. The basic technique requires that the infant be able to crawl and to avoid the "deep" side. All infants, including nonhuman infants, show fear and avoidance of depth by the time they locomote. Recently the technique has been extended downward (Campos, Langer, & Krowitz, 1970) by introducing another response, heart-rate change, recorded when the baby is placed alternately on the deep and shallow sides. Depth discrimination has been documented in this way in infants as young as 3 months. In an extended series of investigations, Bower (1965, 1971) provided very striking demonstrations of depth perception and visually directed reaching in infants at least as young as 30 days of age. In one study, for example, 4-week-old infants are seated in front of a rear projection screen while wearing polarizing goggles. Sometimes a solid object was presented, and on other occasions a three-dimensional version of it appeared on the screen, having the illusion of being placed between the subject and the screen. Infants reached and touched the real object. Upon reaching for the "illusion," they were surprised and often cried, seemingly annoyed that the apparent object was absent.

Audition

Two studies relating sound intensity and heart-rate change have demonstrated that cardiac acceleration in the newborn is a function of sound intensity (Bartoshuk, 1964;

Steinschneider, Lipton, & Richmond, 1966). Although in such studies heart-rate change can be secondary to the startle response, it has been estimated that the threshold for cardiac acceleration in newborns is about 40 decibels, much below the everyday environmental sounds in the newborn's environment (Steinschneider, 1967). The audible frequency range for infants is not yet well known (Eisenberg, in press), in part because of the confounding influence of loudness. Although equal-loudness tones can be presented based on adult loudness judgments at different frequencies, it cannot be assumed with certainty that the loudness functions are equivalent in adults and infants.

Upon intrusion of auditory stimulation during infant sucking, exteroceptive stimuli will tend, especially if intense, to interrupt the sucking pattern (Bronshtein et al., 1960; Semb & Lipsitt, 1968), and in some instance habituation of such sucking disruption will occur. Using this method, the absence of deafness can be quite definitively documented, but the technique has not been sufficiently refined as to enable psychophysical gradients for individual infants.

Sound localization has been successfully documented in procedures involving habituation of response to an auditory stimulus, followed by presentation of that stimulus in an alternative locale (Leventhal & Lipsitt, 1964; Wertheimer, 1961). When recovery of the habituated response occurs upon presentation of the stimulus in the alternate location, auditory localization is assumed.

Using a habituation paradigm, and capitalizing on the proclivity of infants to suck in order to make sound occur, Eimas, Siqueland, Jusczyk, and Vigorito (1971) showed that 1-month-old infants perceive speech sounds categorically. Recovery from habituation of the sucking response was greater when the post-habituation stimulus was from a different phonemic category than when it was an equal distance from the familiarized stimulus but in the same phonemic category. In a study of the neonatal response to natural sounds, while lying quietly, newborns were administered the taped sound of another newborn crying or a computer-simulated cry (Simner, 1971). The cry stimulus was found to elicit much restlessness and crying in the stimulated babies. That the computer simulation did not produce much of the same behavior suggests that the response is not driven by the intensity of stimulus, but rather that there is something about the human voice and the cry that results in a kind of early imitation or "empathetic" response. A study (Ashmead & Lipsitt, in preparation) has shown that the human female voice is a reliable elicitor of cardiac deceleration in the newborn, and that the human male voice uttering the same sounds did not produce comparable attending or observing responses.

Taste

The human newborn is sharply and critically responsive to minimal alterations in the chemical constituency of fluids on the tongue. Newly developed procedures for recording tongue movement (Nowlis, 1973; Weiffenbach & Thach, 1973) and various parameters of sucking behavior (Lipsitt, 1974) have enabled the documentation of fine discriminations that infants make. Subtle sucking changes have been documented when the infant controls his or her own taste stimulus input, as in real-life situations in which the infant may suck slowly or quickly, may take more or less rest periods, may invest greater or lesser numbers of sucks in each sucking burst, and so on. A sucking apparatus connected to a polygraph and then to a computer (Crook & Lipsitt, 1976; Lipsitt, Reilly, Butcher, & Greenwood, 1976) has been used for recording the infant's sucking behavior under conditions in which the presentation of drops of fluid is made contingent on sucking behavior. The "criterion sucks" that exceed a minimal amplitude required for triggering the pumps cause one or another fluid to be ejected. The apparatus can be preset to yield drops of fluid, contingent on each criterion suck, varying in magnitude from 0.01 to 0.04 ml per suck. Because relatively small amounts of fluid per suck are involved, sucking and taste can be studied over a fairly long period of time without appreciably affecting ingestion.

The rate at which newborns suck and the patterning of their bursts and pauses are different depending on whether fluid is delivered. When sucking on a blank nipple, the infant sucks in short bursts separated by long pauses, and sucking within those bursts is quite rapid. When a sweet fluid, such as 15% sucrose, is delivered contingent on sucking, the infant engages in more sucks per minute, invests more sucks per burst, takes shorter rest periods, and sucks more slowly within each sucking burst. Moreover, all of these parameters are affected by sweetness along a continuum from 0 through 15% sucrose, as well as by the amounts of fluid received per suck (Crook, 1976; Crook & Lipsitt, 1976). Thus with either increasing concentrations or amounts of sucrose, infants tend to suck more slowly within bursts. Interestingly, heart rate seems paradoxically affected in these situations, in that despite the slowing down of sucking within bursts with the greater incentive values of the fluid for which the infant is sucking, heart rate is increased. This effect has been demonstrated even under conditions in which appropriate controls have been introduced for differential durations of sucking bursts. It is presumed from these results that the human neonate hedonically monitors oral stimuli and signals the pleasantness of such stimuli with the heart rate as an indicator response.

It also has been documented that swallowing behavior is implicated in the sucking rate changes that occur with different concentrations of sugar (Burke, 1977). Careful measurement of the differences in interresponse times for those sucks coinciding with swallows, and a comparison with sucks not associated with swallows, revealed that swallow and sucking rate are correlated. Sucking and swallowing, and perhaps tongue movement as well, are under hedonic control, with slower sucking and more swallowing occurring together in the presence of increased pleasure.

Crook has capitalized on the sensitivity of sucking parameters, such as length of sucking burst, to study the neonate's response to mildly aversive as well as pleasant taste stimuli (Crook, 1978). By administering three drops of either a sweet or salty fluid, one drop at a time, and recording the length of the immediately subsequent sucking burst, Crook was able to demonstrate that increasing concentrations of sweet fluid produced larger sucking bursts, whereas increasing concentrations of salt produced shorter bursts. The technique has considerable potential for the careful study of the psychophysics of taste in infancy.

The taste of the fluid, for which the neonate sucks, affects the baby's later sucking behavior, at least for a short time (Kobre & Lipsitt, 1972). Three groups of normal neonates were studied over a 20-minute period. One group received a 15% sucrose solution for sucking; a second group received a comparable drop of water for each suck. A third group was alternated between sucrose and water from one 5-minute period to the next, beginning with sucrose. It was found that when the infants in the third group were switched from sucrose to water, their sucking rates dropped appreciably below the level of the infants who, during the same period, sucked for water throughout the 20-minute session. This so-called negative contrast phenomenon shows that the neonate "chooses to suck" for water less after having the opportunity to suck for a sweet fluid. The phenomenon is an example of the way in which early experience even during the neonatal stage may affect subsequent behavior. More is said about learning processes of neonates in a later section of this chapter.

Smell

In a well-controlled study using "real-life stimulation," Macfarlane (1975) positioned two breast pads above infants lying supinely in their cribs. One of the pads was that of the infant's own mother; the other was an unused, and thus nonodorous, pad. In a counterbalanced design, Macfarlane documented that the infants adjusted their faces and gazes toward the mother's pad. In a second study, two used breast pads from nursing mothers were presented, one at the left and one at the right, counterbalancing that of the child's own mother and that of another. Infants again oriented toward the odor of their own mothers. Such a finding has implications for the capacity of the newborn to detect its own mother, particularly after a few days of experience with her, and to become "attached" to her. Interestingly, Macfarlane found that the effect was not present within the first few days of life; rather, the effect seems to accrue over time and with experience.

To test the olfactory sensory acuity of newborns, odorants have been presented on cotton swabs to infants whose respiration, heart rate, activity, and other parameters were monitored polygraphically. These studies have frequently capitalized on the habituation paradigm, in which the gradual diminution of responses to a repetitively presented stimulus is noted, whereupon a dishabituation or recovery stimulus varying along some dimension from the habituation stimulus is presented. If recovery from the habituated response (e.g., respiratory disruption) occurs, then it is concluded that the infant is capable of detecting the difference between the first presented and the subsequent stimulus. In such studies (Engen & Lipsitt, 1965; Engen, Lipsitt, & Kaye, 1963) it has been shown that newborns respond to odorants such as anise oil and asafetida, and that habituation of response to these stimuli takes place. If habituated to one, the infant will respond subsequently to the alternate. Similarly, if a sufficient amount of time is allowed to elapse following habituation, complete recovery of response occurs. It has also been shown that newborns will not dishabituate to components of mixtures to which they have been initially habituated, suggesting that the infant's appreciation of odors and the habituation of response to these odors are controlled at a cortical level rather than simply at a peripheral level.

Touch

Few studies have been done on the neonatal sense of touch, especially considering the obvious importance of both pleasant and unpleasant aspects of the newborn's tactile contact with the environment in the earliest days. The newborn's individualized responses to the warm or cold hand, to encompassing body contact, to pressure, and to the *sturm und drang* associated with birth and institutional care can have, at least in principle, an effect on the infant's caretakers. Yet little is known about such functions in the newborn.

Some salient responses of the newborn to touch may be described. The rooting reflex, involving ipsilateral head turning in response to relatively light touch at the corners of the mouth, is well known. The importance of such tactual stimulation, and the low threshold of the newborn for response to it, can be demonstrated by rotating the finger completely around the lips in a circle and noting the precise following of such stimulation that many newborns can demonstrate. When the intraoral surface of the mouth is touched, this produces closing of the lips and sucking. Pressure on the palms of the hands often produces head turning to midline, with a gaping response of the mouth; this is called the Babkin reflex.

Some aspects of the newborn's response to tactile stimulation have been noted in relation to the well-coordinated defensive maneuvers of newborns. Defensive responses to tactile stimulation, such as pressure on the chin, have been noted to become increasingly pronounced over the first 2 weeks of life, and often to involve effective arm action of the infant against the intrusive stimulus (Sherman, Sherman, & Flory, 1936). In one of the best standardized tests of neonatal behavior, Graham (1956) included a test item involving the application of a gauze pad or cellophane over the infant's mouth and nostrils with moderate pressure. A good response to the threat of respiratory occlusion and head restraint involves adaptive movement of the head and directed arm movements. Similarly, the Brazelton Neonatal Behavioral Assessment Scale (Brazelton, 1973) has an item testing for "defensive behavior," also involving the placement of a cloth over the face of an infant and holding it in place to record the vigor with which objection to the restrictive stimulation occurs.

Tactile stimulation associated with restraint was described early by Watson (1928, pp. 34, 88–96) under the rubric of infantile "rage." Rage was regarded by Watson to be the natural response to pressure applied in such a way as to constitute motoric restraint. Gunther (1961) suggested that threats of respiratory occlusion, when they occur in the context of such restraint or in the context of feeding, which itself constitutes a constraint on mobility, may lead to severe objections by the infant. Such objection may take the form of turning the head away from the breast on subsequent occasions and refusing to feed. Gunther has described some details of the potentially devastating effect that such interactions can have on the developing relationship between mother and infant.

Lipsitt (1976) suggested that the absence of defensive behavior in the presence of motoric restraint and threats to respiratory occlusion could well be associated with developmental jeopardy, possibly including failure to thrive and sudden unexpected death syndromes. If infants do not have the capacity for engaging in behavioral maneuvers capable of freeing their respiratory passages when threatened with occlusion, they may be at special risk at later developmental ages, particularly after the initial reflex repertoire of the infant has waned, by which time the reflexes are normally supplanted by learned responses under greater voluntary control. That crib death usually occurs between 2 and 4 months of age, a period that is critical as a bridge between subcortically controlled and cortically mediated behavior, tends to support the assumption that sudden infant death might relate in some measure to a learning deficiency based on an initially inadequate sensory process.

Learning processes, in general, refer to changes in behavior that accrue over time and as products of experience. Three different types of such behavioral changes are discussed here: habituation, classical conditioning, and operant learning. Although all three of these processes are noncontroversial as experientially induced behavior changes that involve some fairly permanent change in the condition of the organism, only classical and operant conditioning are considered by some to be "true learning tasks."

Habituation, the argument goes, does not involve the paired presentation of stimuli, and therefore does not involve the development of new mental associations. One should not be concerned here with the subtleties of the distinction. Habituation is a behavioral process involving gradual accretions in behavioral change, and the process of habituation seems to be one in which fairly stable and relatively permanent changes occur.

☐ Habituation

With repetitive stimulation, an initially elicited behavior manifests itself to a lesser and lesser degree until, in some instances, the behavior may disappear entirely. Following such waning or disappearance of the indexed behavior, the response may be called forth again, either by the presentation of an alternative effective stimulus or after the sheer passage of time during which the stimulus is not administered. Progressive response decrement with repetitive presentation of stimuli may be noted in all sensory modalities, but is perhaps most easily noted with respect to auditory and olfactory stimuli.

The literature on habituation in early infancy is extensive, and only exemplary studies may be touched on here. Reviewers of studies on infantile habituation (Kessen et al., 1970) have noted that the phenomenon of habituation is a valuable tool for the study of memory processes. Thus habituation, as well as classical and operant conditioning, can illuminate the extent to which cortical functioning is present in the young human and possibly can reveal behavioral aberrations indicative of central nervous system deficits.

Fantz (1961, 1964) did extensive work on visual habituation of infants. He suggested that the infant's gaze duration can be quantified, and that this measure may be used over repetitive trials to assess the infant's diminishing interest in specific visual stimuli. Although Fantz's early studies suggested that the newborn showed little visual habituation, whereas the infant beyond 10 weeks of age showed much of it, later studies (Friedman, Nagy, & Carpenter, 1970) have demonstrated neonatal visual habituation. Forty newborns were presented with two checkerboard targets, one with 4 squares, the other with 144 squares. Both males and females showed response decrement over trials, but males demonstrated the phenomenon for the less dense visual stimulus, and females for the denser (144 squares) stimulus.

In typical studies of auditory habituation, the stimuli are presented in time-locked fashion, such as once every 30 seconds, with some indicator response serving as the measure of response strength over repetitive presentation trials. It has been shown that acceleration of the heart rate declines with repetitive presentations, more quickly with shorter interstimulus interval, and that dishabituation can be seen in the newborn by an increase in the intensity of the test stimulus over the familiarization stimulus, or by a change in the tonal pattern of the recovery stimulus (Bartoshuk, 1962a, 1962b). Response diminution following repeated stimulation may still be present even after a 1-day interval in newborns.

In one study of neonatal sensitivity to olfactory stimuli, and habituation of response to such stimuli, infants were presented with 10 trials of an odorant, with half of the infants receiving asafetida first and the other half receiving anise oil first. Initial response levels to these odorants based on a combined respiration and stabilimeter index were about 90%, and response levels dropped to about 25% by trial 10. At the conclusion of the 10 habituation trials, the alternate odorant was capable of producing response recovery, although not to the level at which the infant first responded (Engen et al., 1963). In subsequent studies, further refinement in method ruled out sensory fatigue as the basis of the response decrement obtained. This was done by showing that in newborns there can occur a response recovery to odorants that were present in a solution to which habituation had been previously obtained (Engen & Lipsitt, 1965).

Inasmuch as habituation relates to memory function, which is mediated by the brain, it should be possible to refine techniques for improved assessment of impairment of the central nervous system by including indices of habituation (Brazelton, 1973). In fact, Lewis (1967) showed that impaired infantile habituation is related to low Apgar scores and other indices of brain damage. Hydrocephalic and anencephalic infants may show no habituation at all (Brackbill, 1971; Wolff, 1969).

A habituation technique involving the sucking response has been used to document that infants born under conditions of excessive cranial pressure or with the cord around the neck have a deficiency in habituation (Bronshtein et al., 1960). While sucking, the infants were presented a stimulus such as sound. Normal infants interrupted their sucking momentarily when presented with such a stimulus, but on repetitive presentations showed no reduction in such sucking suppression or interruption. In this study it was shown that with infants born at risk, it took many more trials of presentation of the stimulus to habituate the sucking-suppression response.

A study of averaged auditory evoked responses in infants with Down's syndrome showed that relative to normal infants matched in age (from 8 days to 13 months), the infants with Down's syndrome showed no significant response decrement (Barnet, Olrich, & Shanks, 1974). As a by-product of the study, it was also demonstrated that none of the babies under 1 month of age, normal or otherwise, evoked response habituation. Finally, effects of obstetrical anesthesia on the infant have been studied using habituation (Bowes et al., 1970). The infants were examined at 2 and 5 days of age. Infants whose mothers received high dosages of anesthesia required as many as four times more trials to habituate than did those whose mothers received little medication; this difference still existed when the infants were retested 1 month later.

☐ Classical Conditioning

Although habituation is an experiential phenomenon, change in the baby's behavior induced by redundant presentations of a stimulus is not as impressive to the observer as classical conditioning, in which there is an obvious recruitment of a new response to a previously neutral stimulus. The first manifestations of socialization are seen in classical conditioning processes; the young infant may quite quickly respond differently to the way in which the mother holds him or her, or how the mother addresses the infant with her voice just before offering the nipple. Pavlovian conditioning involves the presentation of a neutral stimulus (or conditioning stimulus) in association with an initially effective stimulus (or unconditioned stimulus) over a succession of trials. The conditioning stimulus comes to elicit the response. Considerable work has been done with infants and young children to determine the optimal procedures under which stimulus presentation might be administered. As might be expected, different temporal relationships are optimal for different types of stimuli and for different response systems. It is likely that cortical maturation and dendritic development are important in laying the neurophysiological substrate that will permit the cortical innervations and synaptic connections required for learning.

Denisova and Figurin (1929) learned that infants exhibit anticipatory sucking movements when placed in the feeding position to which they have been accustomed. Many of the Soviet investigations lacked adequate controls for the possibility that the response obtained was a congenital response to unconditioned stimulation rather than a conditioned response. However, the early efforts that led to more precise implementation of conditioning procedures with infants have provided the current knowledge that even newborns are classically conditionable.

Eye blinking and sucking have been successfully conditioned to tactile stimuli. A study by Lipsitt, Kaye, and Bosack (1966) involved a paradigm that differed somewhat from strict classical conditioning. Newborns were presented with an intraoral stimulus, actually a short piece of rubber tubing ¼ inch in diameter, which mimicked a nipple but was known to be a less than optimal stimulus for eliciting sucking (Lipsitt & Kaye, 1965). The aim was to determine whether the sucking response to the tube could be enhanced by the presentation through the tube of a known effective elicitor of sucking. Thus the infant was presented with 5% dextrose solution in association with presentation of the tube. In contrast to control infants who did not receive the pairing of conditioning/unconditioning stimuli, but instead received unpaired presentation of the same stimuli, the experimental or "trained" infants came to respond anticipatorily to the presentation of the tube alone with enhanced sucking responses.

The Babkin response (Babkin, 1960) was successfully conditioned by Kaye (1965). This reflex involves several components, including gaping, sucking, turning the head to midline, raising the head, and in some instances eyelid closure and forearm flexion. The congenital stimulus for this behavior is pressure on the baby's palms. Kaye used tactile-kinesthetic stimulation, involving movement of the arms from the infant's sides up to the head, just before application of the pressure. This procedure resulted in classical conditioning of the Babkin response, a finding subsequently replicated (Connolly & Stratton, 1969). The later researchers successfully demonstrated the acquisition of this response to an auditory conditioning stimulus as well as to kinesthetic stimulation. Although questions remain about the procedures involved in these studies (Sostek, Sameroff, & Sostek, 1972) and much work remains to be done to refine our understanding of the necessary and sufficient conditions for the elaboration of different types of conditioned reflexes, these studies support the contention that cortically mediated alterations in behavior take place in the newborn.

Temporal conditioning involves the passage of time as a conditioning stimulus in conditioning processes. Early studies of temporal conditioning were conducted in connection with feeding schedules. If the infant is put on a time schedule for feeding, such as a 3-hour or 4-hour interval, some of the behavioral disruptions that occur subsequent to elimination of a feeding might be attributable to a temporally conditioned effect. Marquis (1941) did a study in which one group of newborns was changed from a fixed 3-hour schedule to a 4-hour schedule. Their behavior was compared with that of a control group on a 4-hour schedule throughout. Infants whose schedules were changed evidenced more bodily activity and general behavior disruption than did the control group during the fourth hour, when the feed ordinarily would have been given. Of course, infants on a 3-hour schedule may not eat as much as those on a 4-hour schedule, and the effect might be due in part to greater hunger in the switched group (Lipsitt, 1963). However, results of further studies, although not entirely free from artifact, have supported the general finding. Changes of feeding schedules have been shown to induce anticipatory increases not only in responses in bodily activity (Bystroletova, 1954), but in blood leukocyte count as well (Krachkovskaia, 1959).

There is a relative lack of studies using visual conditioning stimuli with very young infants. This is probably due to the fact that although tactual and auditory stimulation is essentially inescapable, visual stimulation is received, at least to some extent, at the "whim" of the observer. Nonetheless, in a study by Kasatkin and Levikova (1935), six infants ranging in age from 14 to 48 days developed stable conditioned visual responses to about 60 days of age. In this study, a colored light was presented in association with the bottle for feeding. After a number of trials, the babies responded to the green light with many of the response components, such as turning the head and making mouth movements, characteristic of the feeding situation itself. Following conditioning to a specific hue, generalized responses did occur to other colors close to the conditioning stimulus, but after a number of trials in which the conditioning stimulus and the alternate color were successively presented, response differentiation took place. Very stable classically conditioned differentiation was present between the ages of 88 and 116 days for all infants in the study.

Auditory stimuli have been used successfully in classical conditioning with newborns. Marquis (1941) used the sound of a buzzer preceding the offering of a bottle nipple during the first 10 days of life. Within 5 days of training, the 10 infants studied were making sucking responses to the sound of the buzzer. Kasatkin and Levikova (1935) were able to demonstrate conditioned differentiation of tones by the time infants in their experiment were 2 to 3 months of age.

Lipsitt and Kaye (1964) presented a low-frequency loud tone (93 decibels) in association with the insertion of a nipple in the mouths of infants 3 and 4 days old. Sensitization effects were controlled through the use of a control group to whom the tone and nipple were presented noncontiguously. On every fifth trial, the tone was presented alone as a test for conditioning. After training was completed all babies received a series of extinction trials with the test tone alone. Evidence was found for classical conditioning, although the effects of training did not manifest themselves until the extinction condition. Other investigators have also been able to obtain such conditioning (Abrahamson, Brackbill, Carpenter, & Fitzgerald, 1970).

A practical application of the classical conditioning technique was introduced by Aldrich (1928), who sounded a bell while stimulating the sole of the infant with a pinprick. After 12 to 15 such pairings, Aldrich found that the sound of the bell was effective alone in producing a response. He suggested that such behavior could provide a definite test of deafness. A number of studies demonstrate classical aversive conditioning not unlike that represented by the Aldrich study. Failures to obtain aversive conditioning, which have also been reported, may perhaps be attributed to the possibility that rather intensive noxious stimulation must be used to obtain the effect, and these conditions are seldom implemented in the laboratory.

The extent to which the newborn is capable of retaining memories of experienced pain is, or should be, a matter of clinical import for the neonatologist. That we do not recall 20 years later, or even 5 years later, painful experiences in the first few days of life does not mean that painful neonatal experiences have no effects. It is logically and empirically possible for an infant to experience a painful episode in, for example, the third day of life that could have an effect on perception of subsequent events in the same day or in the next. These altered perceptions could then influence the effects of other experiences. Yet by the time several days or years have passed, although none of the experiences may be remembered specifically, the painful episode and its sequelae nonetheless might have altered the organism in special ways. This is not to say that unremembered painful experiences are necessarily deleterious, for indeed it is possible that early stress and the recruitment of physiological and psychological resources for coping with that stress may even have a beneficial effect on the child's later ability to handle stress. Very little is known about this sort of thing, first because pain perception and its significance have not been studied much in the very young infant, and second, because investigators would be loath to administer unnecessary and intensive pain stimulation. Nonetheless, in the natural course of caring for newborns, unusual levels of aversive stimulation sometimes are administered, as in circumcision, venipuncture, or excision of a supernumerary digit. Researchers would do well to capitalize on these rather routine hospital procedures to explore aspects of pain perception in the newborn and the possible effects that such procedures may have on the infants' reciprocal relationships with caretakers in the immediately subsequent hours and days.

☐ Operant Conditioning

In contrast to classical conditioning, which involves the development of a new association or memory based on the pairing of a neutral and an effective stimulus, operant learning is the consequence of response-contingent stimulation (reward or punishment), which has the effect of altering the response-probability following the response-contingent experience. Operant learning forms the basis for many examples of therapeutic intervention, often called behavior modification. Operant conditioning or behavior modification procedures have been used in the treatment of a wide variety of childhood disorders, including, for example, in the case of an eating phobia in a 15-month-old girl (Davids, 1974). Much remains to be discovered about the principles and processes underlying operant conditioning in young children, but considerable progress has been made over the past two decades.

Several studies described by Sameroff (1972) show that the subsystems of the general sucking pattern of infants can be altered by specific environmental conditions. He showed that when the delivery of fluid is made directly contingent on the negative pressure component of the sucking response, this results in the infant using more negative pressure than when this contingency is not in effect. Such a demonstration is possible because there are two major components of sucking behavior in the newborn, one of these consisting of negative pressure in the buccal cavity, and the other simply the positive pressure created by gum action. The Sameroff study showed that these two components may be reinforced differentially to enhance one or the other of them.

Brown (1972) used a nonnutritive reinforcer, a blank nipple, to show that sucking in newborns can be brought under operant control even without using feeding. She based her study on the hypothesis put forth by Premack (1965) that a response that is higher in the habit hierarchy, or greater in strength, may be used to reinforce a weaker response. As Lipsitt and Kaye (1965) had shown that nipples of certain shapes serve to optimize the sucking stimuli, Brown had infants of 2 and 3 days of age suck on one nipple, either a regular commercial nipple or a blunt variation thereof, in order to obtain access to another nipple, either regular or blunt. On the second day of conditioning, the rate of sucking on the regular nipple in the "nipple followed by blunt" group was reliably lower than the rate of sucking on the regular nipple in the "nipple followed by nipple" group. Sucking rates for the blunt oral stimulus in the "blunt followed by nipple" group, moreover, were significantly higher than such sucking in the "blunt followed by blunt" group.

A similar effect was found by Kobre and Lipsitt (1972) in a study of negative contrast that showed that newborns suck less to receive water after having experienced the taste of sugar than they do if they have been sucking merely for water during a comparable period of time. Although this was a short-term study, as was Brown's, the implication is that a basic memorial process is already available to the infant, and that learning to behave on the basis of differential incentive conditions is possible.

Some studies of infant learning have involved elaborations or modifications of traditional operant conditioning procedures, with good effect. One such study (Siqueland & Lipsitt, 1966) capitalized on conditioned head-turning techniques first reported by Papoušek (1959, 1960). The Siqueland and Lipsitt (1966) elaboration of the procedure studied the effect of contingent reinforcement on the response of ipsilateral head movements. The departure from traditional operant conditioning was that instead of awaiting the natural or spontaneous occurrence of head turning, the head turns were elicited by a touch at the side of the infant's mouth. Such stimulation typically produces the head-turning part of the rooting reflex on about 30% of the preconditioning trials. In three studies, nutritive reinforcement in the form of a 5% dextrose solution was administered contingent on the elicited head-turning movements, with the effect that such responses were enhanced considerably by the reinforcement condition.

In one of these studies, each infant served as his or her own control in order to obviate the possibility that the apparent conditioning effect obtained could be attributed to changes in state rather than changes in cognitive or memorial factors. The study involved the use of two different auditory stimuli or tones. On alternate trials the stimulus for head turning was a different tone–touch combination. On positive trials, the neonate received one of the tone–touch combinations to the left cheek, whereas on the other half of the alternated trials, a different tone–touch combination on the same cheek was used as the negative stimulus. On the positive trials, appropriate head turns were reinforced by opportunity to suck for dextrose, whereas on negative trials, no such opportunity was provided. The results of the study indicated that the positive stimulus combination facilitated the rise of responding from 30 to 83%, whereas on negative trials the response probability remained essentially the same as at the beginning. The total training effort required 30 minutes. The effect was reliable. Following this period of conditioning, the positive and negative stimulus conditions were reversed, such that the stimulus combination that was previously reinforced no longer was, and the previously negative stimulus combination was made positive. A gradual behavioral shift took place in accord with the circumstances of the changed stimulus, producing a reliable effect once again of the contingent reinforcement condition. The reversal of behavior was significant. This and other studies demonstrate clearly that the contingent application of reinforcement may alter even reflexive behaviors typical of infants within the first few days of life.

Visual reinforcement of high-amplitude sucking responses has been used to study operant learning in infants from 1 to 4 months of age (Milewski & Siqueland, 1976; Siqueland & DeLucia, 1969). In such studies, a screen is used for showing slides of varying illuminations, with the illumination being controlled by an operant behavior of the infant, specifically sucking responses. Under these conditions of so-called "conjugate reinforcement," infants show typical acquisition and extinction effects, in which they suck to receive visual reinforcement, and stop sucking either when the screen no longer provides contingently presented visual stimulation or after becoming bored with, or habituated to, the stimuli. The habituation aspects of the typical responses obtained enabled the researchers to capitalize on the familiarization phenomenon to study the discriminability of very similar stimuli. A procedure implemented by Milewski and Siqueland (1975) showed that infants as young as 1 month of age can discriminate between familiar and novel stimuli on the basis of both color and pattern, and that there is an increase in the reinforcing effectiveness of visual stimuli concomitant with an increase in their novelty.

The contingent reinforcement paradigm and the sucking response have been used to study the effect of auditory stimuli on very young infants as well. In one such study (Eimas et al., 1971), it was demonstrated that young infants will suck to hear auditory stimuli up to a certain point, whereupon interest lags and sucking wanes or even ceases. At that point a slight change in the auditory stimulus, such as from *ba* to *ga*, can be made and will cause a significant recovery of the sucking response relative to control infants for whom no such change in auditory stimulus is introduced.

Another response that has been shown to increase as a result of novel or interesting visual reinforcers, such as pictures of checkerboards, color patches, triangles, bull's-eyes, and so on, has been head turning (Caron, 1967; Levison & Levison, 1967). Reinforcers combining several different modalities, such as visual and tactual, have also yielded positive results (Bower, 1965; McKenzie & Day, 1971).

☐ Imitative Behavior of Infants

Several interesting studies have demonstrated that very young infants are capable of engaging in rudimentary imitative behaviors in response to a visual model. In such studies it has been shown that infants even as young as 2 to 3 weeks of age may respond with enhanced tongue movement and tongue thrusting when another person, in appropriate visual range and after assuring the infant's visual attention, sticks the tongue out. In a pioneering experiment of this sort, in which controls were introduced to assure that the "imitative behavior" was not merely the result of enhanced arousal, Maratos (1973) simultaneously recorded a number of different responses in infants 7 to 8 weeks of age, while serving as a model performing only one of these responses at a time (e.g., thrusting of the tongue, movement of the fingers, vocalization). When the model engaged in tongue thrusting, tongue movement on the part of the infant was increased, and when the model engaged in finger waving, the infant's finger movement was enhanced.

In replications of the Maratos study, under different conditions and with even younger infants, it has been asserted that such imitative behavior is present by 3 weeks of age (Meltzoff & Moore, 1977) or even by 10 days of age (Bower, 1977). Meltzoff (1977) has even reported that babies as young as 21 days of age can hold in memory the imitated model for at least 2½ minutes. He first demonstrated tongue thrusting to the infants while they were sucking on a pacifier and presumably were thus inhibited from engaging in the imitative tongue thrusting. After an interval of 150 seconds following the demonstration, the pacifier was then removed from the infant's mouth, whereupon a significant amount of imitative tonguing was seen to occur.

☐ The Significance of Early Learning

Although much of the behavior of young organisms is generated endogenously, early human behavior is also elicited and modified by environmental stimulation, some of it planned and deliberate (as in playing mouth-opening games) and some inadvertent (as with the noise accompanying the closing of a door). The baby and its caregivers control each other's behavior. Each responds reciprocatingly, and each thus serves as a stimulant of the other in a continuing flow of communications involving sights, sounds, and touches. Such stimulation is often accompanied by affect in others as well as the pleasures of stimulation inherent in the experiences themselves. Thus the infant has best opportunities for learning about his or her own feelings of satisfaction in the presence of selected sensory stimulation and of other people.

The essence of babyhood sometimes has been characterized as a period of dependency, involving passive assimilation of environmental inputs. The contrary view is taken here that the infant is an active participant in a fairly constant flow of reciprocating gestures, evoking response from others as much as reacting to their stimulation. It is in the context of mutually satisfying, often pleasant, transactions that the infant acquires coping skills and gestures, the capacity for increasingly complex manipulations of the environment and other people, and the learned "social graces" that are shaped by environmental rewards and punishments.

The early months of life are also a proving ground for the adequacy of the infant's congenital response repertoire, the eventual embellishment of which results from early practice. Even some types of learning disability and psychopathological conditions may well have their earliest origins in the interplay between constitutional and experiential factors impinging on the baby from the first days. Our knowledge about these processes remains woefully inadequate today.

Studies reviewed elsewhere (Lipsitt, 1983) have suggested that some of the first manifestations of developmental disability may be found in the earliest days of life. Many of these have their roots, of course, in events surrounding birth, such as maternal anemia, oxygen deficit, jaundice, and, in general, conditions that jeopardize respiration and adequate blood circulation to the brain. Infants who are born prematurely, who are small and require prolonged administration of oxygen at birth, or who are floppy or limp (or overly tense and tight) do less well, physically and behaviorally, during the first year of life and in later years than infants whose histories are not marked by these indicators (Sameroff & Chandler, 1975). Many prenatal and neonatal birth-risk conditions have their most debilitating effects on the sensory systems and on central nervous system functioning. Behavioral deficits, and learning problems in particular, are therefore increased in such populations.

☐ Rage and Learned Anger in the Newborn

Aversive or avoidance behavior is much in evidence in newborn children. Moreover, babies in the first few days of life may be seen to engage in quite effective defensive behaviors against bright lights, loud noises, and threats to their respiration. Some of these responses, particularly when intense, have a quality of anger about them, and the close observer of babies soon appreciates that these patterns of aversion and protest must have real adaptive significance.

Mavis Gunther, the noted British pediatrician, described how the "feeding couple," as she called the mother-and-suckling pair, affect one another in subtle ways that may have enduring consequences (Gunther, 1961). She noted that the newborn, quite naturally, can occasionally become smothered for brief moments during the course of feeding. The infant's nostrils are very close to the mother's breast and sometimes are occluded while the baby has a tight latch on the nipple. This causes difficulty in breathing, at least for a few moments. The infant objects to this, often strenuously, and this frequently causes quiet (often undisclosed) tension in the mother. When briefly deprived of its air supply, the baby turns its head back and forth and pulls back from the nipple. The arms flail, the face reddens, and rather as a last resort if the respiratory blockage continues, there is a burst of crying. This throws the nipple from the baby's mouth with a force and decisiveness that often cause chagrin in the mother. The mother may become quite annoyed with herself after a few such occasions, frequently not knowing what has started this cycle of discontent and feeling herself a failure in coping with her baby's needs and frustrations.

From her extensive observation of newborns with their mothers, Gunther outlined some simple behavioral maneuvers that the mother can adopt to adjust herself posturally and to present the nipple in such a way as to minimize respiration blockage in the infant. Bottle-fed as well as breast-fed babies can be plagued by the awkward-stimulation problem, because the shield of the artificial nipple can come against the baby's nostrils while feeding. When respiratorily occluded, the newborn usually goes through the described pattern of behavior, culminating in releasing itself from the nipple by crying out, then taking in air, and regaining physical and behavioral stability. Paradoxically, perhaps, this is a high-incentive consequence, or a pleasurable experience, and thus some learned changes in the baby's behavior may occur (Lipsitt, 1979a, 1979b). Indeed, it is very likely some aspect of this process through which babies by 10 days of age become remarkably adept at moving their heads about the breast in such a way as to prevent anything more than very brief respiratory occlusion. The learning process involved results from the fact that the baby's aversion to occlusion produces escape from the breast and is thereby rewarded. The next time that the baby is put to the breast, the position will be found less desirable than previously, and the baby may adaptively decline another opportunity to be smothered!

Gunther's simple instructions to the mother concerning the necessity of helping the infant keep its air passages clear usually produce rapid change, first in the behavior of the mother and then in the satisfaction of the baby. Too few studies provide helpful information about these critical early moments of mother–infant interaction and about the possible lasting consequences of critical experiences with powerful hedonic overtones.

Until quite recently, the literature of child development and pediatrics seemed to suggest that the newborn child is an essentially decorticate organism. Myelination was presumed to be developed to such an insufficient extent that little more than rudimentary sensory and motor responses could be expected (Peiper, 1963). For the prediction of possible developmental deficit, therefore, scales of perinatal hazard (Hobel, Hyvarinen, Okada, & Oh, 1973; Prechtl, 1968) tended to concentrate more on the prenatal condition of the mother, specific birth hazards that the infant endured, and the traditional neurological examination of the newborn than on behavioral or psychophysiological assessment.

Although cortical insult and deficit are most likely to be reflected in the behavioral functioning of the baby, relatively little attention has been paid to the refinement of psychophysiological assessments as compared with assessments of early motor function (Amiel-Teson, 1968). Recent studies indicate that the newborn child may have more precocious neurological and behavioral development than was previously suspected. Purpura (1975) demonstrated the presence of dendritic spines, presumably the sites of synaptic contact, not only in the full-term newborn, but in the premature infant as well. Electrophysiological analysis of regional cortical maturation (Vaughan, 1975) now shows promise for the plotting during development of the emerging anatomical permissions that make increasingly mature behavior possible, and such studies tend to show that there is a considerable amount of functional cortex present at birth.

Supporting the new anatomical and electrophysiological findings are the results from studies of behavioral assessment, many of them cited earlier, that have documented rather "mature" sensory discrimination and learning processes in the neonate. These studies indicate clearly, too, that there are reliable individual differences at birth in sensory-motor functioning and that at least some of these differences can be related to perinatal hazards, such as prematurity and/or small size, the need for oxygen administration at birth, low Apgar scores, or drugs used during delivery.

This new expertise in the elaborate assessment of the newborn cannot but have an effect on the ability to identify, and perhaps identify for special follow-up, heretofore undetected deficits. Reason for even greater optimism in this direction is the possibility of carrying out extensive polygraphic assessments with the newborn, which will reveal signs that are not of themselves "deficit conditions" but that presage a condition of developmental jeopardy yet to be realized (Lipsitt, 1976). For example, an infant with no or minimal adverse perinatal signs might be seen on close testing to have difficulty in defending against respiratory occlusion when suckling or when moving about the crib. The response might be weak rather than absent and for that reason might not be regarded as a critical sign. The presence of that response insufficiency, however, could become critical in the ensuing months when the infant ordinarily has so many opportunities for coping with or parrying threats of respiratory occlusion, as when the nasal passages are blocked by mucus. The infant who is "unprepared" by experience for coping with such blockages might be in special jeopardy between 2 and 4 months of age, when so many previously automatic reflexes wane and are supplanted by voluntary responses that become established through important experiential input. Thus the infant with an innocuous deficit at birth might actually be demonstrating a precursor of a very serious condition once the initial deficit is compounded by failure of the environment to provide compensatory experience.

The scenario just described is quite possibly relevant to certain types of developmental disorder, perhaps especially those that remain rather a mystery, such as failure to thrive and crib death. Both of these syndromes are marked by a "failure to behave" in a life-preserving way. The thrust of research into the mechanisms by which infants succumb to such anomalies must be in the behavioral direction (Lipton, 1962; Naeye, Messmer, & Specht, 1976).

Amazing progress has been seen in the fields of developmental psychophysiology, fetology and neonatology over the past decade. Small premature infants who would not have had 1 chance in 2,000 for survival just two decades ago now survive routinely.

A great deal is now known about the ontogeny of the human sensorium, and about the influences of experience on the young organism, that was unknown until recently.

The newborn comes into the world with all sensory systems functional. There is convincing evidence that the neonate responds discriminatively to exteroceptive stimulation and that sensory preferences already are present in the first few days of life. Moreover, the neonate may learn to respond differentially based on sensory preferences and reinforcement contingencies, and in less than 1 hour of training may come to turn his or her head more in one direction than another, or more in response to one sound than another, or even open his or her mouth in response to one stimulus and not another. All of this must have enormous implications for the condition of behavioral reciprocity that characterizes the early interactions of mother and infant.

Parents and professional caretakers of infants are increasingly interested in providing a milieu that will tend to develop the potentialities of babies, and that caters to the burgeoning capabilities of the infant. The plethora of books on the market today encouraging parents and professionals to make the most of infancy attests to the extent to which people have become sensitized to the young child's capacities and developmental horizons. All of this attention, directed differently to different children by different adults, will probably have the effect of increasing the range of human behavioral and cognitive potential. The situation is not very different from that of the world of athletics, in which technology, human aspirations, competitiveness, and increased professionalism all conspire to promote record-breaking performances year after year. One cannot have such a stretch of human potential at one end of the continuum without affecting the other; the meaning of developmental disability must shift as well.

Another factor promoting greater variation in human potential, for better or worse, is related to the increasing survival rates of smaller and smaller babies. Although amniocentesis and elective abortion are reducing the incidence of certain types of congenital development anomalies, technological advances in both fetology and neonatology now permit the survival of infants who heretofore would have been destined for demise as "pregnancy wastage." The so-called continuum of reproductive casualty remains, but the cutoff point for survival has shifted greatly. Evidence suggests (or better, insists) that while many of the very small, very premature babies will grow up to be fully functioning humans, a large number will have developmental deficits. The full impact of recent progress in this area has not yet been felt. One thing is certain, however. The next technological advances must be in the realm of servicing the injured survivors, and this will require the development of even greater knowledge about the capacities of the developing human, perhaps especially about the potential of individuals with various constitutional or congenital deficiencies. The behavioral scientist, the developmental psychophysiologist, and the early-intervention specialist are uniquely trained to bring quantitative discipline and methodological rigor to the study of individual differences in human development under a large variety of environmental conditions. Efforts in this direction should yield advances in the detection of subtle developmental deficits, and in the application of experiential interventions or other remedial procedures that might diminish the tragedy of the disability. The task is largely an educational and psychological one.

☐ Concluding Comments

When a baby is born, the principal concern of parents and relatives and of professional caregivers is with the infant's survival. The concern for survival of the infant and mother and protection of their biological comfort quite naturally tends to overshadow the behavioral, psychophysiological, and psychodynamic features of early life, even those involving interactions of the mother and infant. Attention sometimes does get drawn, however, to the relationship of the mother and infant to the baby's psychological functions. This has become increasingly so as perinatal technological expertise has increased, thus rendering the birth process less hazardous than in years past. For example, observers can see the mother and quite probably the infant as well; one mother was heard saying, "Come on, baby. Open your eyes. I know you're in there." Acknowledgment and recognition of the baby's "personhood" is an immense achievement for the mother and presages the eventual necessity for the child to become autonomous, a task on which he or she will be working throughout the first year, if not the rest of life. From the moment of these first interactions, the capacity of the infant for experiencing pleasures and annoyances is operative and will become exceedingly important in impelling and sustaining learning. Many of these learned behaviors will be based on fundamental biological reflexes, some of them involving approach to positive, desirable stimulation (like tastes) and others of which will be put to the service of enabling the infant to escape from noxious experiences.

Only relatively recently in the history of medicine and the biomedical sciences have sensory and behavioral features of infants been noted carefully and credited with relevance to later life outcomes. It has been suggested here that the infant's sensory and learning capacities have important roles in assuring the infant's survival. Indeed, it has been proposed that crib death and other critical conditions of infancy might result from a concatenation of risk factors, all conspiring to create a major deficit at the critical period of about 2 to 4 months of age. The initial deficits are considered in their origins to be constitutional, but with increasing experience during development they become clearly psychobiological. In any event, they can be lethal in their effects, and much more needs to be discovered about the psychodynamics of infancy in relation to initial constitutional markers.

☐ References

Abrahamson, D., Brackbill, Y., Carpenter, Y., & Fitzgerald, H. E. (1970). Interaction of stimulus and response in infant conditioning. *Psychosomatic Medicine, 32,* 319.

Aldrich, C. A. (1928). A new test for hearing in the newborn: The conditioned reflex. *American Journal of Diseases of Children, 35,* 36.

Amiel-Tison, C. (1968). Neurological evaluation of the maturity of newborn infants. *Archives of Disease in Childhood, 43,* 89.

Babkin, P. S. (1960). The establishment of reflex activity in early postnatal life. In *The central nervous system and behavior* (U.S. Department of Health, Education, and Welfare, Public Health Service, Trans., pp. 24–32). Washington, DC: U.S. Government Printing Office.

Barnet, A. B., Olrich. E. S., & Shanks, B. L. (1974). EEC evoked responses to repetitive stimulation in normal and Down's syndrome infants. *Developmental Medicine and Child Neurology, 5,* 612.

Bartoshuk, A. K. (1962a). Human neonatal cardiac acceleration to sound: Habituation and dishabituation. *Perceptual and Motor Skills, 15,* 15.

Bartoshuk, A. K. (1962b). Response decrement with repeated elicitation of human neonatal cardiac acceleration to sound. *Journal of Comparative and Physiological Psychology, 55,* 9.

Bartoshuk, A. K. (1964). Human neonatal cardiac responses to sound: A power function. *Psychonomic Science, 1,* 151.

Bower, T. G. R. (1965). Stimulus variables determining space perception in infants. *Science, 191,* 88.

Bower, T. G. R. (1971). The object in the world of infants. *Scientific American, 225,* 30.

Bower, T. G. R. (1977). *A primer of infant development.* San Francisco: Freeman.

Bowes, W., Brackbill, Y., Conway, E., et al. (1970). The effects of obstetrical medication on fetus and infant. *Monographs of the Society for Research in Child Development, 35,* 55.

Brackbill, Y. (1971). The role of the cortex in orienting: Orienting reflex in an anencephalic human infant. *Developmental Psychology, 5,* 195.

Brazelton, T. B. (1973). *Neonatal behavioral assessment scale.* Philadelphia: J. B. Lippincott.

Bronshtein, A. I., Antonova, T. G., Kamenetskaya, A. G., Luppova, N. N., & Sytova, V. (1958). On the development of the functions of analyzers in infants and some animals at the early stages of ontogenesis. In *Problems of evolution of physiological functions. U.S.S.R. Academy* (U.S. Department of Health, Education, and Welfare, Trans. of PTS Report No. 60-61066). Moscow: Academy of Science.

Brown, J. (1972). Instrumental control of the sucking response in human newborns. *Journal of Experimental Child Psychology, 14,* 66.

Burke, P. M. (1977). Swallowing and the organization of sucking in the human newborn. *Child Development, 48,* 423–431.

Bystroletova, G. N. (1954). The formation in neonates of a conditioned reflex to time in connection with daily feeding rhythm. *Zhurnal Vysshei Nervnoi Devatel'nosti imeni I.P. Pavlova, 4,* 601.

Campos, J. J., Langer, A., & Krowitz, A. (1970). Cardiac responses on the visual cliff in prelocomotor human infants. *Science, 170,* 195.

Caron, R. F. (1967). Visual reinforcement of head turning in young infants. *Journal of Experimental Child Psychology, 5,* 489.

Chase, W. B. (1937). Color vision in infants. *Journal of Experimental Psychology, 20,* 203.

Crook, C. K. (1976). Neonatal sucking: Effects of quantity of the response-contingent fluid upon sucking rhythm and heart rate. *Journal of Experimental Child Psychology, 21,* 539.

Crook, C. K. (1978). Taste perception in the newborn infant. *Infant Behavior and Development, 1,* 52–69.

Crook, C. K., & Lipsitt, L. P. (1976). Neonatal nutritive sucking: Effects of taste stimulation upon sucking rhythm and heart rate. *Child Development, 47,* 518.

Davids, A. (1974). *Children in conflict: A case book.* New York: John Wiley and Sons.

Dayton, G. O., Jr., Jones, M., H., Aiu, P., Rawson, R. A., Skele, B., & Rose, M. (1964). Developmental study of coordinated eye movements in the human infant. I. Visual acuity in the newborn human: A study based on induced optokinetic nystagmus recorded by electrooculography. *Archives of Ophthalmology, 71,* 865–870.

Denisova, M. P., & Figurin, N. L. K. (1929). Voprosu o pervykh sochetatelnykh pishchevykh refleksakh u grudnykh detei. *Voprosy Genet. Refleks. Pedologii, 1,* 81.

Dobbing, J. (1975). Human brain development and its vulnerability. *Mead Johnson Symposium on Perinatal and Developmental Medicine, Biological and Clinical Aspects of Brain Development, 6,* 3–12.

Dobson, V. (1976). Spectral sensitivity of the two-month infant as measured by the visually evoked cortical potential. *Vision Research, 16,* 367.

Eimas, P. D., Siqueland, E. R., Jusczyk, P., & Vigorito, J. (1971). Speech perception in infants. *Science, 171,* 303.

Engen, T., & Lipsitt, L. P. (1965). Decrement and recovery of responses to olfactory stimuli in the human neonate. *Journal of Comparative and Physiological Psychology, 59,* 312.

Engen, T., Lipsitt, L. P., & Kaye, H. (1963). Olfactory responses and adaptation in the human neonate. *Journal of Comparative and Physiological Psychology, 56,* 73.

Fantz, R. L. (1961). The origin of form perception. *Scientific American, 204,* 66.

Fantz, R. L. (1964). Visual experiences of infant: Decreased attention to familiar patterns relative to novel ones. *Science, 146,* 668.

Fantz, R. L., & Miranda, S. B. (1975). Newborn infant attention to form of contour. *Child Development, 46,* 224

Friedman, S., Nagy, A. N., & Carpenter, C. C. (1970). Newborn attention: Differential response decrement to visual stimuli. *Journal of Experimental Child Psychology, 10,* 44.

Globus, A., & Scheibel, A. B. (1967). The effect of visual deprivation cortical neurons: A Golgi study. *Experimental Neurology, 19,* 331–345.

Graham, F. K. (1956). Behavioral differences between normal and traumatized newborns. I. The test procedures. *Psychological Monographs, 70* (427).

Gunther, M. (1961). Infant behavior at the breast. In B. M. Foss (Ed.), *Determinants of infant behavior.* New York: Wiley.

Haith, M. M. (1969). Infrared television recording and measurement of ocular behavior in the human infant. *American Psychologist, 24,* 279.

Hershenson, M. (1964). Visual discrimination in the human newborn. *Journal of Comparative and Physiological Psychology, 58,* 270.

Hobel, C. J., Hyvarinen, M. A., Okada, D. M., & Oh, W. (1973). Prenatal and intra-partum high-risk screening. *American Journal of Obstetrics and Gynecology, 117,* 1.

Hubel, D. H., & Wiesel, T. N. (1970). The period of susceptibility to the physiological effects of unilateral eye closures in kittens. *Journal of Physiology, 206,* 419–436.

Jacobson, M. (1978). *Developmental neurobiology* (2nd ed.). New York: Plenum Press.

Jeffrey, W. E. (1980). The developing brain and child development. In M. C. Wittrock (Ed.), *The brain and psychology.* New York: Academic Press.

Karmel, B. Z. (1969). The effect of age, complexity, and amount of contour on pattern preferences in human infants. *Journal of Experimental Child Psychology, 7,* 339.

Karmel, B. Z., & Maisel, E. B. (1975). A neuronal activity model for infant visual attention. In L. B. Cohen & P. Salapatek (Eds.), *Infant perception: From sensation to cognition. Basic visual processes* (Vol. 1, pp. 77–131). New York: Academic Press.

Kasatkin, N. I., & Levikova, A. M. (1935). On the development of early conditioned reflexes and differentiation of auditory stimuli in infants. *Journal of Experimental Psychology, 18,* 1.

Kaye, H. (1965). The conditioned Babkin reflex in human newborns. *Psychonomic Science, 2,* 287.

Kessen, W., Haith, M. M., & Salapatek, P. H. (1970). Human infancy: A bibliography and guide. In P. H. Mussen (Ed.), *Carmichael's manual of child psychology* (pp. 287–445). New York: John Wiley and Sons.

Kobre, K. R., & Lipsitt, L. P. (1972). A negative contrast effect in newborns. *Journal of Experimental Child Psychology, 14,* 81.

Krachkovskaia, M. V. (1959). Reflex changes in the leucocyte count of newborn infants in relation to food intake. *Pavlov Journal of Higher Nervous Activity, 9,* 193.

Leventhal, A. S., & Lipsitt, L. P. (1964). Adaptation, pitch discrimination, and sound localization in the neonate. *Child Development, 35,* 759.

Levison, C. A., & Levison, P. K. (1967). Operant conditioning of head turning for visual reinforcement in three month old infants. *Psychonomic Science, 8,* 529.

Lewis, M. (1967). The meaning of a response, or why researchers in infant behavior should be oriental metaphysicians. *Merrill-Palmer Quarterly, 13.*

Lipsitt, L. P. (1963). Learning in the first year of life. In L. P. Lipsitt & C. C. Spiker (Eds.), *Advances in child development and behavior* (Vol. 1, pp. 147–195). New York: Academic Press.

Lipsitt, L. P. (1974). The synchrony of respiration, heart rate, and sucking behavior in the newborn. *Mead Johnson Symposium on perinatal and developmental medicine: Biological and clinical aspects of brain development, 6,* 67.

Lipsitt, L. P. (1976). Developmental psychobiology comes of age. In L. P. Lipsitt (Ed.), *The significance of infancy.* Hillsdale, NJ: Lawrence Erlbaum Associates.

Lipsitt, L. P. (1979a). Critical conditions in infancy: A psychological perspective. *American Psychologist, 34,* 973–980.

Lipsitt, L. P. (1979b). Learning assessments and interventions for the infant born at risk. In T.

Field, A. M. Sostek, S. Goldberg, & H. H. Shuman (Eds.), *Infants born at risk: Behavior and development* (pp. 145–169). Spectrum.

Lipsitt, L. P. (1983). Infant behavior, birth risk, and development. In J. Calhoun (Ed.), *Environment and population: Problems of adaptation* (pp. 82–84). New York: Praeger.

Lipsitt, L. P. , & Kaye, H. (1964). Conditioned sucking in the human newborn. *Psychonomic Science, 1.* 29–30.

Lipsitt, L. P., & Kaye, H. (1965). Change in neonatal response to optimizing and non-optimizing sucking stimulation. *Psychonomic Science, 2,* 221–222.

Lipsitt, L. P., Kaye, H., & Bosack, T. N. (1966). Enhancement of neonatal sucking through reinforcement. *Journal of Experimental Child Psychology, 4,* 164–168.

Lipsitt, L. P., Reilly, B. M., Butcher, M. J., & Greenwood, M. M. (1976). The stability and interrelationships of newborn sucking and heart rate. *Developmental Psychobiology, 9,* 305–310.

Lipton, E. L. (1962). Developmental aspects of rate and rhythm in young infants. *Psychosomatic Medicine, 24,* 517.

Macfarlane, A. (1975). Olfaction in the development of social preferences in the human neonate. In *Parent–infant interaction, CIBA Foundation Symposium 33* (pp. 103–117). Amsterdam: Elsevier.

Maratos, O. (1973). *The origin and development of imitation in the first six months of life.* Unpublished doctoral dissertation, University of Geneva, Geneva, Switzerland.

Marquis, D. P. (1941). Learning in the neonate: The modification of behavior under three feeding schedules. *Journal of Experimental Psychology, 29,* 263.

McKenzie, B., & Day, R. H. (1971). Operant learning of visual pattern discrimination in young infants. *Journal of Experimental Child Psychology, 11,* 45.

Meltzoff, A. N. (1977, May). *Gestural imitation in early infancy: Some implications for Piaget's theory of representation.* Presented at meetings of the Jean Piaget Society, Philadelphia.

Meltzoff, A. N., & Moore, M. K. (1977). Imitation of facial and manual gestures by human neonates. *Science, 198,* 75–78

Milewski, A. E., & Siqueland, E. R. (1976). Discrimination of color and pattern novelty in one-month human infants. *Journal of Experimental Child Psychology, 19,* 122.

Naeye, R. L., Messmer, J., & Specht, W. (1976). Sudden infant death syndrome temperament before death. *Journal of Pediatrics, 88,* 511.

Nowlis, G. (1973). Taste elicited tongue movements in human newborn infants: An approach to palatability. In J. F. Bosma (Ed.), *Oral sensation and perception: Development in the fetus and infant* (pp. 292–303). Bethesda, MD: U.S. Department of Health, Education and Welfare.

Papoušek, H. (1959). A method of studying conditioned food reflexes in young children up to the age of six months. *Pavlov Journal of Higher Nervous Activity, 9,* 136.

Papoušek, H. (1960). Conditioned motor digestive reflexes in infants. II. A new experimental method for the investigation. *Czechoslovenka Pediatrie, 15,* 981.

Peiper, A. (1963). *Cerebral function in infancy and childhood.* New York: Consultant's Bureau.

Pratt, K. C. (1933). The neonate. In C. Murchison (Ed.), *A handbook of child psychology* (2nd ed.). Worcester, MA: Clark University Press.

Pratt, K. C. (1946). The neonate. In L. Carmichael (Ed.), *Manual of child psychology.* New York: John Wiley & Sons.

Prechtl, H. F. R. (1968). Neurological findings in newborn infants after pre and para-natal complications. In J. H. P. Jonix, H. K. A. Visser, & J. A. Troelstra (Eds.), *Aspects of prematurity and dysmaturity.* Leiden: Stenfert Kroese.

Premack, D. (1965). Reinforcement theory. In D. Levin (Ed.), *Nebraska Symposium on Motivation.* Lincoln: University of Nebraska Press.

Pribram, K. H. (1971). *Languages of the brain: Experimental paradoxes and principles in neuropsychology.* Englewood Cliffs, NJ: Prentice Hall.

Purpura, D. P. (1975). Neuronal migration and dendritic differentiation: Normal and aberrant development of human cerebral cortex. *Mead Johnson Symposium on Perinatal and Developmental Medicine, Biological and Clinical Aspects of Brain Development, 6,* 13–27.

Salapatek, P. (1975). Pattern perception in early infancy. In L. B. Cohen & P. Salapatek (Eds.), *Infant perception: From sensation to cognition, Vol. 1. Basic visual processes* (pp. 133–248). New York: Academic Press.

Sameroff, A. J. (1972). Learning and adaptation in infancy: A comparison of models. In H. W. Reese (Ed.), *Advances in child development and behavior* (vol. 7, pp. 169–214). New York: Academic Press.

Sameroff, A. J., & Chandler, M. (1975). Reproductive risk and the continuum of caretaking casualty. In F. Horowitz, M. Hetherington, S. Scarr-Salapatek, & G. Siegel (Eds.), *Review of child development research* (Vol. 4, pp. 187–244). Chicago: University of Chicago Press

Schapiro, S., & Vukovich, K. R. (1970). Early experience effects upon cortical dendrites: A proposal model for development. *Science, 167,* 292–294.

Semb, C., & Lipsitt, L. P. (1968). The effects of acoustic stimulation on cessation and initiation of non-nutritive sucking in neonates. *Journal of Experimental Child Psychology, 6,* 585.

Sherman, M., Sherman. I., & Flory, C. D. (1936). Infant behavior. *Comparative Psychology Monographs, 12,* 1.

Simner, M. L . (1971). Newborn's response to the cry of another infant. *Developmental Psychology, 5,* 136.

Siqueland, E. R ., & DeLucia, C. A. (1969). Visual reinforcement of nonnutritive sucking in human infants. *Science, 165,* 1144.

Siqueland, E. R., & Lipsett, L. P. (1966). Conditioned head turning in human newborns. *Journal of Experimental Child Psychology, 3,* 356.

Sostek, A. M., Sameroff, A. J., & Sostek, A. J. (1972). Evidence for the unconditionability of the Babkin reflex in newborns. *Child Development, 43,* 509.

Steinschneider, A. (1967). Developmental psychophysiology. In Y. Brackbill (Ed.), *Infancy and early childhood: A handbook and guide to human development* (pp. 3–47). New York: Free Press.

Steinschneider, A., Lipton, E. L., & Richmond, J. B. (1966). Auditory sensitivity in the infant: Effect of intensity on cardiac and motor activity. *Child Development, 37,* 233.

Trincker, D., & Trincker, I. (1955). Die ontogenetische Entwicklund des Helligkeits und Farbensehens beim Menschen. I. Die Entwicklund des Helligkeitssehens. *Albrecht v. Graefes Archives of Ophthalmology, 156,* 519.

Vaughan, H. G., Jr. (1975). Electrophysiologic analysis of regional cortical maturation. *Biological Psychiatry, 10,* 513.

Walk, R. D. (1966). The development of depth perception in animal and human infants. *Monographs of the Society for Research in Child Development, 31*(5), 82–108.

Watson, J. B. (1919). *Psychology from the standpoint of a behaviorist.* New York: Lippincott.

Watson, J. B. (1928). *The psychological care of infant and child.* New York: W.W. Norton & Co.

Weiffenbach, J. M., & Thach, B. T. (1973). Elicited tongue movements: Touch and taste in the newborn human. In J. F. Bosma (Ed.), *Oral sensation and perception: Development in the fetus and infant* (pp. 232–243). Bethesda, MD: U.S. Department of Health, Education and Welfare.

Wertheimer, M. (1961). Psychomotor coordination of auditory and visual space at birth. *Science, 134,* 18.

Winick, M. (1973). Effects of prenatal nutrition upon pregnancy risk. *Clinical Obstetrics and Gynecology, 16,* 1.

Wittrock, M. C. (1980). *The brain and psychology.* New York: Academic Press.

Wolff, P. H. (1969). *What we must and must not teach our young children from what we know about early cognitive development. Planning for better living.* New York: S.I.M.P. William Heinemann Medical Books.

William P. Fifer

The Fetus, the Newborn, and the Mother's Voice

As is evident throughout this volume, the development of early infant–mother interactions is a complex and multifaceted issue. My considerations of Baby XXI will focus on one particular aspect of this complicated and fascinating developmental process: the effects of prenatal experience on the response to the maternal voice. My interest in this specific capability grew out of questions relating to how the young infant is able to make sense of his or her early environment. That is, how is the newborn equipped to deal with this mandate to interact and adapt to the ex utero world and how has fetal experience shaped the development of the requisite equipment? The baby, faced with a myriad of stimuli, must learn to pay attention to some kinds of stimulation and learn to ignore others. My belief is that the newborn's preferential response to the mother's voice may aid in this early learning task, and that the development of this capability is a model for the sculpting effects of experiences in utero. This chapter focuses on our research attempts to characterize this early preference and to understand whence it came. I would also like to take this opportunity to speculate on how continued exploration of these issues could affect both Baby XXI and Fetus XXI.

☐ Newborn Response to Voice

Mills and Meluish (1974) and Mehler, Bertoncini, and Barriere (1978) showed that young infants (3–4 weeks of age) would respond preferentially to their own mother's voice. Anthony DeCasper and I began to investigate whether newborns with only minimal postnatal experience would behave in a similar fashion (DeCasper & Fifer, 1980). We developed experimental procedures in which newborns could selectively listen to recordings of their own mother's voice by means of changing the patterns of their nonnutritive sucking behavior. Even the youngest of the newborns tested, under 24 hours of age, were able to demonstrate a discrimination of, and in fact a preference for, the maternal voice. I would like to briefly describe a series of experiments, conducted by Christine Moon and myself, in which new techniques were developed to follow up this earlier finding and begin to investigate the origins, attributes, and functions of this early capacity.

Our experimental procedure is as follows: Newborns between 24 and 72 hours of age were brought to a quiet room, adjoining the neonatal nursery. Once awake, comfortably fitting headphones were placed on the infant's head and a nonnutritive pacifier (connected to a computer) was placed in the mouth (see Moon & Fifer, 1990, for a more complete description of the procedure). Infants were first presented with an alternation of syllables that served as signals for different voices. For example, in one experiment, the infant would hear a 4-second recording of "pat, pat, pat" followed by "pst, pst, pst." For half of the infants, sucking during the "pats" would result in the infant's hearing a recording of their own mother's voice; sucking during the "pst" would be followed by a period of silence.

This syllable pairing was reversed for the remaining infants. These periods of "voice" or "silence" would last as long as the sucking burst continued. At the end of the burst, the syllable alternations would begin again and would remain on until the next burst of sucking occurred. Testing sessions lasted 18 minutes, unless infants cried or fell asleep, in which case they were returned to the nursery.

In the first series of experiments using this protocol, our aims were to investigate whether newborns prefer their mother's conversational speech over silence, whether an unfamiliar female voice is preferred over silence, and lastly, whether the original finding for preference of mother's voice over an unfamiliar female voice (DeCasper & Fifer, 1980) could be replicated using this procedure. Three separate groups of infants age 33–64 hours participated in one of the three experiments described next. In Experiment 1, infants were presented with the choice of hearing their own mother's voice or a period of silence. By the final third of the session, infants sucked more often to the signal for the mother's voice over silence. In Experiment 2, infants could hear an unfamiliar female voice or silence. Infants sucked more often for the unfamiliar female voice over silence (the female voice used was different for each child). In the third experiment, infants were presented with the choice of their own mother's voice or an unfamiliar voice. Infants sucked more often to the signal for the maternal voice than to that for an unfamiliar female voice.

There are several interesting questions that arise from these findings. One line of investigation follows from the fact that infants in these experiments have had minimal postnatal experience with the mother's voice. We therefore decided to first investigate the possible in utero origins of maternal voice preference. Fetuses have had experience with the mother's voice in utero during the last trimester of gestation (Querleu, Renard, Boutteville, & Crepin, 1989). Transmission of voices is apparently not substantially masked by intrauterine background noises. The maternal voice is transmitted both internally and externally to the fetus, with considerably less attenuation than nonmaternal speech. If the preference for the maternal voice is based on prenatal experience, then newborns might be expected to prefer the sound of the mother's voice, as heard in utero.

In one experiment, 16 infants less than 48 hours of age were presented with the choice of listening to their own mother's voice or a version altered to be similar to the intrauterine voice. That is, infants could hear a "normal" recording of the maternal voice or an altered recording filtered to progressively attenuate frequencies above 500 Hz. Additionally, the altered version was presented with a background recording of intrauterine heartbeat sounds. The experimental procedure was identical to the one described above, except that the syllable signals used in this experiment were "/a/ (ah)" and "/I/ (ee)."

Infants sucked more often to the signal for the altered, in utero version of their mother's voice. Though we may conclude that newborns demonstrate a preference for our "uterine" version of the maternal voice, the background heartbeat noise may have been the salient feature for the infant. A second experiment was conducted for another group of infants, to test whether heartbeat sounds were necessary for this preference to be demonstrated. Infants now heard either the mother's voice or her filtered voice without background heartbeat sounds. Infants again sucked significantly more often to the signal for the filtered version over the extrauterine unfiltered maternal voice.

Using the same paradigm, we asked infants if they preferred to listen to the language they heard in the womb in order to continue exploring the intrauterine origins of voice preferences (Moon, Cooper, & Fifer, 1993). We presented 16 newborns with pairs of female voices either conversing in the language that they heard in utero or another language. Eight infants, who were born to monolingual Spanish speakers, were presented with female voices conversing either in Spanish or in English. Eight infants born to monolingual English speakers were presented with the same recordings. The results showed that newborns responded to the sounds of the language that they heard in utero. This preference may have been partially shaped by postnatal experience during the first hours after birth. However, the newborn is more likely responding to some general property (e.g., intonation pattern) of the native language that they heard in utero.

Historically, the study on the effects of sound stimulation in utero has focused on either consequences of noise in the workplace or the fetal response to high intensity stimulation, that is, the vibroacoustic stimulation (VAS) used in clinical tests of fetal reactivity (Abrams, 1995; Kisilevsky, 1995; Leader, 1995; Lecanuet, 1995). The fetal response has been found to range from transient heart rate changes which rapidly habituate to prolonged alterations in state of arousal depending on the intensity, duration and sleep state in which the stimulus is presented. In our hands, VAS stimulation induced marked changes in heart rate, breathing and body movements in preterm fetuses (Zimmer et al., 1993).

We designed another study to more closely examine the effect of vibroacoustic stimulation on the near-term fetus. Fetal bladder volumes were examined serially by ultrasound 5 and 1 minutes before and 1 and 5 minutes after vibroacoustic stimulation or a sham stimulation. In the VAS stimulated group the mean bladder volume decreased from 21.7 ml 1 minute before stimulation to 12.8 ml 1 minute after the VAS stimulation. Twenty of 21 fetuses emptied their bladders following stimulation, demonstrating a previously unexamined, and perhaps undesirable, stress response to VAS. More recently, a number of investigators have begun to study the fetal response to less intense, as well as more naturally occurring, sources of stimulation, speech sounds, and voices.

The contingent sucking paradigm is not a viable alternative in investigations of fetal responsiveness to voice. However, cardiorespiratory reactivity may provide a rich source of psychophysiological correlates of attention and information processing throughout the perinatal period. We and others have shown that newborn infants show a reliable cardio-respiratory change to speech sound stimulation (Clarkson & Berg, 1983; Fifer & Moon, 1994). Lecanuet has reported that in the near-term fetus, low-intensity and low-frequency sounds evoke a decelerative heart rate response (Lecanuet, Granier-Deferre, & Busnel, 1989). These observations are consistent with studies of infants where the direction of heart rate change was dependent on the type of sound stimulus (Berg & Berg, 1987). Loud sounds were typically associated with heart-rate accelerations, while low-intensity stimuli induced mainly heart-rate decelerations.

External sounds, including speech sounds, are minimally masked by background uterine noise and are transmitted in utero with relatively little attenuation (Querleu et al., 1989). Morphological and anatomical studies of the human cochlea, as well as studies of auditory brainstem evoked potentials, have shown that the fetus is capable of responding to sound as early as 25 to 26 weeks gestation (Birnholz & Benacerraf, 1983; Pujol, Lavigne-Rebillard, & Uziel, 1990). In addition, premature infants show reliable auditory evoked responses to speech sound stimuli (Kurtzberg, Hilpert, Kreuzer, & Vaughan, 1984).

We investigated the response of the preterm fetus to speech stimuli in 41 healthy pregnant patients at 26–34 weeks of gestation (Zimmer et al., 1993). Speech stimuli consisted of repeated syllables ("ee" and "ah") presented externally over the maternal abdomen at 100, 105, or 110 decibels. Sound stimuli were delivered during periods of both high and low fetal heart rate (FHR) variability. During periods of low FHR variability, a decrease in fetal heart rate and an increase in the standard deviation of heart rate were found.

During periods of high FHR variability, no significant change in either fetal heart rate or standard deviation was observed. This is the first clear demonstration of responses to speech stimuli in the premature fetus. As is the case in the near-term fetus, this response is dependent on baseline heart-rate variability, which is the primary determinant of fetal state.

We next investigated whether the mother's naturally occurring speech would elicit a fetal attentional response. That is, are there detectable changes in fetal heart rate when the mother is actually speaking? Mothers repeated a 10-second rehearsed phrase of adult-directed speech, at least six times. These trials were alternated randomly with "whisper trials" in which mothers whispered the same phrases. Data were collected in fetal state 1F (Nijhuis, Prechtl, Martin, & Bots, 1986), the fetal analog to quiet sleep. Fetuses showed a significant heart rate (bpm) decrease from baseline during the last 5 seconds of the periods in which mothers were speaking.

During periods of whispering, in which fetuses received similar vestibular and tactile stimulation from maternal breathing movements, no significant response was detected. These data provide evidence for fetal heart-rate change in response to a salient naturally occurring stimulus and may offer a unique probe for studying both the immediate and the enduring effects of stimulation during the perinatal period.

☐ Questions for Baby and Fetus XXI

There are several "maternal voice" questions that I would like to ask, or would have others ask, of Baby XXI. The answers could help us understand the role of experience in the emergence of the infant mind, for the care of infants who have atypical early experiences, and for the development of more sensitive assays of well-being throughout the perinatal period. For example, when and in what contexts does the newborn begin to prefer the "normal" extrauterine maternal voice? When does the preference for other caretakers' voices (e.g., father's, adopted parent's) emerge? Does this early preference affect other early aspects of the infant's behavior or infant–parent interaction? For example, are the infant's early emotional responses affected by the presence or absence of the mother's voice? Does this attention to her voice facilitate later aspects of language development? Does the presence of voice affect the newborn's ability to interact with the rest of his or her environment or to attend to other sensory input?

Current baby lore suggests that newborns are soothed more by the maternal voice than other kinds of stimulation, and that early feeding interactions are strongly influenced by the qualities and timing of maternal speech. Furthermore, it is believed that older infants are better able to explore their environment when some "aspect" of their mother is available for attachment or engagement at a distance. Perhaps the newborn's earliest explorations of the environment are facilitated when the sounds of the mother's voice are available. Finally, babies have some of their earliest experiences with the emotional states of others by way of voices. These vocal emotional cues may play an important role in the earliest social interactions.

Although I believe fetal experience with the maternal voice profoundly affects the developing brain, it may very well be that this experience is neither necessary nor sufficient for later attachment to voices. Perhaps only limited postnatal experience may be needed for early "attachment" to voices and the early cognitive, emotional, and social development that this may afford. Many experiments, including our own, have shown that babies like to hear voices, not just the maternal voice, and that early on infants become attached to voices of significant others. But what of those infants whose early experience with voices is so atypical—the severely premature infant who has had limited pre- and postnatal experience with the maternal voice? I hope "Preemie" Baby XXI will continue to be asked not only how to improve the overall sound environment of the newborn intensive care unit (NICU), but also how to incorporate the parents' voices into his or her care. Questions regarding the quality, quantity, and timing of this "supplementary" experience should keep researchers and babies very busy in the next century.

One of my fondest wishes for Baby XXI is that he or she has a relevant clinical history. That is, Baby XXI will not supply the first data point for assessing progress along important developmental trajectories. Rather, can we more fully exploit the mother's voice as a unique probe into the development of Fetus/Baby XXI? For example, how does fetal experience with the mother's voice actually affect brain development? Neuronal systems are being constantly reshaped during this time of rapid growth, and the auditory system is no exception. Moreover, the autonomic nervous system is responding to many of these auditory experiences. Will the cardiorespiratory response to voice offer useful markers for the effects of various clinically relevant perturbations, such as hypoxia, growth restriction, or drug therapies on central nervous system function?

A related set of questions for the fetus of the twenty-first century could help to unravel the effects of other maternal–fetal interactions. For example, how does the pregnant woman respond physiologically to various kinds of stressors? How and when are these changes transduced to the fetus? How is the healthy fetus buffered from these maternal physiological changes? What are the immediate and enduring consequences of these "interactions"? That is, when is maternal stress fetal stress? How can we better educate parents as to what is, or is not, a potential fetal stress? For example, current prenatal extra stimulation programs for the unborn infant, which have no scientific evidence to support their claims and are taking advantage of anxious parents who want the best for their infants, may also be stressful for the fetus.

We are currently engaged in studies on the fetal and neonatal autonomic response to speech sounds as a function of a range of maternal risk factors. For example, do fetuses who are at risk for developmental disorders because their mothers are smokers, anemic, or too young have different autonomic responses to sound stimulation? Our speculation, and our hope, is that these and other studies investigating the fetal behavior in general, and the response to the highly salient sound of mother's voice in particular, will provide some answers, as well as better questions for both Baby XXI and Fetus XXI.

☐ References

Abrams, R. M. (1995). The fetal sound environment. In J. P. Lecanuet, N. A. Krasnegor, W. P. Smotherman, & W. P. Fifer (Eds.), *Fetal development: A psychobiological perspective*. Hillsdale, NJ: Lawrence Erlbaum Associates.

Berg, W. K., & Berg, K. M. (1987). Psychophysiological development in infancy: State, startle, and attention. In J. Osofsky (Ed.), *Handbook of infant development* (2nd ed., pp. 238–317). New York: John Wiley & Sons.

Birnholz, J. C., & Benacerraf, B. R. (1983). The development of human fetal hearing. *Science, 222,* 516–518.

Clarkson, M. G., & Berg, W. K. (1983). Cardiac orienting and vowel discrimination in newborns: Crucial stimulus parameters. *Child Development, 54,* 162–171.

DeCasper, A. J., & Fifer, W. P. (1980). Of human bonding: Newborns prefer their mothers' voices. *Science, 208,* 1174–1176.

Fifer, W. P., & Moon, C. M. (1994). The role of mother's voice in the organization of brain function in the newborn. *Acta Paediatrica Supplementa, 397,* 86–93.

Fifer, W. P., & Moon, C. M. (1995). The effects of fetal experience with sound. In J. P. Lecanuet, N. A. Krasnegor, W. P. Smotherman, & W. P. Fifer (Eds.), *Fetal development: A psychobiological perspective*. Hillsdale, NJ: Lawrence Erlbaum Associates.

Kisilevsky, B. S. (1995). The influence of subject and stimulus variables on fetal response to sound and vibration. In J. P. Lecanuet, N. A. Krasnegor, W. P. Smotherman, & W. P. Fifer (Eds.), *Fetal development: A psychobiological perspective* (pp. 263–278). Hillsdale, NJ: Lawrence Erlbaum Associates.

Kurtzberg, D., Hilpert, P. L., Kreuzer, J. A., & Vaughan, H. G., Jr. (1984). Differential maturation of cortical auditory evoked potentials to speech sounds in normal fullterm and very low-birthweight infants. *Developmental Medicine and Child Neurology, 26,* 466–475.

Leader, L. (1995). The potential value of habituation in fetus. In J. P. Lecanuet, N. A. Krasnegor, W. P. Smotherman, & W. P. Fifer (Eds.), *Fetal development: A psychobiological perspective* (pp. 383–404). Hillsdale, NJ: Lawrence Erlbaum Associates.

Lecanuet, J. P. (1995). Development of human auditory perception. In J. P. Lecanuet, N. A. Krasnegor, W. P. Smotherman, & W. P. Fifer (Eds.), *Fetal development: A psychobiological perspective* (pp. 421–429). Hillsdale, NJ: Lawrence Erlbaum Associates.

Lecanuet, J., Granier-Deferre, C., & Busnel, M. (1989). Differential fetal auditory reactiveness as a function of stimulus characteristics and state. *Seminars in Perinatology, 13*(5), 421–429.

Mehler, J., Bertoncini, J., & Barriere, M. (1978). Infant recognition of mother's voice. *Perception, 7,* 491–497.

Mills, M., & Melhuish, E. (1974). Recognition of mother's voice in early infancy. *Nature, 252,* 123–124.

Moon, C., & Fifer, W. P. (1990, April). *Newborns prefer a prenatal version of mother's voice.* Poster presented at biannual meeting of International Society of Infant Studies, Montreal.

Moon, C. M., Cooper, R. P., & Fifer, W. P. (1993). Two-day-olds prefer their native language. *Infant Behavior Development, 16*(4), 495–500.

Nijhuis, J. G., Prechtl, H. F. R., Martin, C. B., & Bots, R. S. G. M. (1982). Are there behavioral states in the human fetus? *Early Human Development, 6,* 177-195.

Pujol, R., Lavigne-Rebillard, M., & Uziel, A. (1990). Physiological correlates of development of human cochlea. *Seminars in Perinatology, 14,* 275–280.

Querleu, D., Renard, X., Boutteville, C., & Crepin, G. (1989). Hearing by the human fetus? *Seminars in Perinatology, 13*(5), 409–420.

Zimmer, E. Z., Fifer, W. P., Kim, Y., Rey, H. R., Chao, C. R., & Myers, M. M. (1993). Response of the premature fetus to stimulation by speech sounds. *Early Human Development, 33,* 207–215.

CHAPTER

J. Kevin Nugent

The Cultural Context of Child Development: Implications for Research and Practice in the Twenty-First Century

As this century comes to a close, an examination of global demographic trends reveals a world in which more and more societies are characterized by cultural heterogeneity. In the twenty-first century, there will be fewer and fewer ethnically homogeneous or so-called "ethnically pure" societies. Indeed, the very concept of homogeneous national cultures is in a profound process of redefinition (Bhabha, 1994; Said, 1993; Takaki, 1994). Even today, almost every society can be described as multicultural, populated by different cultural groups, who have moved to that region for reasons that may be economic, social, or political. What then are the implications of these dramatic population changes for research and practice in the progressively multicultural world of the twenty-first century?

☐ The Culture of the "In-Between"

A recent report from the Institute for Population Studies revealed that for the first time, the majority of the world's families can be classified as migrants, headed by parents who are living in diasporic situations or cultural settings other than those where they themselves were brought up. These parents are caught between cultures, born into one but living in another. Moreover, there is no evidence that the worldwide movement of families from rural to urban centers, often crossing national boundaries, that has characterized this century will be reversed in the new century. It is likely that every society will, in a very real sense, be multicultural, and most parents in the twenty-first century will be facing the task of bringing up their children in a milieu that is alien to them.

According to the recent Research and Policy Committee for Economic Development report, in the United States, by the year 2000, 38% of U.S. children under 18 years will be non-White, non-Anglo. In fact, it is clear that in the twenty-first century, ethnic diversity will characterize more and more countries and the ethnic composition of societies will become increasingly more diverse. In this new multicultural setting, the challenge for parents is to bring up their children in a way that is consistent with their own cultural belief system and at the same time in a way that promotes the child's successful adaptation to the new culture. The parents are in an "in-between cultural milieu" and their parenting is characterized by cultural discontinuity. Because their traditions, customs, and worldview are different from those of the dominant "host" country, these parents are even more likely to feel isolated and alone in their parenting roles, cut off from traditional support systems and unsure of their cultural and personal identity. Their philosophy of child rearing may be in conflict with that of the new society in which they are bringing up their children. This condition will be normative for the twenty-first century.

As we prepare for the next century, researchers and clinicians have to take a closer look at the cultural context of parent–child development and must begin to address the liminality of the parenting experience. We must see culture as the primary organizer of family experiences so that the research challenge is to shift the focus of our research from the child or family in isolation to the study of the child and family in context. We need to study the child in the "culture of the in-between," parent–child relations in a diasporic situation.

☐ Research on Child and Family Development: Lessons from the Twentieth Century

A careful examination of the existing canon of research on child and family development, the very canon on which the principles and guidelines for working with children and families is based, reveals that much of our information on child development is based on norms that are almost exclusively Western and middle class. Most of the studies that provide the foundation for theory and practice have been conducted in Western settings and can scarcely be said to be representative of the world's population. As such, this body of research has perpetuated "a middle-class, Western and male centered view of the universe" (Greene, Chap. 12, this volume). The classic dominant research tradition in child development tells us little about how children develop in many parts of the world and indeed has little to tell us about how children develop in the so-called minority cultures in Western societies (LeVine, 1988; Valsiner, 1989).

We must question not only the representativeness of our current research but also the very nature of the research process itself. Much of the research on child development has been conducted within the classic empirical tradition and reveals little about the dynamic nature of child–culture relations or the social or political context of child and family development. The scientific method, with its emphasis on the child and family in a controlled experimental environment, does not allow for the study of the child in context or for the study of the developmental process itself. Bronfenbrenner has described this endeavor as "the science of the strange behavior of children in strange situations with strange adults for the briefest possible periods of time" (Bronfenbrenner, 1979). As such, most empirical studies provide us with little information about the range of variability in children's patterns of development and the role of the specific environmental variables in shaping development and thus provide us with few reliable guidelines for understanding the developmental needs of children and families from different cultures. One of the goals of research in the field of child and family development is to describe the process of development by examining the process of child–environment transactions (Sameroff & Chandler, 1975). By examining the child's development in a variety of settings, and by examining the social and cultural context of development, research can provide the clinician with valid and trustworthy guidelines for meeting the needs of children and families. This is the challenge for the researcher in the twenty-first century. As we stand on the threshold of the twenty-first century, it is incumbent on us to expand the phenomenology of childhood by supporting research in a wider range of cultural settings and by expanding our research efforts to a range of cultures and populations that better represent the world of this century.

☐ Culturally Inclusive Research: A Model for the Twenty-First Century

Culturally inclusive research can serve as a model for the kind of research we need to adequately address the critical questions facing children and their families in tomorrow's world. Studies that examine the child in context provide researchers and clinicians with three critical principles that can serve to support and direct research and practice for the twenty-first century. First, although studies of child development in different cultural settings are essential in contributing to our appreciation of the rich diversity of child rearing practices and belief systems across the globe, they also serve to challenge our own assumptions about the very nature of child development and in turn help to free us from whatever residual nostalgia we may have for the primacy or superiority of our own cultural worldview. Second, research that considers culture as the main organizer of the child's development reminds us that experimental-controlled studies are by no means the only source (or even the chief source) of data collection or information gathering about child development. Alternative ethnographic qualitative research paradigms must be incorporated into mainstream child development research. Third, research that focuses on the cultural context of development forces practitioners, program designers, advocates, and policymakers to question the appropriateness of every program goal and the validity of every assessment tool in the light of the cultural background of the children and families whom they serve.

Taking a cultural-developmental approach to research will have serious implications for clinicians serving families from different cultural backgrounds. In the absence of systematic information on the child-rearing philosophies of different ethnic groups, the ethnographic approach of the cross-cultural tradition has immediate applicability to the study of different cultures about which we have little systematic information. Even in Western countries, there are still few ethnographically based studies of children and their families from the so-called minority cultures. This means that many outreach programs may be based on a priori goals that bear little relation to the cultural background of the families in which the programs are set. By emphasizing the primacy of context, this approach leads us to question the appropriateness of program goals and to reexamine the kinds of assessment tools we use to evaluate children, in the light of the cultural background of the children and families in the program. From this perspective, the clinician becomes the data gatherer, and each program must challenge itself to develop a set of strategies to meet the unique culturally mediated goals of the population being served and ultimately to develop program goals that are inclusive and culturally comprehensive.

☐ Research in Context: Challenging Conventional Assumptions about the Nature of Development

The classic cultural tradition guiding the study of child development has been the cultural transmission approach. It is an approach that has as its focus the description of socialization practices and examines the effects of different child-rearing practices on personality. However, although this tradition has provided a rich description of socialization practices in different cultures, it is essentially unidirectional in its thrust, with the child seen as a passive receptor of cultural messages. "Personality is culture writ large," as Ruth Benedict (1946) argued. Cultural practices are seen to shape behavior, and child-rearing practices determine it. The underlying assumption is that the study of child-rearing practices is the key to understanding the child.

A more recent approach to the study of cultural differences in behavior has been to examine the contribution of the child to the developmental process and to examine development as a dynamic interaction between the organism and culture in which it is embedded (Rogoff, 1989; Super & Harkness, 1980; Valsiner, 1989). The socialization process is seen as an active coconstruction process in which the developing child reconstructs cultural messages from the very beginning. This perspective is bidirectional, and socialization is understood as an active reconstruction of the parent's culture by the child. We have conducted a series of studies using the Brazelton Scale, from a wide range of cultural settings, and the data clearly demonstrate that the child has a role in shaping and directing the socialization process itself from the very beginning (Nugent, Lester, & Brazelton, 1989, 1991, 1995).

Chisholm's study of the Navajo culture and the effects of cradle-boarding on the child's development provides an illuminating example of this perspective (Chisholm, 1989). The cultural transmission approach would suggest that the reportedly shy, withdrawn behavior of Navajo children was the result of the custom of cradle-boarding. The "swaddling hypothesis" suggested that carrying the infant on a cradle board served to inhibit the child's movements, and this in turn was instrumental in promoting a quiet, shy, withdrawn disposition among Navajo children. Chisholm suggested that an alternative hypothesis could be that this view may rather be a reflection of the projection of Anglos, who would like to see the Navajo as a submissive people. Using the Brazelton Scale, Chisholm discovered that at birth the Navajo infants had a unique behavioral repertoire: They displayed well-modulated state organization, they cried little, they had generally low activity levels, and these qualities were present at birth. These were the very capacities that made it easy for Navajo mothers to carry them on cradle boards. In this case, it was the behavior of the child that contributed to shaping the behavior of the parent, so this provides an example of socialization as a dynamic interactive process from the beginning.

Guided by the notion of socialization as a coconstruction, I now briefly describe three studies, conducted in three different cultural settings, that produced results that serve to challenge our assumptions about the nature of development by yielding results that could be called counterintuitive.

☐ The Need for Ethnography: The Effects of Maternal Marijuana Use on Neonatal Outcome in a Jamaican Sample

In a study of maternal marijuana use during pregnancy in Jamaica, which was conducted along with Melanie Dreher and Rebekah Hudgins (Dreher, Nugent, & Hudgins, 1994), we examined the effects of maternal marijuana use on behavioral outcome in the newborn period. A series of studies conducted in North America have demonstrated the deleterious effects of prenatal marijuana use on newborn outcome. Fried and Makin (1987), for example, reported that moderate levels of marijuana use in pregnancy were related to poorer habituation scores, higher irritability levels, and more tremors and startles, as measured by the Brazelton Scale. Similarly, Coles, Platzman, Smith, James, and Falek (1992) found that infants whose mothers used marijuana in pregnancy demonstrated depressed Orientation scores at 14 days and had poorer Range of State at 1 month, compared to a matched group of unexposed infants.

Our study of 33 marijuana-using mothers and 27 nonusers and their newborn infants was conducted in the southeastern part of Jamaica, in which there is widespread use of marijuana. Consistent with the working class in other parts of Jamaica, residents in this community view marijuana not only as a recreational drug but also as one that has ritual and medicinal value. It is valued for its health-promoting functions and is consumed as a tea by family members for a variety of illnesses and to maintain and promote health. Rastafarians endorse marijuana as a sacred substance and may smoke ritually on a daily basis. Although women traditionally prepared marijuana in teas and medicines, female marijuana smoking is a new phenomenon. If they were Rastafarians they were called Roots Daughters, described as women with a purpose, who think, reason, and smoke like a man (Dreher, 1987). They are considered self-reliant and dignified. Many of these women smoked marijuana on a daily basis and continued to smoke during pregnancy and the breast-feeding period. Marijuana use is not necessarily indicative therefore of a mother's lack of concern for her baby. Supported by the folk belief that it has health-giving properties, women use it to deal with the difficulties of pregnancy. Nineteen of the women in our sample reported that it reduced nausea, and 15 said that it reduced fatigue and improved their appetites during pregnancy. Postnatally they reported that marijuana helped alleviate postpartum depression. All reported that it was good for themselves and their families. In general, however, it should be pointed out that these women are a minority and most women in Jamaica refrain from smoking marijuana during pregnancy.

An ethnographic design combining community and household naturalistic observations was employed. Field workers lived for up to 2 years in the parish, and local midwives were part of the team and helped recruit the women. The final samples were matched and consisted of 33 users and 25 nonusers. The users were divided into three groups:

Heavy users (n = 10): smoked daily: 21 cigarettes/week.
Moderate users (n = 9): smoked 3–4 times/week: 11–20 cigarettes/week.
Light users (n = 12): used tea only or smoked less than 10 cigarettes/week.

In this study, marijuana use was uncontaminated by any other drugs. Results revealed no differences between the infants of users and nonusers on Brazelton Scale scores at 3 days. However, there were differences at 30 days: Babies of marijuana users had better physiological stability and required less examiner facilitation to reach alert states. In the comparison of heavy users the results were more striking. The infants of heavy users were more autonomically stable at 30 days than the infants of the light users and the nonusers. On the Supplementary items of the Brazelton Scale they showed better quality of alertness, were less irritable, needed less examiner support, had better self-regulation, and were judged to be more rewarding for caregivers.

Conventional wisdom and the existing data suggested that not only would the infants of heavy users be negatively affected by the maternal marijuana use, but heavy users would be less likely to provide an optimal caregiving environment postnatally. In an effort to interpret these counterintuitive results, we were forced to look in more depth at our ethnographic data. In our post hoc analysis of the data we found that the environments of these infants were in fact more optimal, despite the fact that they were matched on global socioeconomic status (SES) ratings. The SES rating did not, however, reveal significant but subtle differences that were present between the environments of the heavy-using mothers and those of the nonusers. It seems that the heavy users, the Roots Daughters, were better educated and their households had fewer children. In other words, they had more adults living in their households and fewer children to compete for parental attention. Thus, these differences may well be the result of environmental influences that overrode the drug effects.

Studies of the effects of prenatal drug use in the United States reveal that not only are drug-using mothers more likely to use other drugs and consume insufficient nutrients during pregnancy, but the mothers themselves are more likely to have a history of interpersonal trauma and abuse than nonusing mothers. Due to the great number of social, medical, and psychological factors associated with prenatal drug use, the exposed infants are more likely to have caregivers who are at higher risk for parenting failure (Parker et al., 1988). The role of the caregiving environment therefore becomes increasingly important in predicting the effects of drug use during pregnancy.

In this study in Jamaica, maternal marijuana use is but one of many variables that may influence the infant's risk status from the beginning, and thus the absence of any differences between the exposed and nonexposed groups suggests that the better scores of the marijuana-exposed infants are traceable to the cultural positioning and social and economic characteristics of mothers using marijuana that select for the use of marijuana but also promote neonatal development. If we had not studied the cultural context of drug use and had not used an ethnographic approach to study the value system and the cultural worldview of that particular cultural setting in Jamaica, our data analysis and interpretation of the results would have yielded an incomplete description of the effects of maternal marijuana use on neonatal behavior.

☐ The Cultural Construction of Risk: A Study of Unmarried Mothers and Their Infants in Ireland

There has been a dramatic increase in the percentage of infants born to unmarried mothers in Ireland over the last decade. For the first 50 years of this century, 2% of all registered births were to single mothers. In 1975 the figure had risen slightly to 3.7%. Within 10 years it had risen to 8.5% and in 1996 the figure stood at 18%. We conducted a study to examine this phenomenon by examining the contraceptive practices of Irish women. Sheila Greene, Marie-Therese Joy, Paul O'Mahony, and I concluded that increased rates of sexual activity among unmarried couples, lack of information on family planning, and unavailability of artificial birth control contributed to this sharp increase (Greene, Joy, Nugent, & O'Mahony, 1989). Historically, there is evidence to suggest that at least since the beginning of the middle of the last century attitudes toward unmarried mothers in Ireland have been overwhelmingly negative. We were interested therefore in studying the effects of this cultural milieu on the experience of single mothers in their transition to parenthood in contemporary Ireland. Did the culture act as a buffer or as a risk factor in this process? In the North American-based literature on the effects of maternal marital status on child development outcome, there is a general consensus that infants born to unmarried mothers are at increased risk for negative developmental outcome (Garfinkel & McLanahan, 1986). Data on young single mothers suggest that these mothers are less responsive to their infants and are at risk for interactional failure (Culp, Applebaum, Osofsky, & Levy, 1986). We decided to test this out in an Irish cultural setting by studying a sample of unmarried mothers and their young infants.

We studied 200 first-time working-class Irish (Dublin) mothers, half of whom were unmarried and half of whom were married. They were first interviewed during the third trimester of pregnancy (Nugent et al., 1993). Consistent with our social-historical analysis and consistent with results from similar studies in North America, our results demonstrated that during pregnancy, the unmarried mothers had significantly less social support than married mothers and were significantly more depressed than the married mothers. On the basis of these findings, we expected that the unmarried mothers and their infants would be at risk for interactional problems.

One hundred and eight of these mothers and their infants were observed in their home settings at 1 month after delivery. We studied mother–child play in an effort to assess the quality of the mother–infant relationship and to assess the incidence of interactional failures. At the home visit, we compared the married and unmarried mother–infant dyads on the Belsky et al. assessment of mother–infant play (Belsky, Taylor, & Rovine, 1984). We found no differences in the quality of mother–infant play between the two groups on the six global dimensions. In fact, on a closer examination of the patterns of interaction, we found that the unmarried mothers showed more positive affect than the married mothers; they stimulated their infants more and looked at them more during the play sequence. We found no evidence of interactional failure among the unmarried mother–infant dyads. In addition, we found that the unmarried mothers as a group were no longer clinically depressed in the postpartum period, as they had been during pregnancy.

We concluded that this counterintuitive outcome was mediated by cultural factors. The disappearance of the depressive symptomatology in unmarried mothers may be due to the fact that the cultural rejection experienced by the unmarried mothers during pregnancy was replaced by a general cultural acceptance of mother and infant, which characterizes Irish societal attitudes to mothers and babies. These findings demonstrate that what constitutes risk in one setting may not in another. Definitions of risk are inevitably cultural constructions by virtue of the fact that they are derived from specific circumscribed empirical data sets that often have limited application across cultural settings. These results demonstrate the danger of using a priori categories of risk and the importance of collecting baseline data on the population with whom we work. Definitions of risk must be context specific in order to provide appropriate guidelines for clinicians and policymakers who are trying to meet the needs of infants and families in at-risk settings.

☐ Culture and Development: An Example from Japan

Although sleep disturbances are the most common concern among parents of young infants today in North America and in other industrialized countries (e.g., Brazelton, 1990a; Dawes, 1989; Lozoff , Wolf, & Davis, 1984), sleep problems and night waking are less commonly reported as clinical concerns in Japanese settings. Over the past 10 years Berry Brazelton and I have been working with colleagues Tomitaro Akiyama, Chisato Kawasaki, and Tsurusaki and Shoseo Ohgi on a longitudinal study of infants born on the Goto Islands off the coast of Nagasaki. Recently we have been studying the sleep arrangements of infants in two Japanese settings (Kawasaki, Nugent, Miyashita, Miyahara, & Brazelton, 1995). We found that up to 3 years of age none of the infants in our rural Goto Islands sample (n = 21) slept alone. Eighteen of the infants (86%) slept with their parents and the remaining three (14%) slept with their grandparents or siblings. In a study of 45 children between the ages of 4 and 28 months in Nagasaki itself, we found that 73% slept in the same bed as their parents. The remaining 24% slept in the same room but on a separate mat. No infant slept alone in either sample.

Sleeping arrangements with the management of sleep in young infants is one of the ways in which a culture attempts to achieve its goals for its children. In Japan, parents want their children to develop a sense of what can be loosely translated as dependence or obedience from the very beginning. Doi refers to this as *amae*, and in a recent study of Japanese fathers and mothers, we found that parents valued this characteristic above all others as the primary goal of socialization (Doi, 1990; Takahashi et al., 1994). The sleeping arrangements in Japanese society seem to have evolved to promote the development of *amae* in Japanese infants and to foster the development of a close, dependent relationship between children and parents, especially mothers.

It is tempting to suggest that this sleeping arrangement, which provides the infant with continued close physical contact with the mother, also results in an absence of sleep problems. However, from a more dynamic constructivist perspective, we recognized that the interpretation must lie in an examination of the interactions of the infant with the environment. In fact, when we examined the Japanese infants on the Brazelton Scale, we found that these infants showed little state lability and were especially able to deal with environmental perturbations while asleep (Akiyama et al., in press). However, we also found that these Japanese infants had a specific threshold for incorporating stimulation, and once that threshold had been crossed, the infants became extremely distressed and very difficult to console. Together these two sets of data suggest that the behavioral repertoire of the Japanese newborn with his or her capacity for shutting out negative stimuli while asleep, as well as the baby's relatively low tolerance for excessive levels of stimulation, serves as an enabling predisposition that ensures that the baby can deal with negative unpredictable stimuli when asleep but needs parental support when this stimulation becomes excessive, for his system at least. Together these help to reduce the possibility of problems with sleep or night wakefulness. We hypothesized that the behavioral disposition of the Japanese infants combined with sleeping arrangements that promote extensive close physical contact with parents may together result in fewer sleep problems.

The sleeping arrangements we observed in Japan challenged our assumption of what in Western societies is conventionally considered to be the "normative" or more optimal practice of having the baby sleep on his or her own from birth on (Brazelton, 1990a). In the United States at least 89% of infants sleep alone in a separate room apart from their parents (Shand, 1981), and parents believe that this facilitates the separation-individuation process in the young child and will in turn promote the child's independence and successful adaptation in society (LeVine, 1988). It is clear that neither the Japanese or the U.S. approach is a better or worse strategy of child rearing. Both practices are culturally based solutions to a specific child-care issue, and they are guided by separate cultural belief systems that have evolved over time in response to very different social environments, in two societies that have very different sets of goals for their children.

☐ Implications for Researchers and Clinicians

The heuristic value of this kind of approach to research goes beyond the simple description or documentation of different patterns of child rearing in strange or exotic cultures. The exposure to research from different cultures enables us to broaden our appreciation of cultural differences in the socialization process. Studies of child development in context can reveal the universals and the specifics of human behavior, what may be biologically based and unchangeable, and what is environmentally induced and therefore by nature variable. They may tell us what is phylogenetically programmed and what is culturally programmed, what is "bred in the bone" and what is shaped by parents and society. They can extend our understanding of the clinical process, since the goal of cross-cultural research is to expand the range of variability of what is considered to be normative behavior. Cultural studies in turn help us identify the particular kinds of experiences that affect health and development, the role of poverty and economic instability, the role of mothers and fathers in the socialization process in societies where a larger family network is responsible for child care, and the role of different kinds of discipline or child-rearing practices, and in general help us to describe the range of settings in which development takes place.

However, the study of development in context serves to challenge the validity of our current assumptions about human behavior and to free us from our own unconscious ethnocentrism. This form of ethnocentrism can be called unconscious or latent because it is not readily accessible to our conscious reasoning and it plays a subtle and often unconscious role in our interactions with families from cultures other than our own. The clinical goal of conducting contextual research is to challenge our core assumption about the nature of development, about what we think of as "good" or what is "optimal," what is "normal" or what is "abnormal." The concepts of normality and risk are therefore seen as cultural constructions that may not have validity in cultures other than in the one in which the concept was constructed.

These three studies conducted in very different cultural settings demonstrate that the notion of risk is a cultural construction, so that we always have to examine the validity of the data bases on which many of our at-risk categories and diagnoses are based. Risk categories have to be contextualized, and the only valid risk inventories are those that emerge from and are constructed from the communities that we serve. Listening to and searching for the authentic voices of these communities through conducting ethnographic research is the first step for the culturally sensitive clinician (Finn, 1994). Engagement with children and families from other cultures can have a disequilibrating effect on our clinical worldview and may yield counterintuitive feelings. These counterintuitive feelings in turn may turn out to be our most sensitive gauge for action, because in our engagement with families from other cultures, we may find the opposite of what our previous experience led us to expect. Cross-cultural experiences can serve to challenge the very essence of our beliefs about what we are doing and the efficacy of our interventions.

Studies of the child and family in context also serve to challenge the hegemony of logical positivism, which has been the dominant research approach of the twentieth century. We need to question the traditional primacy of experimental-controlled studies in our efforts to study and understand the nature of child development and meet the needs of families from a wide range of cultural backgrounds. When Berry Brazelton points to the risk of "throwing out the baby when we throw out the bathwater" in our search for objectivity (Brazelton, 1990b), he is suggesting that it may be the "bathwater" or the so-called interfering or contextual variables of the experimental paradigm that may well be the source of the most significant information on the cultural-environmental influences that shape the child's behavior. If we throw this out in our search for objective "generalizable" data, we may be left with little information on the specific environmental practices that influence the child's development. A cultural-contextual approach to clinical research forces us to examine behavior in context, to examine the ecology of development, and to come to an appreciation of the historical and cultural antecedents of the behavior under study (Bronfenbrenner, 1979; Bronfenbrenner, Kessel, Kessen, & White, 1986; Valsiner, 1989).

In sum, studies of child–family relations in different cultural settings serve to challenge our assumptions about the nature of development. They urge introspection as they force us to examine our own belief systems, and to unmask our own cultural biases by reviewing our attitudes toward children and toward families. It goes without saying that without an awareness and appreciation of our own culture or without a firm sense of identity with our own culture, it will be extremely difficult to be sensitive to or open to the nuances of another culture. It will be equally difficult to have access to our own biases and prejudices. Paradoxically, it is only in our engagement with other cultures that our understanding of our own culture is refined and our appreciation of other cultures is simultaneously enriched.

☐ References

Akiyama, T., Kawasaki, C., Goto, Y., Tsurusaki, T., Ogi, S., Nakamura, M., Kawaguchi, Y., Brazelton, T. B., & Nugent, J. K. (1995). The relationship between neonatal behavior and developmental outcome at seven years of age in a sample of Japanese infants in the Goto Islands. In J. K. Nugent, B. M. Lester, & T. B. Brazelton (Eds.), *The cultural context of infancy* (Vol. 3). Norwood, NJ: Ablex.

Belsky, J., Taylor, D. G., & Rovine, M. (1984). The Pennsylvania Infant and Family Development Project, II: The development of reciprocal interaction in the mother–infant interaction dyad. *Child Development, 55*, 706–717.

Benedict, R. (1946). *The chrysanthemum and the sword.* Boston: Houghton-Mifflin

Bhabha, H. (1994). *The location of culture.* London: Routledge.

Brazelton, T. B. (1990a). Parent-infant co-sleeping revisited. *Ab Initio, 2*(1), 1–2.

Brazelton, T. B. (1990b). Saving the bathwater. *Child Development, 61*(6), 1661–1671.

Bronfenbrenner, U. (1979). *The ecology of human development.* Cambridge, MA: Harvard University Press.

Bronfenbrenner, U., Kessel, F., Kessen, W., & White, S. (1986). Toward a critical social history of developmental psychology. *American Psychologist, 41*(11), 1218–1230.

Coles, C. D., Platzman, K. A., Smith, I., James, M. E., & Falek, A. (1992). Effects of cocaine, alcohol and other drug use in pregnancy on neonatal growth and neurobehavioral growth and status. *Neurotoxicology and Teratology, 14,* 22–33.

Chisholm, J. (1989). Biology, culture and the development of temperament: A Navajo example. In J. K. Nugent, B. M. Lester, & T. B. Brazelton (Eds.), *The cultural context of infancy* (Vol. 1). Norwood, NJ: Ablex.

Culp, R., Applebaum, M. I., Osofsky, J. D., & Levy, J. D. (1988). Adolescent and older mothers: Comparisons between prenatal and maternal variables and newborn interaction measures. *Infant Behavior and Development, 11,* 353–362.

Dawes, D. (1989). *Through the night: Helping parents and sleepless infants.* London: Free Association Books.

Doi, T. (1990). *The anatomy of dependence.* Tokyo: Kodansha International.

Dreher, M. (1987). The evolution of a roots daughter. *Journal of Psychoactive Drugs, 19,* 165–170.

Dreher, M., Nugent, J. K., & Hudgins, R. (1994). Prenatal marijuana exposure and neonatal outcomes in Jamaica: an ethnographic study. *Pediatrics, 93*(2), 254–260.

Finn, C. (1994, September). *Irish mothers' perception of parenting a handicapped infant.* Presented at the 14th Annual Conference of the Society for Reproductive and Infant Psychology. Dublin.

Fried, P., & Makin, J. E. (1987). Neonatal behavioral correlates of prenatal exposure to marijuana, cigarettes and alcohol in a low risk population. *Neurotoxicology and Teratology, 9,* 1–7.

Garfinkle, I., & McLanahan, S. (1986). *Single mothers and their children: A new American dilemma.* Washington, DC: Urban Institute Press.

Greene, S., Joy, M. T., Nugent, J. K., & O'Mahony, P. (1989). Contraceptive practices of married and single first-time mothers. *Journal of Biosocial Science, 21,* 379–385.

Kawasaki, C., Nugent, J. K., Miyashita, H., Miyahara, H., & Brazelton, T. B. (1994). The cultural organization of infants' sleep. *Children's Environments, 11*(2), 135–141.

LeVine, R. A. (1988). Human parental care: Universal goals, cultural strategies and individual behavior. *New Directions for Child Development, 40,* 3–12.

Lozoff, B., Wolf, A. W., & Davis, A. W. (1984). Co-sleeping in urban families with young children. *Pediatrics, 74*(2), 172–182.

Muret-Wagstaff, S., & Moore, S. (1989). The Hmong in American: Infant behavior and rearing practices. In J. K. Nugent, B. M. Lester, & T. B. Brazelton (Eds.), *The cultural context of infancy* (Vol. 1, pp. 319–339). Norwood, NJ: Ablex.

Nugent, J. K., Greene, S., Wieczoreck-Deering, D., Mazor, K., Hendler, J., & Bombardier, C. (1993). The cultural context of mother-infant play in the newborn period. In K. Macdonald (Ed.), *Parent–child play* (pp. 367–389). Albany, NY: State University of New York Press.

Nugent, J. K., Lester, B. M., & Brazelton, T. B. (1989). *The cultural context of infancy* (Vol. 1). Norwood, NJ: Ablex.

Nugent, J. K., Lester, B. M., & Brazelton, T. B. (1991). *The cultural context of infancy* (Vol. 2). Norwood, NJ: Ablex.

Nugent, J. K., Lester, B. M., & Brazelton, T. B. (1995). *The cultural context of infancy* (Vol. 3). Norwood, NJ: Ablex.

Parker, S., Greer, S., & Zuckerman, B. (1988). Double Jeopardy: the impact of poverty on early child development. *Pediatric Clinics of North America, 35,* 1227–1240.

Rogoff, B. (1989). The joint socialization of development by young children and adults. In A. Gellatly (Ed.), *Cognition and social worlds.* Oxford: Oxford University Press.

Said, E. W. (1993). *Culture and imperialism.* New York: Alfred A. Knopf.

Sameroff, A. J., & Chandler, M. J. (1975). Reproductive risk and the continuum of caretaking casualty. In F. D. Horowitz, M. Hetherington, S. Scarr-Salapatek, & G. Siegal (Eds.), *Review of child development research* (Vol. 4). Chicago: University of Chicago Press.

Shand, N. (1981). The reciprocal impact of breast-feeding and culture form on maternal behavior and infant development. *Journal of Biosocial Science, 13*(1), 1–17.

Super, C. M., & Harkness, S. (1982). The infant's niche in rural Kenya and metropolitan America. In L. L. Adler (Ed.), *Cross-cultural research at issue* (pp. 45–55). New York: Academic Press.

Takahashi, S., Nugent, J. K., Kawasaki, C., Greene, S., Wieczorek-Deering, D., & Brazelton, T. B. (1994, September). *Parents' socialization goals and father involvement in caregiving in Japan and some comparisons with Ireland*. Presented at the 14th Annual Conference of the Society for Reproductive and Infant Psychology, Dublin.

Takaki, R. (1994). At the end of the century; The "culture wars" in the U.S. In R. Takaki (Ed.), *From different shores: Perspectives on race and ethnicity in America* (pp. 296–299). New York: Oxford University Press.

Valsiner, J. (1989). *Development and culture*. Lexington, MA: Lexington Books.

THE ONTOGENY
OF THE PARENT–CHILD
RELATIONSHIP

Hanus Papoušek
Mechthild Papoušek

Parent–Infant Speech Patterns

This book offers a rare opportunity to reconsider whether the enormous progress in scientific knowledge, in the potential for rational intervention, and in the resulting tendency to manipulate and direct biological processes are still in an acceptable balance with the laws of Nature. Whether we like it or not, human reproduction, babies' births, and early child care that leads to good health and mental development still depend on those laws to a degree that easily escapes the attention of politicians and administrators but should never be underestimated by scientists. Baby care may be influenced by ever-changing fashions or superstitions: North American parents visit prenatal classes, and mothers listen to selected musical records during pregnancy and read texts to 2-month-old babies without asking how they themselves could have possibly developed mentally and emotionally during the dark period of ignorance two or three decades before. However, such short-lived fashionable interventions do not significantly affect the course of human processes that are based on organic forces and result from Nature's experiments, spread over thousands of generations.

In infancy research, we can observe a remarkable conceptual development, the transition from stimulus–response studies on isolated babies to research on babies in natural systems that include not only the entire family but also the ecological and sociocultural environment. Moreover, the progress in infancy research necessitates consideration of yet another dimension, namely, time in terms of evolutionary processes. In this perspective, the infant is not only a part of this generation's ecology and culture, but also a part of a system with a long evolutionary history, during which anatomical and physiological predispositions, intrinsic motivations, and behavioral tendencies have developed and, for good reasons, persist until now. These determinants may have evolved prior to the evolution of cultures, religions, or political ideologies, may be older but not less significant, and may not be without scientific concepts. System theories that encompass such complex and highly dynamic systems teach us how difficult it is to detect vector space and direction of movements within such systems and how dubious it is to restrict analyses to simplified testing of a mere few factors.

Students of infancy have successfully overcome the pitfalls of former conceptual dichotomies in interpretations of developmental processes, concerning, for instance, the roles of genetic versus environmental factors, cognitive versus emotional regulation of behavior, or continuity versus discontinuity in developmental changes. Typically, dichotomies were replaced with the concept of organisms embedded in networks of dialectic interrelationships among subsystems within the organism and other systems within biological and cultural environments. In relation to human baby care, we should not underestimate the nature–culture dichotomies that still persist in the background of controversies among various psychological or educational theoreticians.

To a great degree, the overemphasis on either nature or culture is also an artifact of conceptual simplification, due to a lack of biological thinking in one case, and ecological in the other. Sometimes a tendency to look for animal models of human behavior leads to overemphasizing the similarities between humans and other animals and to underestimating the sociocultural aspects.

At the same time, problems related specifically to present circumstances can reduce the interest in the biological past of human behavior and in comparative research. Moreover, studying behavioral evolution is difficult and hardly thinkable without interdisciplinary cooperation. Like all living organisms, humans represent complex dynamic systems with available self-regulation that differentiates them from physical systems. In its fundamental form, self-regulation is based on genetic transfer and has been selected during evolution under a long-lasting influence of ecological circumstances. In humans, self-regulation has reached an unparalleled complexity and adaptive relevance because it has evolved under the influence of both nature and culture.

The border between nature and culture is marked less distinctly than many people assume. It is true that in its present form—intimately interrelated with the use of words as abstract symbols—human culture is a unique phenomenon. However, the roots of human culture reach to precursors and capabilities that are common to many mammals. Special skills transferred by animals from one generation to another by learning can be viewed as a simple form of precursors of culture. These special skills include dialects in communication among birds or monkeys, and travel routes and home ranges used by mountain sheep or caribou. There are well-documented examples of precultural phenomena in the Japanese macaque, who invented and learned by imitation how to wash sand off potatoes (Kawai, 1963) and dig up peanuts (Tsumori, 1967). Van Lawick-Goodall (1971) summarized primatologists' research on tool use in chimpanzees and described a variety of modifications in it. Learning and play were found to be crucial elements for acquiring skills underlying tool use; if a young primate is deprived of opportunities for playing with adequate objects, tool use will develop slowly and remain on a low level.

To infancy researchers, it is particularly important to consider both cultural and biological factors involved in early interactions between infants and their environment. During infancy, social and cultural integration is spurred by the development of playful activities, the emergence of a capacity to process abstract symbols, the acquisition of language, and the ability to leave parents and explore other parts of the child's environment. The development of these abilities represents the beginning of species-specific features of humans; therefore, it deserves special attention for at least two reasons. First, a closer look at the beginning of species-specific abilities during ontogeny helps conceptualize theoretically their evolutionary past. Second, it would be difficult to design any care for Baby XXI if gaps in our knowledge on the most fundamental aspect of human development remained unfulfilled. To the authors, attempts to elucidate the beginning of cultural integration, acquisition of speech, and thus the beginning of humanity during early development have brought about surprising discoveries that are relevant to perspectives of future infant care and are to be explained in this chapter.

☐ Preverbal Communication

Human newborns exert a strange yet powerful influence on caregivers: They trigger speech in them. We can truly say that a word is at the beginning of the newborn's first social experience. The effect is strange inasmuch as the newborn can neither be expected to speak in response to nor to understand verbal messages. However, this effect was carefully documented by Rheingold and Adams (1980) and is easily observable. Another strange aspect of this effect is that it long remained unexplored while so many researchers were observing neonatal behaviors and effects of maternal heartbeats, smiles, holding, touching, and the like. Obviously, preverbal vocal interchanges were underestimated in theoretical concepts on early development and consequently underresearched. Moreover, attention was focused on infant behavior and on the effects of maternal stimulation. Attempts to analyze the earliest preverbal interchanges in the 1970s made it evident how little was known about predispositions and functional mechanisms on both sides of interacting parent–infant dyads. At that time, infant vocalizations were viewed as expressions of mere affective states, and contemporary lists of infant needs did not include more than the vegetative, nutritional, hygienic, and emotional. Parents' behavioral repertoire seemed to be fully controllable by cultural traditions or rational decisions and explorable with the help of questionnaires or interviews. Only affective bonding used to be considered as a biologically determined predisposition and studied in comparative research.

The introduction of microanalytic methods in interactional research revealed several novel and relevant aspects of human parenting (Papoušek & Papoušek, 1978):

1. The existence of a rich repertoire of caregiving behavior in the domain of nonconscious regulations (intuitive parenting in the Papoušeks' terms).
2. The universality of intuitive parenting (across age, sex, and culture), indicating its prevailing biological determination (Papoušek & Papoušek, 1992a).
3. The close interrelationship between intuitive parenting and speech acquisition in the infant, indicating a coevolution of supportive predispositions in the parent (Papoušek, 1989).
4. The close interrelationship between parental supports to communicative and cognitive development in the infant (Papoušek & Papoušek, 1992a).
5. The participation of behavioral patterns that lend the intuitive supports for infant communication or cognition a character of effective didactic intervention (Papoušek & Papoušek, 1987).

The newly revealed aspects of human parenting correspond to the biological evidence that, for the most relevant means of species-specific adaptation, predispositions coevolve on both parental and filial sides with a certain surplus and start functioning early during ontogeny. From the biological perspective, verbal communication represents a very powerful means of adaptation in humans. It is not a mere product of human culture, but like culture, it originated from precursors of speech in animal communication. Conversely, human communication reached a unique level of complexity, brought about the accumulation of knowledge in culture, and increased the probability of survival and resistance against diseases and dangerous environmental risks.

The detection of intuitive parenting helps us understand how infants learn the mother tongue. There is no doubt that they learn it; as cross-cultural adoptions show, infants learn the language of their new environment, although parents cannot explain whether and how they may facilitate infant learning. They do so unwillingly and unconsciously.

Research on nonconscious learning, cognition, and behavioral regulation has recently increased in connection with studies on hemispheric lateralization in the brain. However, unlike former speculative interpretations of subconscious mental processes in psychoanalytic approaches, contemporary interpretations of nonconscious regulation are based on neuroscientific and verifiable concepts. In studies on intuitive parenting, the authors have used two criteria to identify nonconscious forms of parental interventions: the lack of conscious awareness as evident in prestructured interviews, applied at the end of observations, and the length of latency in parental responses to infant cue signals. For example, parents tend to reach visual contact with the newborns or young infants and use a set of auxiliary behaviors for this purpose; having reached the visual contact, they carry out a "greeting response"—one of the first contingent displays controllable by the infant (Papoušek & Papoušek, 1979a, 1987). Yet parents are unaware of those behaviors, and the latency between the achievement of visual contact and the beginning of the greeting response is in most cases under or around the limit of 500 ms, which is the minimum duration of direct cortical brain stimulation necessary for aware perception. Naturally, conscious decision making requires substantially more time than 600 ms.

Interestingly, the system of intuitive caregiving guarantees an easygoing display of models for producing vocal sounds and their use in preverbal communication. Under favorable conditions, caregivers guide the infant toward higher levels of vocal communication in playful ways and adjust to the infant's momentary behavioral/emotional states and level of communicative competence like an experienced teacher. The intuitive character of this guidance guarantees a regular and repetitive delivery of behavioral patterns that facilitate integrative processes in infants—detection of contingency, conceptualization, prediction, expectance, control of caregiving, and anticipatory coping with interactional sequences that concern highly relevant adaptive capabilities and thus are associated with a strong intrinsic motivation and expressive emotionality in both infants and caregivers (Papoušek & Papoušek, 1981, 1987).

In hardly any other case has a coevolution of human predispositions in parental and filial subjects been documented as distinctly as in the case of preverbal communication and thought. Detailed studies on infant learning and concept formation (H. Papoušek, 1967, 1969), vocal development (M. Papoušek, 1994), and hemispheric differentiation (de Schonen & Mathivet, 1989) have gradually revealed astonishing fits.

For example, parents use the earliest convenient modulations in infant vocalization—the melodic contours—to deliver the first categorical messages and thus prepare the infant to use words as abstract symbols (Papoušek, Papoušek, & Bornstein, 1985). Prior to the appearance of reduplicated, canonical syllables, parents typically support processing of procedural messages, such as models for imitation and production of vocal sounds, consonants or syllables, for turn-taking or other dialogic skills, and for the skill of rhythmic movements. At the time of a developmental spurt in the speech-dominant hemisphere, the emergence of canonical syllables elicits parental transition from procedural to declarative guidance—a tendency to use each form of reduplicated syllables as a potential protoword, to give it a meaning, and associate it with some object in the infant's intimate environment (H. Papoušek, 1989; M. Papoušek, 1994).

The acquisition of the first infant words seems to open the avenues for cultural integration. Members of the infant's social environment start using verbal explanations and instructions with a strikingly increased frequency. The first words usually come together with the infant's first unsupported steps and tendency to leave caregivers and explore the newly opened horizons. Such exploration often leads to interactions or conflicts with new social and cultural environments and calls for confrontation with cultural traditions and rules. Caregiving increasingly mediates cultural impacts in comparison with the preceding intuitive didactics, based on biological predispositions. The new tendencies increasingly include the conscious and rational use of verbal mediation.

The first intuitive, melodic word seems to disappear and make way for the consciously used, rational word. Very soon, however, it will reappear when the infant becomes a child and meets another baby. At the age of 2 or 3 years, children display the features of an infant-directed speech very much like adult caregivers. This is another piece of evidence that adaptively relevant predispositions develop rather early during ontogeny.

☐ Implications for the Care of Baby XXI

The existence of a biologically determined system of caregiving capabilities, as it was just briefly described, seems to safely guarantee that even the next generations of babies are going to be so well supported in the most relevant directions of development that no improvements are to be needed. Unfortunately, this impression is delusive.

As in all biological predispositions, in intuitive caregiving universality does not eliminate variability. Minor variations in genetically mediated predispositions allow for the identification of individual caregivers. However, major variations may reduce the effectiveness of intuitive caregiving and cause failures in expected competencies. Conversely, intuitive caregiving partly depends on cue signals coming from the infant, and the expressivity of infant behavioral signals also shows a remarkable biological variation. Incidentally, a low expressivity on one side may meet a low responsiveness on the other side, and together this may cause failures in interactional communication. The incidence of unfavorable biological variations is relatively stable and need not be higher in the next century than it is now. However, the authors' clinical experience indicates an alarming increase in interactional and communicative failures and calls for increased attention to both parental competencies and ecological factors.

Human families are part of physical and social environments, with which they may have good or bad relations, and the state of these relations can affect parent–infant interactions. The aforementioned strong intrinsic motivation for communicative interchanges brings about correspondingly intensive fluctuations in the regulation of fundamental adaptive functions (Papoušek & Papoušek, 1979b) in the sense of either activation or inhibition, and such fluctuations may lead to different effects. On the one hand, they may increase pleasant emotional experience during interactions and resistance against unfavorable environmental agents; on the other hand, they may cause opposite effects, reduce the pleasure of parent–infant interactions, and increase the risks of failure. Intuitive processes require certain conditions to function successfully.

In general, the functioning of intuitive processes depends, for instance, on a relaxed and stress-free state of mind (Bastick, 1982). This seemingly simple requirement is increasingly difficult to fulfill in the modern world in which the available space and time for parenting have been widely reduced beyond acceptable limits. The former assistance of a larger family has been eliminated in many nuclear families, and mothers have often been left with the exclusive responsibility for infant development under problematic conditions. To look for help from the flood of unverified recommendations for family life and infant rearing may increase the risk of failure, because exaggerated rational guidance may harm intuitive processes (Bastick, 1982). Consequently, the adaptive role of primary parenting can easily reverse into maladaptive vicious cycles, including pathogenetic mechanisms that may cause depressive states or aggressive child abuse in parents, and retardation or developmental disorders due to parental rejection in the child (Papoušek & Papoušek, 1979b, 1992b).

Furthermore, unfavorable factors often accumulate. Thus, general life conditions in overpopulated and/or overexploited areas may be so stressful that they cause deficient intrauterine development of the fetus. Unwanted pregnancy is frequently associated with marital problems, drug use, or alcoholism. Additional difficulties usually result from hostile attitudes in the social environment. Under such conditions, primary parental attempts can fail to establish satisfactory communication with the infant, particularly if they are disturbed by additional difficulties from the infant, such as sleep disorders, nutritional problems, or excessive crying.

Deviations in interactional processes between parents and progeny, elicited by social or cultural circumstances, may fluctuate in frequency much more irregularly than the variation in biological predispositions. Conversely, they can also be positively affected in the therapeutic sense by improved social or cultural conditions. Here appears the main impetus for consideration of factors that codetermine the care for Baby XXI. With all respect to the merits of existing theories on early human development, the reader may realize that these theories do not cover the entire problem as long as they do not pay attention to biological aspects, particularly to the proper functioning of predispositions for communicative and integrative development. To reduce the roles of parenting to the issue of emotional bonding means to reduce access to explanation of interactional failures, to reduce ways to treat such failures, and to reduce the society's responsibility to the exclusive maternal responsibility. In a similar way, if supportive interventions in favor of infant health and mental development are to be considered, it may be problematic to reduce the forms of interventions to rational recommendations or commercial offerings of "educational aids." The authors strongly believe that the rational way should lead to the rescue of what Nature has selected in the form of primary, intuitive parenting.

To conclude, we wish Baby XXI two things. First would be the full scientific attention of interdisciplinary and well-supported research teams to the broad, unlimited spectrum of factors affecting early development. Much has already been detected and verified in infancy research, but just as much or more is still to be done. Second is a full public attention to the question of how scientific knowledge is applied in political and administrative decisions concerning family and child care.

☐ Acknowledgment

The authors' research and preparation of this publication have been kindly supported by the "Alexander von Humboldt Foundation."

☐ References

Bastick, T. (1982). *Intuition. How we think and act.* New York: Wiley & Sons.

de Schonen, S., & Mathivet, E. (1989). First come, first served: A scenario about the development of hemispheric specialization in face recognition during infancy. *Cahiers de Psychologie Cognitive 9*, 3–44.

Kawai, M. (1963). On the newly acquired behaviors of the natural troop of Japanese monkeys on Koshima Island. *Primates, 4*, 113–115.

Papoušek, H. (1967). Experimental studies of appetitional behavior in human newborns and infants. In H. W. Stevenson, E. H. Hess, & H. L. Rheingold (Eds.), *Early behavior: Comparative and developmental approaches* (pp. 249–277). New York: Wiley.

Papoušek, H. (1969). Individual variability in learned responses during early postnatal development. In R. J. Robinson (Ed.), *Brain and early behavior. Development in the fetus and infant* (pp. 229–252). London: Academic Press.

Papoušek, H. (1989). Coevolution of supportive counterparts in caretakers: A potential contribution to the hemispheric specialization during early infancy. *Cahiers de Psychologie Cognitive. European Bulletin of Cognitive Psychology, 9*, 113–117.

Papoušek, H., & Papoušek, M. (1978). Interdisciplinary parallels in studies of early human behavior: From physical to cognitive needs, from attachment to dyadic education. *International Journal of Behavioral Development, 1*, 37–49.

Papoušek, H., & Papoušek, M. (1979a). Early ontogeny of human social interaction: Its biological roots and social dimensions. In M. von Cranach, K. Foppa, W. Lepenies, & D. Ploog (Eds.), *Human ethology: Claims and limits of a new discipline* (pp. 456–478). Cambridge, UK: Cambridge University Press.

Papoušek, H., & Papoušek, M. (1979b). The infant's fundamental adaptive response system in social interaction. In E. B. Thoman (Ed.), *Origins of the infant's social responsiveness* (pp. 175–208). Hillsdale, NJ: Erlbaum.

Papoušek, H., & Papoušek, M. 1987. Intuitive parenting: A dialectic counterpart to the infant's integrative competence. In J. D. Osofsky (Ed.), *Handbook of infant development* (2nd ed., pp. 669–720). New York: Wiley.

Papoušek, H., & Papoušek, M. (1992a). Early integrative and communicative development: Pointers to humanity. In H. M. Emrich & M. Wiegand (Eds.), *Integrative biological psychiatry* (pp. 45–60). Berlin: Springer-Verlag.

Papoušek, H., & Papoušek, M. (1992b). Beyond emotional bonding: The role of preverbal communication in mental growth and health. *Infant Mental Health Journal, 13*, 43–53.

Papoušek, M. (1994). *Vom ersten Schreizum ersten Wort: Anfange der Sprachentwicklung in der vorsprachlichen Kommunikation.* Bern: Huber.

Papoušek, M., & Papoušek, H. (1981). Musical elements in the infant's vocalizations: Their significance for communication, cognition and creativity. In L. P. Lipsitt (Ed.), *Advances in infancy research* (Vol. 1, pp. 163–224). Norwood, NJ: Ablex.

Papoušek, M., Papoušek, H., & Bornstein, M. H. (1985). The naturalistic vocal environment of young infants: On the significance of homogeneity and variability in parental speech. In T. Field & N. Fox (Eds.), *Social perception in infants* (pp. 269–297). Norwood, NJ: Ablex.

Rheingold, H. L., & Adams, J. L. (1980). The significance of speech to newborns. *Developmental Psychology, 16*, 397–403.

Tsumori, A. (1967). Newly acquired behavior and social interactions of Japanese monkeys. In S. A. Altmann (Ed.), *Social communication among primates* (pp. 207–219). Chicago: University of Chicago Press.

van Lawick-Goodall, J. (1971). *In the shadow of man.* Boston: Houghton Mifflin.

CHAPTER 9

Hubert Montagner

The Ontogeny of the Baby's Interactions over the First Year

The attachment theory proposed by Bowlby (1958, 1960, 1969, 1973, 1980) strongly influenced the clinical and experimental studies performed in the 1970s and 1980s on the "nature" of the interactions that form the basis for and nourish affective links between babies and their mothers. The theory is predictive, and deterministic in some respects, and researchers increasingly tried to identify the indicators that reflect in children a few months or a few years old the establishment of a "secure" attachment to their mothers or, in contrast, difficulties of attachment. This is the case, for example, of the experimental work of Ainsworth (1973, 1974, 1979a, 1979b; Ainsworth & Bell, 1969; Ainsworth, Bell, & Slayton, 1971). Her procedure consists of seven 3-minute periods for the objective examination and quantification of the behavior of 1-year-old children in the presence of their mother (or father) and then with an unknown person who joins the parent. The parent then leaves and returns as the other person goes, and so on. Ainsworth makes a distinction here between three categories of children.

1. Those who have established a "secure" attachment to their mother and seek proximity, contact, or interaction at a distance according to the context. They do not display distress, anger, or avoidance when the mother leaves or returns.
2. Those who display avoidance, that is, who tend to ignore or avoid their mothers.
3. Those who are resistant, that is, whose behavior displays anger or rejection of their mothers, especially when they return, but who at the same time seek closeness and contact.

The reactions of the children in categories 2 and 3 are considered to be indicators of uncertain, nonsecure attachment to the mother. In spite of sometimes severe criticism (Lamb, Thompson, Gardner, Charnov, & Estes, 1984), Ainsworth had the considerable merit of having developed a methodological tool that enables researchers to validate, refute, and/or make progress in one of the most pertinent theories available for studying the development of children and developmental disabilities. This type of method enables the factual search for correlations, congruence, or agreement between what clinicians and researchers observe in a particular child at a particular age and what they observe in interactions between the same child and its mother (and other partners) during the first days and weeks. This can reveal the temporal continuities and discontinuities that give meaning to observations, to clinical analyses, and to the data provided by experimental research.

However, the procedure used by Ainsworth and other workers seeking temporal continuities and discontinuities in the development of young children can only be truly pertinent if it is based on precise assessment—as complete as possible—of the "initial" capabilities of the baby, that is, at birth (the abilities of the fetus are not discussed here). The most functional evaluation (which is also multifactorial) available is probably given by Brazelton's Neonatal Behavioral Assessment Scale (NBAS) (Als & Brazelton, 1975; Als, Lester, Tronick, & Brazelton, 1979, 1982; Als, Tronick, & Brazelton, 1977, 1981; Brazelton, 1973a, 1973b, 1979, 1981; Nugent, Lydic, & Burke, 1986; Pedro, 1988). The scale combines physiological, psychophysiological, and behavioral variables in infants. The NBAS enabled Brazelton, his colleagues, and many other clinicians and researchers to perform accurate studies of how a baby can use its capabilities in adjusted interaction with its mother according to the specific features of one or the other of the two people and in relation to cultural and ethnic influences. The scale is also used to analyze how specific difficulties may occur during early development of the child, especially when interactions with the mother appear to lack adjustment and attunement (in the sense used by Stern, 1985), and also to analyze the building up of interactions between babies "at risk" and their mothers, and between mothers "at risk" and their babies (Als & Brazelton, 1973, 1982; Als et al., 1979; Brazelton, Kolowski, & Main, 1974; Brazelton & Lester, 1983; Brazelton & Tronick, 1980; Brazelton, Tronick, Adamson, & Wise, 1975; Brazelton & Yogman, 1985; Brazelton, Yogman, Als, & Tronick, 1978; Nugent at al., 1986; Pedro et al., 1988; Tronick, 1982; Tronick, 1978; Tronick, Als, & Brazelton, 1977). In spite of the quality of the studies and concepts of Brazelton, Als, Tronick, Nugent, and Pedro and of many other clinicians and researchers, we still lack clinical and quantitative information on the continuities and discontinuities that may exist between the different features of a baby from one moment to the next in its development according to its special features and those of its mother (and more generally of its family). Further "longitudinal" studies are required for better identification of the moment(s) in development and the contexts, circumstances, mechanisms, and processes associated with various disturbances, difficulties, or dysfunctioning that may appear in young children according to whether they display certain skills and whether attachment to the mother is "secure" or "nonsecure." Better understanding is also needed of why and how disturbances, difficulties, or dysfunctioning decrease or disappear in babies who display signs of insecurity and somatic anomalies (including those of genetic origin) and behavioral and/or interactive anomalies—sometimes very marked in the early weeks.

Accumulation of clinical and fundamental research in these fields is indispensable for the scientific community to be able to propose to mothers, families, and society pertinent, operational, and non-guilt-making strategies to enable the emergence of children's skills that are hidden, buried, masked, or inhibited. With his or her skills recognized, every baby can then discover, consolidate, or restore the mechanisms and processes forming the basis of adjustment and attunement of interactions with its mother and its other partners. This will establish the conditions for affective, relational, and probably cognitive development without major difficulties even when early development is difficult.

☐ The Major Obstacles to Knowledge of Child Development and Its Problems

It is still necessary to collect as much data as possible on developmental processes in the young child, and especially on the phenomena that regulate the adjustment and attunement of interactions with the mother and the other people in its environment. Research can provide families and society an increasing body of reliable information in this field and thus modify their attitudes, decisions, and behavior so that every child can develop with all his or her potential and gain new skills. However, certain obstacles hinder or prevent progress in scientific and medical knowledge. It seems to me to be necessary to identify them in this book, which is devoted to future evolution of the family. I mention four obstacles that seem to be particularly important.

1. The difficulty of setting up longitudinal studies to monitor a child and family at regular intervals using controlled procedures under reproducible conditions.
2. The lack or inadequacy of interaction between clinicians and researchers engaged in fundamental work in order to clarify their concepts and theoretical frameworks and to combine or make compatible their respective methods.
3. The difficulty of defining indicators enabling an objective approach to the "quality" of the attachment between mother and child and then its changes as the weeks go by according to child developmental factors and the changes that take place in the mother and the family. These are often still too general or vague to be identified in the same way by different researchers and subjected to unequivocal qualitative analysis or quantitative study. In other cases they are divided into such an array of items that they cannot be of any functional value.
4. The still insufficient development of research and consideration of the human and physical environment that can bring out, consolidate, and enrich the skills of a young child in its family context and also outside it, thus changing positively the attitude, representation, and practices of the parents.

☐ Our Research

My colleagues and I have attempted to develop research that meets these requirements. Its backbone consists of a longitudinal study of several dozen children who were 3 to 5 days old at the start of the research. The approach combines child psychiatric and ethological methodology (i.e., observation of subjects during free activity and without limiting their motricity and without social taboos or conditioning). The children were filmed continuously during the study sessions and were monitored by a child psychiatrist and an ethologist on the double-blind principle (no exchange of information). Discussions with the mother (collection of clinical data) and the sessions filmed with the family (collection of ethological data) were held when the children were 1, 4, 8, 12, 18, and 24 months old. It is thus possible to perform interactive gathering of clinical data on the history, experience, images, and plans of the mother and of the family, the gathering of quantitative data on the child's behavior and skills, and the gathering of clinical and quantitative data on the interactions between child and mother (and the other persons in the family environment). Correlations, agreement, and congruence can then be sought between variables concerning the child and those concerning the mother (and the family) at each of these ages and from one age to another. Some of the variables may then stand out as pertinent indicators of processes of attachment, nonattachment, and difficulty in attachment (or detachment) between child and mother (and the other persons in the family). They may simultaneously accompany or herald developmental features, especially when it is possible to arrange comparative monitoring of risk babies and control babies, risk mothers and control mothers, and risk dyads and control dyads ("controls" should be understood as babies, mothers, and dyads with no objectively identifiable somatic, behavioral, or psychic disorders). This was performed during the longitudinal studies using low-weight, premature, and control babies. There was also a follow-up of babies with feeding difficulties and mothers with psychological and/or social difficulties.

The main line of research enabled us to identify some of the mechanisms or processes that play a significant role in the emergence and development of adjusted or nonadjusted interactions between baby and mother and, in parallel, in the phenomena of attachment, nonattachment, and difficulty in attachment (or "detachment") between the two persons (Montagner, 1993). However, this was not enough for understanding the "nature" and the features of the abilities (or skills) that the child can or should use as a resource to establish attachment to his or her mother and thus set up the basic conditions for the mother to become attached to the baby or not to become detached from the baby. In particular, this study alone did not reveal the basis or foundation enabling a baby to develop as an interactive, social and cognitive being over the days and months as he or she grows and through the range of influences to which he or she is subjected. Indeed, phenomena of masking, inhibition, defense, and/or time lag between the perceptual and cognitive capabilities of the baby and mother and the difficulties of functional adjustment between their respective repertoires (discussed later) may hinder or prevent the emergence and development of skills in the child. This led us to the idea that babies and young children should be studied in other interactive systems with partners other than the mother. This should paradoxically lead to a better understanding of their relational difficulties and their personal difficulties.

This is why we instigated research on the establishment and regulation of the behavior and interactions of young children with another child of the same age, that is, with another human being who a priori shares the same perceptual, tonico-postural, motor, emotional, and cognitive skills but with whom there is no shared experience, history, or imprinting. It shows that from the age of at least 4 or 5 months old, a child objectively possesses a varied range of capabilities that he or she does not display under other conditions and with other partners, including the mother. The skills "demonstrated" in this way appear to form the foundation of the child's emotional, interactive, social, perceptual, and cognitive development, especially with regard to maternal influence, even if these are not completely or clearly objectifiable during interaction with the mother. Their emergence or nondevelopment may be pertinent indicators of difficulties in development and the adaptation of the child from one age to another in different environments.

☐ From Research to Practical Proposals That Can Enhance Child Development and Family Life at the Same Time

I discuss first the five core skills revealed by our experimental studies on interactions between children 4 to 7 months old and children of the same age. This is followed by a description of the complex behavior shown in the "normal" child in a group of peers and whose creation and regulation seem to take place—throughout the first 3 years at least, around and from the five core skills. Comparative study of children with various developmental problems, and especially autists and children suffering from cerebral palsy, did not reveal either the five core skills of the first year or behavior seeming to become organized around and from these skills in the second year. I then discuss the contribution of the results to the analysis of interactions between a baby and its mother, especially when these are related or correlated with difficulties, disturbance, or dysfunctioning of development of the child. They lead to proposing strategies and organization of space for the various living areas of a child, and not only the family environment, so that everybody can acquire and develop all its possibilities and skills and so that in parallel the family can recognize them completely in a context of positive interaction. I feel that families and society will develop with this prospect of early "opening up" of the child to the world outside the family and of the creation of new settings and new living areas designed to enhance perceptual, motor, interactive, and cognitive emergences, which is not always possible in the family "niche" alone.

☐ The Core Skills That Appear to Emerge from Study of Interactions Between a 4- to 7-Month-Old Child and a Peer

Description of the Study

Interaction between a child 4 to 7 months old and a child of the same age was studied in an experimental situation making it possible to "free" them from the constraints related to tonico-postural immaturity. Their mothers dressed each in a jacket that contained their body masses, and they were then installed in a specially designed seat that kept them in a stable, unwavering sitting position in which their heads did not oscillate. Two straps attached to the clothing and linked to the back of the seat by a buckle prevented them from falling forward or sideways. The two seats were mounted on a system of rails and rack bar and could be approached, withdrawn, and angled in relation to each other and in relation to the mothers according to a procedure consisting of eight 3-minute phases (Montagner, 1993; Montagner et al., 1993a, 1993b, 1994). Remote operation was from a control console.

The aim of the study was to verify the hypothesis that young children placed under conditions that "compensate" their tonico-postural immaturity reveal motor, interactive, and cognitive capacities that are not observed when they are in an unstable sitting position and when they cannot themselves regulate the position of their head. The hypothesis is based on the work of Grenier (1981) and on our observations over a 6-

year period during our longitudinal studies. Grenier showed that when 2-week-old to 2-month-old babies are seated on the edge of a bench with the pediatrician holding their head with one hand and supporting the abdomen with the other, they display "liberated" motor capability and an enhanced capacity to hold their observation and scan with their eyes in comparison with other situations. We have regularly observed in our own studies that when children display substantial difference in timing (from the mean) in the emergence of regulation enabling unwavering carriage of the head, passage from a position on the stomach to a position on the back (and vice versa), and a fairly stable sitting position without help, they also display considerable difference in the development of gestures, especially in grasping objects, and in their interactive and social behavior. There appear to be functional and ontogenetic correlations between these different processes.

As the same child–child dyads were filmed continuously under the same conditions for four sessions, each lasting 30 minutes at weekly intervals (study of one dyad thus lasted for a month), the research produced new data, the most significant of which can be summarized as follows (for more details, cf. Montagner et al., 1993a, 1993b, 1994).

1. The frequency and duration of directions of gaze are significantly greater when the target is the face, hands, eyes, or feet of the partner child rather than any other target, including the spatial sector in which the mother remains continuously.
2. They can diversify and adjust their gestures in relation to the partner child. They can extend their arms, not only with pronation (lateral or oblique) but also in supination position; they can rotate their hand from pronation to supination position and can also grasp and shake the hand of the other child and develop structured manual interactions.
3. They can reproduce the movements and utterances of the other child.
4. They display sometimes considerable modifications in behavior and utterances between the first and second sessions or between the second and third sessions. This includes very significantly increased frequency of gestures with arm outstretched in the direction of the other child and pronation or supination. The same applies to the frequency of manual contacts (especially those continuing with the taking of the partner child's hand) and utterances. The duration of movements of the torso toward the other child increases, and they display items not seen in the preceding session. Familiarization with the partner and the experimental situation is thus accompanied by various modifications not only in the frequency and/or duration of certain items but also in their behavioral and vocal "repertoire." Qualitative and quantitative analysis of the behavior and interactions of 30 children led to suggesting that the capabilities displayed in this dyad situation are based on five core skills that cannot fail to be observed during the first year if there are no developmental anomalies (we do not prejudge the role of genetic factors and programming in the emergence or nonemergence of these core skills; we consider them overall as anthropological universals, which obviously remains to be verified).

The Core Skills

Capacity for Sustained Visual Attention.   Numerous clinical and experimental studies show the early emergence and the importance of the eye-to-eye contact and interaction in attachment phenomena between mother and baby. However, none seem to have stressed the more or less sustained character of the visual attention that the child pays to its mother and its other partners in the building up of its interactive and cognitive systems. In addition, there is no well-established information on the differences that may exist during their development between young children who appear able to fix their gaze onto a target—especially a person—and others who avoid eye contact with their partner(s). Our research on interactions between two children kept in a stable sitting position in experimental seats shows that from 4 to 5 months onward they are capable of developing both considerable mobility of directed vision and uninterrupted, long-duration visual targeting (sometimes for longer than one or two minutes) of the partner child. The body areas most frequently and longest drawn by their gaze are those that play a major role in the expression of human emotions: the face, eyes, and hands. The hypothesis can be put forward that the early emergence and development of sustained visual attention capability during the early months are essential for the emergence, development, and regulation of the child's emotional systems by enabling it to perceive (i.e., receive, memorize, and compare current and engrammed information) its partner's emotions, test the reactions that it induces according to its own emotions, and adjust its responses to those of the partner. The more it is capable of sustained mobilization of its visual attention capacities in the direction of a partner who possesses approximately the same skills as itself, the more it is likely to give a meaning to what the other perceives, does, and "thinks." It can thus develop, refine, and adjust in an integrated manner the emotional and cognitive components of its relations with another person without the processes being slowed or inhibited by shared history (as can be the case in relations between mother and child). However, the visual scanning of the face of the other child and/or the avoidance of its gaze does not enable a child to decode the changes in look, mimicry, attitudes, and gestures of its partner and hence give them a meaning and adjust to them (and to attune to them in the meaning given by Stern, 1985). Later in this chapter, we examine what light this can shed on difficulties of attachment between babies and mothers and on questions of developmental difficulties in children.

"Hunger" for Interaction.   In our experimental conditions, children display very marked élan for interaction when they are in an interaction situation (they lean forward; they switch their gaze toward the partner as soon as the latter changes its behavior or its utterances; they approach their hands to make contact; they touch their partner or take its hand when they are mechanically able to do so; they make modulated utterances in its direction, especially when it turns its head). Neither of them holds an object (except in the final phase of the procedure), and nothing leads to thinking that their behavior is part of a cognitive strategy for taking an object held by the partner or for "dominating" this partner. Each child seems to behave as if it sought to approach and contact the other child, that is, to display attachment behavior (in the meaning used by Bowlby). The hypothesis can thus be put forward that the child hungers for interaction with its peers, at least when it can understand their "register," and provokes adjusted or nonexclusive reactions that are independent of any genetic or historical affiliation. The concept of interaction does not thus seem to only (or exclusively) depend on the initiation of relations between the baby and its mother or any other person with whom it has a "historical" attachment. It may also show movement toward any living being whose initiatives and responses are based on the same system of signs. In other words, there may be search and mutual recognition of signs that enable communication and not only the consequence or effects of early interactions and of attachment or of the affective relationship with the mother. This movement might not be specific in the sense of being reserved for human beings. It may be observed in a child in the presence of a pet cat or dog, even if it takes other forms and is regulated differently. As a result, the hypothesis that one of the bases of the development of children is the emergence of a core skill that stimulates interaction, whatever the "category" of the partners, leads to a fresh view of the initiation, dynamics, and regulation of ontogenic processes. In particular, it puts into perspective the determinist aspect of the theory of attachment and of psychoanalytical theory, even if attachment and the sexualized affective relation between baby and mother play an incontestable role in the emotional, relational, social, and probably the cognitive development of the child. It makes it possible to complete the clinician's assessment scales through observation of children at risk or in difficulty during interactions and relations with various partners, and not only the mother and close family.

Affiliative Behavior. Affiliative behavior refers to any behavior and any combination of behaviors and utterances that appear to result from empathy with the behavior and utterances of the partner and to any link between behaviors and combinations of behavior and utterances resulting from each other (created mutually) in the two children. These are socially positive behaviors that do not lead to self-centered behavior or the avoidance or refusal of interaction or crying or reactions which could be interpreted as distress or insecurity patterns. The behavior consists of smiles, nonfugacious eye-to-eye contact, modulated utterances (that are neither moans nor grunts), advance of the torso toward the partner accompanied or followed by extension of the arm and hand in the same direction, hand contacts between the two children, hand sliding, and mutual grasping. There is a strong probability (threshold $< .01$) that these types of behaviors and vocalizations bring responses of the same kind which may be simultaneous or synchronous. Self-centered behavior, refusal, and avoidance (the child turns its head away from its partner and keeps it turned away) are different, as is behavior that can be interpreted as related to insecurity or distress (the mimicry that generally precedes crying, erratic agitation of hands and/or feet accompanied by moans or grunts, or crying), nonresponse to the behavior of the other (the child's gaze remains fixed and turned away from the partner's face and the body is motionless) and behavior that can be interpreted as aggressive (gripping, pinching or striking the other's hand, or causing moaning or crying).

Affiliative behavior forms over 80% of the objectifiable behavioral and vocal "repertoire" of the children in an interaction situation with a peer in the experimental seats (less than 10% of the 35% of directing of gaze in a direction other than that of the partner child was directed at the mother). In contrast, self-centered behavior totaled less than 3% of all behavior observed; directing of gaze toward their body (they look at their hands, feet, or their jacket) also totaled less than 3% of orientation or reorientation of gaze in various sectors of space. Very few instances of avoidance or refusal to interact were observed (such occurrences are not quantifiable in our study—at least for statistical analysis—as they were too rare and too brief). Very little behavior that can be interpreted as related to insecurity, distress, or nonresponse to the signs of the partner was observed. In addition, we never observed the pushing away of the partner child's hand or behavior that could be interpreted as being aggressive.

In the second session, when children and mothers met for the second time 1 week later, the frequency and duration of most of the affiliative behavior of the children were two to five times greater (Montagner et al., unpublished observations). This was the case for smiles, nonfugacious directing of gaze, forward movement of the torso accompanied or followed by extension of the arm and hand in pronation or supination position, contacts, and finding or grasping of the hands of the two children. The children thus chose to reduce the distance and establish contact between them, that is, to develop attachment behavior, as defined by Bowlby. In addition, each child displayed at the second or third session—varying according to the child—behaviors, utterances, or combinations of physical behavior and utterances not observed during the first session. Most of the "new patterns" were displayed by the partner in the first session. Children at least 4 or 5 months old thus showed themselves able to add to their repertoire the behavior and utterances of a child of the same age, with whom they have developed familiarity in the previous week, or to reveal the same features that were hitherto hidden, buried, masked, or inhibited—in any case not expressed—before they met a partner of the same age who could bring out the behaviors and give them a meaning.

Affiliative behaviors thus seem to be both indicators of the so-called normal development of a child and the core or foundation of its affective, interactive, social, and cognitive constructs.

Other forms of affiliative behavior emerge during the second half of the first year and during the second year: offering, postural and manual requests, finger pointing, exchange of objects, and mutual aid (Montagner, 1988, 1993; Montagner et al., 1988a, 1988b, 1993a, 1993b). These are also indicators and cores of child ontogenetic processes.

Targeted Organization of Gestures.   Under the conditions of our research, children 4 to 5 months old are capable of accurate, adjusted arm and hand movements in the direction of the partner's hand. They can then rotate their hand from pronation to supination position without resting the forearm on the arm of the seat. They thus show that they already control the gestures forming the basis of prehension or grasping and also manual request movements (extension of the arm with the hand in pronation position not attaining the object or without grasping it), offering, and pointing that are observed at the end of the first year or the beginning of the second.

They thus reveal not only well-structured motor abilities and coordination, but also core patterns forming the framework of more elaborate behaviors required for handling objects and for the development of social and cognitive processes. We have called these *behavioral organizers* (Montagner, 1988; Montagner et al., 1988a, 1988b).

Imitative Behavior.   The two 4- to 5-month-old children can already reproduce not only the form but also the rhythm of each other's gestures and utterances. They can follow imitation of an act or a succession of acts—for example, rhythmic beating of the feet on the lower part of their seats or scratching their jackets—to the imitation of an utterance or vice versa. However, their behavior is flexible; the imitator can continue with other behaviors or utterances and in turn induce imitation of its acts by the other child, in a different register and at a different rhythm.

Children 4 to 5 months old thus appear to be capable of imitating a partner of the same age even if, with the exception of tongue pulling, they do not imitate adults, including their mothers, perhaps because their behavioral movements, utterances, and language are too complex; they can also bring adults to imitate their behavior and utterances. These skills seem to be cores for the adjustment of the emotional states of the two partners who have approximately the same capacity for decoding emotions.

☐ The Complex Behaviors that Appear to Become Established During the First 3 Years on the Basis of the Core Skills of the First Year

Fitting a setting in which a peer group of children can use the third dimension of space without limiting the scope of their locomotion and interactions and without taboos enables comparison and monitoring at regular intervals of the behaviors of children with no objectifiable deficiency or anomaly (so-called normal children taken by two day-care centers) and children with various behavioral or developmental difficulties, such as those attending a medical nursery, or autistic children and children suffering from cerebral palsy (Montagner, 1993; Montagner et al., 1993a, 1993b, 1994).

Groups of six children were filmed continuously during free activity in 30-minute sessions once a week or once a fortnight according to the procedure chosen. The same children were monitored for 1 or 2 years. Two staff members were present at all times. The instructions were that there should be no intervention except when a child was in difficulty. The films were analyzed either on a 1-second or a $^1/_{10}$-second time step according to the objectives.

As the results have been reported elsewhere (Montagner, 1993; Montagner et al., 1993a, 1993b, 1994) or are in press, some of the main conclusions can be summarized here.

Children from the Day-Care Centers

Filmed from the age at which they acquired locomotor autonomy by reptation (creeping) or crawling on all fours (between the ages of 7 and 9 months), the children displayed greater precocity and greater complexity in motor skills than previously reported in scientific publications and indicated on developmental scales. For example, half of the children succeeded in climbing the whole of a spiral staircase at the age of 13 months and all succeeded at 17 months.

At the age of 12 or 13 months, some of the children displayed a varied range of already complex social behaviors, for example, repeated multimodal interaction (consisting of series of gazes directed at a partner, smiles, mimicry, gestures, touching and utterances; the partition with holes of various shapes and sizes and with a "porthole" was a preferred site for these interactions), imitation, and behavior involving cooperation and anticipation of the movement and behavior of the partner in the interaction. However, the frequency of these affiliative behaviors increased considerably from 13 to 17 months (at 17 months, it was 2.5 times higher than at 13 months for multimodal interactions, 5 times higher for imitations, and 6 times higher for cooperation) or fluctuated at relatively high levels (anticipation behavior). At the same time, the frequency of "elementary" social behaviors (offering, requests, pointing) increased and aggressive behavior was still infrequent. These simultaneous changes coincided with the emergence of new motor skills and the dominant use of the standing position during climbing and descending vertical structures.

In a more general manner, the moments in development characterized by the emergence or significant reorganization of motor skills were also marked by the emergence, increased predominance, and/or accelerated development of one or other or all of the affiliative behaviors identified. It was as if in the first 2 years of life there are functional and ontogenic links between the emergence and mastery of new motor skills and those of new affiliative behaviors.

The 17 children monitored regularly and whose behaviors were quantified for at least 1 year all displayed patterns that appear to form the five core skills defined earlier:

1. They were all capable of sustained visual attention. This was particularly clear during the multimodal interactions that developed on either side of the pierced wall. Such interaction often lasted more than 10 seconds and could exceed a minute, especially when interactions between the partners followed each other without interruption.
2. They sought interaction with one or other of their peers at all times, sometimes with periods of requests to the two attendants or periods of "refuge" with them. Periods of isolation from their peers were infrequent and short, except on days when they were crying when they arrived at the experimental installation. The frequency and duration of their interactions did not decrease significantly from the start to the end of the observation sessions, although fluctuations were observed. It was as if the children had a sustained desire for interaction.
3. Although the frequency and duration of self-centered behavior, crying, behavior that appeared to indicate fear and aggressive acts were slight, the frequency and duration of affiliative acts were almost always at high levels throughout the latter part of the first year and then throughout the second and third years. These behaviors continued from the age of 20 to 24 months, varying according to the child, by mutual aid behavior, symbolic activities, and role games, during or at the end of which isolation, crying, fear, and aggression were rarely observed.
4. The children developed all the gestures and manual activities adapted to their target, especially in relation to the face, hand, or another part of the body of the partner with whom they interacted through the pierced wall. As we have reported, the controlled, targeted extension of the arm appears to organize various behaviors displayed toward objects and persons. It formed in particular the "framework" of many types of behavior in exchanges during the second year.
5. They displayed increasing imitation of the acts, movements, and utterances of their peers in all sectors of the space. Imitations were increasingly alternated, with each partner imitated after imitating. Reciprocal imitation developed.

Children Displaying Behavioral or Developmental Disturbances

Although quantification has not yet been completed for the children from the medical nursery, the autists and children suffering from cerebral palsy monitored under the same conditions and with the same procedure as those from the day-care centers, the data show that:

1. Most (and all the autistic children) have varyingly marked deficiencies in visual attention capacity (not catching or avoiding the "partner's" gaze; visual scanning of the partner's face without stopping; fleeting glances at the partner and especially its face; rapid fluctuations of gaze from one target to another, especially when the target is a face).

2. Most did not display desire for interaction. They did not seek sustained, repeated interaction with one or other of their peers; they avoided looks or faces and moved aside or went away at the approach of or contact with another child; they did not respond to the behavior, utterances, and speech of the others; they froze and remained unsmiling and expressionless in a face-to-face position; they kept apart from their peers and did not attempt to participate in their activities; they remained alone and adopted closed body position, sometimes in the sites of activity of the others (e.g., one of the children curled up in a site generally used for play); they made circular, to-and-fro or hairpin movements, as if they were trying to avoid the others.

3. The dominant behaviors were self-centered behavior: acts revealing fear, starts or aggression (self-aggression or aggression toward others), and in some children combinations or sequences of these patterns. In contrast, affiliative behaviors were rare or infrequent and sometimes not observed at all (as in some autists). This was the case for smiles, offering, manual and postural requests, and pointing. Cooperation, repetitive interactions, and anticipation behavior did not occur, with rare exceptions (quantification in progress).

4. In children less than 1 year old, arm and hand movement is of the enveloping type. The arm and hand generally remain against the body when an object is offered to the child. It is grasped "weakly" (the fingers do not close around the object or it is not well grasped or supported) and dropped. No frontal, adjusted, well-targeted extension of arm and hand is observed (reaching behavior) leading to taking the object (grasping behavior) and then handling it or presenting it to another child. In older children, deficiencies remain in control of grasping, prehension, and handling of objects and exchange with others; grasping is still "weak" and the object is soon dropped or abandoned; prehension is inaccurate and tentative, proceeds in fits and starts, and is accompanied or followed by falls; the object is held with full palm contact and not with the tips of the fingers, and drawing and writing cannot be mastered; the object is more often dropped or thrown than offered to a partner child. In autists and children with severe developmental difficulties, the failure to master or the tentative beginnings of the reaching–grasping sequence are frequently accompanied by acts without meaning or apparent function (irrelevant acts and acts without detectable function) and/or stereotypes ("puppet movements," swinging arms, glider movement, etc.). It was as if the nonmastery of structured, organized targeting of reaching with arm and hand, that is, the failure to emerge and to develop a fundamental organizer of handling and social behaviors, is accompanied by the nonstructuring or parasitizing of the whole of gestural activity. Stereotype behavior might thus be the "product" of absence of functional and ontogenic structuring of the "initial" gestures that organize and regulate interactions with objects and persons, against a background of other difficulties.

5. Most of the children who display behavioral and/or developmental disturbances do not perform either gestural, vocal or verbal imitation behavior. They would appear to not have or no longer have the capacity to reproduce actions by one or more partners and hence to not or no longer be able to display their links with the emotions, intentions, or plans of others.

One might wonder whether this "deficiency" is related to or correlated with a "deficiency" in perceptual abilities, such as in the ability to compare the data received during interaction with itself and with stored (memorized) data, in cognitive abilities (more or less linked with perceptual abilities) recognizing and giving a meaning to information in interactive abilities, in decision-making abilities, or in the ability to prepare for action and for the reproduction of the actions of another person.

In practically all cases, the children in difficulty displayed substantial deficiencies, anomalies, and/or age lags in the five core skills. The genesis of these deficiencies, anomalies, and lags would appear to be based on functional and also ontogenetic (interactive at any moment and from one moment to the next during development) links between these skills. This is suggested in particular by observation of children 1 to 3 years old.

However, the monitoring of children with behavioral and developmental disturbances, especially autists and children suffering from cerebral palsy, shows that under specific human and spatial conditions (Montagner et al., unpublished observations), they may at one time or another reveal more or less sustained visual attention skills, élan for interaction, affiliative behavior, targeted organization of gestures, and imitative behavior that had hitherto been hidden, buried, masked, or inhibited. This leads to proposing that, subject to full analysis of the data, one of the objectives of fundamental and clinical research on developmental difficulties and pathologies should be the design of living areas in which there is a strong probability of the emergence and development of the core skills that appear to be the foundation for the regulation and the future of emotional, affective, interactive, relational, social, and cognitive systems in children.

One should also examine the genesis of nonemergence, degradation, and disappearance of patterns, functional "deviations," "substitution" processes, resistance, and inhibitions that may be related to or correlated with the nondifferentiation of the child's core skills. Are there predominant factors inherent in the child itself? (What would be the result of genetic factors, in particular?) How, at what moment(s) in development, and in what contexts could phenomena of maladjustment, nonattunement (Stern, 1985, 1989), "unadjustment," "unattunement," nonsynchronization, desynchronization, or "mutual defense, resistance or avoidance" between mother and baby induce or facilitate nondifferentiation of the core skills in a child?

☐ "Nondifferentiation" of Core Skills During the First Year Could Be a Pertinent Indicator of Developmental Difficulties in a Child, Especially with Regard to Interactions with its Family

Our longitudinal studies on babies that are premature, of low weight, display feeding difficulties, or have a mother or a family considered as bearing or generating risks (in comparison with control babies) led me to the following statements and suggestions in relation to the core skills that appear to emerge from research on children a few months old studied in pairs in experimental seats or in peer groups with freedom of activity.

The Capacity for Sustained Visual Attention

When interactive and relational difficulties are observed and then identified between a mother and her child either from clinical approaches by the pediatrician and the child psychiatrist or from observations by nursery nurses and researchers monitoring the child's development and when they are still observed several months later, especially between 8 months and 12 months, there is a strong probability that the following features will be observed:

1. Failure of the baby's gaze to catch the mother's (and frequently vice versa on a reciprocal basis). This is particularly marked in the 4- to 6-month stage.
2. The nondirecting of the baby's gaze by the mother's gaze. Here again, the 4- to 6-month age range is particularly revealing.
3. Avoidance by the baby's gaze of the mother's gaze and more generally of her face. The 4- to 6-month age range should be noted here again.
4. The fleetingness of the baby's visual attention, especially when it is face to face with its mother. However, in some cases the same baby seems to be able to develop sustained visual attention toward the face of an unknown person, as if it had found the occasion to reveal a skill that it could not or would not display to a mother with whom it had a painful past and thus protected itself against the pain of the person with whom it had its initial attachment. It is therefore possible that the baby might have the ability to withdraw for a few weeks or months from difficulties of adjustment and attunement in interactions with its mother, on condition that it can bring out and develop its visual attention capacities with other people. However, persistent nonengagement of the mother's gaze (and also that of other people), refusal to allow gaze to be directed, avoidance of the gaze of others, and fugacious visual attention during the second year appear to slow or prevent the development of sustained visual attention capacity, whoever the partner in the interaction.

Hunger for Interaction

Babies in difficulty, or whose mothers are in difficulty, also display deficiency in their élan for interaction. This results in:

- Frequent, persistent turning of the baby's head away from its mother's face. This is particularly marked during bottle feeding or in the face-to-face position after breast or bottle feeding during the first 6 months; the baby turns its head away or lowers it and maintains this position.
- Absence or low capacity for facial expression (the baby's face looks sad and "frozen") and especially the absence or deformation (grimace) of its smile.
- No exploration of the mother's face by the baby's hand.
- Absence or strangeness (to the ear) of modulated utterances. Whining, grunts, and crying are dominant.
- No requests to be taken in its mother's arms (arms reaching out to the mother), especially at waking, during the second half of the first year.
- Absence of response or uncertain response of the baby to its mother's gaze, smile, gestures, touches, utterances, and speech.
- Tendency for "fatigue at interaction"; after responding to its mother with a certain

pattern, for example by smiles and speech just after waking, the child appears to lose interest in interaction and simultaneously displays tonico-postural and motor fatigue (discussed later).

Affiliative Behaviors

Affiliative behaviors are rare, infrequent, or nonexistent, or are "replaced" by other behaviors in these babies (this is observed in particular in babies 4 to 12 months old):

- They do not have the "magnetized" or brilliant gaze of babies who have established or are establishing a strong, secure attachment to their mothers.
- They do not smile, as already mentioned.
- They do not wave legs and arms (described as "pedaling") when stimulated by smiles, mimicry, gestures, touches, utterances, or words, especially from their mother.
- They do not offer and exchange objects.
- They do not develop pointing in face-to-face situations.
- Self-centered behaviors are frequent and sustained.
- Crying and whimpering are more frequent than speech.
- They are considered to be difficult to quiet.
- They start when their mother or another person brings their head, and sometimes their hand, close to their face when they are in a sitting position.
- They put their hands to their ears when they are lifted, as if to protect themselves from external solicitation.
- They bring their hands forward in a gesture of protection or defense in contact with their mother's face when she embraces them suddenly or overwhelmingly and then seem to push her away and hide their face in their own hands.
- They often scratch and bite.
- They may scratch, pinch, or bite their partner.

Targeted Organization of Gestures

The babies that appear to have the most difficulties between 4 and 6 months (they avoid their mother's gaze and that of other people, their gaze lacks mobility and seems "empty"; the absence or rarity of their mimicry gives the impression that they are sad and closed; they do not respond to solicitation with a gaze, smiles, utterances, or speech; they display tonico-postural deficiency to the extent that the head lowers as soon as they are taken in the arms of their mother or another person) do not move a hand frontally toward an object brought within their range of vision. They drop objects put into contact with the palm of their hand. They have not developed frontal, adjusted, targeted reaching with arm and hand at 12 months; this is the usual framework for most cases of grasping of an object by children with no deficiency or lag in their developmental process at this age. In the second year, some display grasping actions but with enveloping, fumbling, hesitant and sometimes erratic and almost always clumsy gestures. They display an increasing tendency to fatigue the longer they are awake; the frequency and duration of directing of their gaze toward the objects brought within their field of vision decrease and may become nonexistent; and the same applies to adjusted, targeted reaching with arm and hand and then the grasping and keeping of an object.

When difficulties are slighter, for example, when the catching of gaze between a mother and a 4- to 6-month-old baby is fleeting but without active avoidance of the mother's gaze by the baby, when the baby's face is not very expressive but does not give an impression of profound sadness, when response capacities are little developed and only observed in certain contexts (just after waking, during and just after feeding), and when the baby seems easily tired after bottle feeding (it falls on its side after being installed in a sitting position), it also displays hesitant enveloping, fumbling, and sometimes erratic or mere sketches of gestures when an object is presented. The baby often drops the object a few seconds after grasping or palm contact. The fingers are often folded and the fists closed before and after taking the object. At 10 to 12 months old, depending on the case, these children still display more or less marked deficiencies in the dynamics and effectiveness of their gestures. In addition, they cannot yet control their sitting position, do not bear on their legs when they are placed upright, cannot cease to bear on their arms when they are placed on their front, and cannot reach toward an object presented in front of them when they are lying on their front with their arms folded beneath them. They are easily tired and display deficiencies in the other core skills, especially when their mother is the partner. In parallel, the mothers display dwindling visual attention capacity toward children of this age, increasingly weak, less durable and less marked interaction movements, less frequent affiliative behavior, and little imitation, whereas when the child was 6 months old these features were comparable to those in mothers whose babies displayed no particular difficulty or risk factor.

It was as if the nonelaboration or difficulty of organization of the frontal, targeted arm and hand reaching during the grasping of objects were correlated with the nonemergence or deficiencies in the other core skills identified. These features are all the more marked and persistent at the end of the first year and during the first half of the second year if the child displays marked, durable tonico-postural deficiency "preventing" it from sitting up without aid and then from remaining vertical in standing position. There seem to be functional and ontogenetic relations between these systems, although it is not yet possible to unravel the processes inherent in the child and those related to the nature of the interactions and attachment between the child and its mother, with regard in particular to the mother's psychic life and family difficulties.

Imitation Behavior

Although children with no deficiencies, disturbances, or lags in development display an increasing amount of imitative behaviors of all kinds when they are 6 to 12 months old, and especially in relation to their mothers, this is not the case in those who appear to be in difficulty or whose mother is in difficulty. Indeed, the latter do not seem able to or "do not want" to reproduce the behavior and speech of their partners. They also have deficiencies in other core skills.

☐ Proposals for Strategies to Help Mother and Family to Recognize Core Skills in Young Children and to Thus Enhance Their Development, Based on the Example of Two Children Monitored During the First Two Years of Their Lives

Two Examples

A Boy with Lags and Deficiencies in his Tonico-Postural Systems.   Born with a body weight of 1.250 kg (a low-weight child), the boy displayed no clearly objectifiable deficiency or lag during sessions filmed on day 3 and after 1 month. However, when he was 6 months old, his head flopped when a person took him in his or her arms in a face-to-face position. He did not adopt the "glider" position and his body sagged when he was held at arm's length. He did not roll over from back to stomach and his fists were generally clenched in all situations. When placed in a sitting position, he rolled on the side or the back without any counterbalancing reaction using the hand of the adult supporting him. At 12 months, he still did not remain in a sitting position through his own efforts and did not roll over from stomach to back and vice versa. When placed on the front, resting on his arms, he only changed position by collapsing, with his head striking the underlying surface unless he was held. He did not remain on his legs, which bent as soon as his feet touched the floor. Simultaneously, his head fell forward and his body slumped.

At 4 and 12 months and between these ages, the child displayed deficiencies in the five core skills as follows:

1. Development of visual attention capacity was poor. Gaze holding was fugacious, whether his partner was his mother or another person. Failure to hold his mother's gaze and fugacity of direction of his gaze toward various partners became increasingly marked and frequent as the waking period progressed.
2. Except during the moments following waking, his face was inexpressive and unsmiling. He seemed sad and "closed" and unenthusiastic about interaction with his mother.
3. He did not offer things or make manual or postural requests. More generally, he did not display affiliative behavior with the exception of smiles and laughs only after waking. He displayed a high frequency of self-centered behavior and acts of fear and starts.
4. His gestures were clumsy at all ages. When on his stomach at 12 months, he never displayed adjusted frontal reaching of arm and hand toward an object placed in his field of vision.
5. He did not imitate any of his partners: mother, father, sister, or researcher.

The mother displayed a very strong capacity for attention to the face and look of the child until he was 6 months old. She displayed a strong desire for interaction. She smiled frequently and emitted much speech for her baby. She also caressed him frequently and was always ready for interaction. She often presented objects to the child or placed them in contact with the palm of his hand. Finally, she mimed mouth open-ing, swallowing, and the child's mimicry during feeding. These behaviors, related to the five core skills, gradually decreased in frequency and duration from 6 months on-ward. Some were no longer observed at 12 months, as if the mother had given up communicating with the child or inducing responses to enhance their reciprocal at-tachment. She devoted herself essentially to meeting the overall requirements of the child (food, hygiene, sleep, medical care). The child accumulated tonico-postural, mo-tor, interactive, and cognitive disturbances throughout his second year. He walked at 25 months without yet speaking a single clear word (he nevertheless speaks, but not very audibly and with a third person).

This example shows that the difficulties of attachment and tenderness of a mother toward her child in the first year may be related not "simply" or "only" to a lack of maternal tenderness and love for the child, but also with infantile behavior that does not meet (or no longer meets in other cases) the mother's expectations. It was seen that the child's first year was marked by nonemergence, deficiencies, and lacks (inter-preted by the family as late development) in the five core skills. In parallel, and insofar as the mother did not find the development of the child to be a secure experience (in comparison in particular with children of the same age and especially in comparison with her experience of the child's elder sister), she sought her baby's gaze less and less, smiled at him less frequently, looked at him in a worried manner, solicited him more rarely and for shorter periods of time, and reduced the frequency and duration of all the speech behavior and utterances addressed to the child.

The monitoring of 35 other children showed that when a mother undertakes an attachment process during the first days and weeks and in which she is active and reassuring, she can progressively reduce her attempts to adjust and attune her child to her bodily, vocal, and speech behaviors if the evolution of the child in time does not correspond to her expectations. In parallel, the mother seems increasingly insecure and worried. It is seen in this type of evolution that the child's core skills are only clearly or fully identifiable in certain contexts (mainly when he has just woken up and when he is in an interaction situation with a person other than his mother). As a result, the child's core skills cannot develop in a fully functional manner and form the daily basis for a "secure" attachment of such children to their mothers. This can result in the establishment and aggravation in some mothers and families of affective withdrawal processes from a baby that does not meet their expectations of the moment or their initial attachment. Certain forms of detachment, rejection, and/or mistreatment ("cup-board children," child beating) may develop in this way.

The Hypertonic Boy Who "Did Not Look At" His Mother. Born at 9 months after a normal pregnancy and weighing 3 kg, this child displayed neither any defi-ciency nor objectifiable lag at 3 days old. In regular contact with a doctor from the mother and child care administration ("Protection Maternelle et Infantile") and a child psychiatrist, his 19-year-old mother displayed considerable psychological and social vulnerability. Unmarried, unemployed, and with no family, she had been in a children's home during preadolescence and adolescence and had had an abortion 2 years previ-ously.

At 4 to 7 months, the child appeared to be hypertonic (held at arms' length, he stiffened, extended his arms and legs, and displayed good control of head posture). He displayed deficiencies in four out of five core skills but only during interaction with his mother:

1. He actively avoided his mother's gaze (he turned his head or eyes away and kept them away in spite of caresses, generous kisses, and much talking from his mother), whereas he accepted and enhanced eye contact with other persons present by means of smiles and insistent gaze (especially a girlfriend of his mother and a researcher whom he had never met before).
2. He showed no desire for interaction with the mother (no smiles, mimicry, utterances, gestures toward her face, or touches). He even displayed rejection when she came close to his face to kiss him. In contrast, he displayed all the usual patterns of desire for interaction in situations with other people.
3. He did not develop any affiliative behavior with his mother but stressed self-centered behavior and acts of retreat (he held his face in two hands on several occasions at 4 months). His face was sad, closed, and scratched (self-inflicted scratches). In contrast, he smiled, produced speech, and explored the face of a partner when this was another person.
4. At 7 months, no imitation of his mother's behavior or speech was noted, except with the telephone, which the child put to his ear after seeing his mother do this. However, he developed a number of imitations of the nursery nurses and of other children at the children's home where his mother left him for 3 or 4 days a week.

Only the "targeted organization of gesture" core skill was well developed in all contexts when the child grasped objects. However, offering, solicitation, finger pointing, and exploration of the body of a partner were observed at the children's home but not at the mother's home.

The child seemed to protect or defend himself from interactions with his mother, or reserved his skills for persons other than his mother. Mistreatment by a massively affectionate mother could be feared (she caressed, embraced, and spoke to the child very much when interacting with him); she displayed disappointment ("He's sulking") when she observed that his behavior was very different with other people.

However, considerable changes modified mother–child relations from 9 to 12 months. At 12 months, the child "agreed" to use all his skills as resources in adjusted (and apparently attuned in the sense used by Stern, 1985) interactions with his mother and no longer only with other people. The mother herself seemed adjusted and attuned in her interactions with the child. She had "discovered" an essential key to interaction and communication: She sought the gaze of the child and waited for his action before modifying her behavioral, vocal, and language register. In other words, she had discovered the importance of interactive loops (me to you and back to me, you to me and back to you). She henceforth matched the requirements enabling the functional and operational development of the child's five core skills.

The combined analysis of clinical data collected by the child psychiatrist and the quantitative results obtained by the research team at different ages did not result in the establishment of correlations between the double development of the child and his mother with regard to each other and the events that occurred to them both. It is possible that the monitoring of both persons by the mother and child care doctor, the child psychiatrist, and the research team, combined with many interactions with other children and professionals at the children's home, may have enhanced better adjusted and attuned relations between mother and child.

In any case, this example shows the merits of the core skill concept, as the features of a difficult attachment between mother and child in the early months can be objectified and also because it enables the revealing of the true capabilities of the child when it is in an interaction situation with other partners who have not shared this difficult attachment. (If we had established this before monitoring this dyad, all the professionals involved might not have been so concerned by the nonadjusted and apparently nonattuned interactions observed between mother and child.)

Proposals for Families in 2000 to Benefit from More Appropriate Conditions for the Development of Child Skills and the Security of All Concerned

The research just reported above and the two examples described led to suggesting a set of strategies and measures that are likely to prevent the establishment of misunderstanding, disappointment, worry, lack of interest, rejection, abandonment, and mistreatment of young children, especially when there are risk factors with the child, mother, or family. The measures and actions listed here could be used.

Proposal 1.   Make it possible for mothers-to-be, mothers, and anyone else to meet professionals well trained in the knowledge and recognition of the signs and indicators of nonemergence, deficiency, anomalies, and lags in the various types of child skills. (Brazelton's NBAS, the core skills that we have defined, and the other developmental chronologies and scales could be combined to form an even more reliable, pertinent, and predictive appraisal tool than the methods generally used to assess developmental difficulties in children.)

For this, in addition to removing the obstacles that impede knowledge of ontogenic processes (cf. introduction to this chapter), I feel that it is essential to set up information and consultation centers open to all and that are not fundamentally medically oriented but that also serve social and educational functions. At such centers, people would be able to meet pediatricians, child psychiatrists, special teachers, social workers, mothers, and researchers who, in an atmosphere of positive interaction, know how to bring out the hidden skills in a baby, while explaining the reality to each visitor, reassuring him or her, and relieving him or her of guilt.

This type of structure already exists at least in partial form in an increasing number of hospitals and centers specialized in child care and children's activities (such as those under the responsibility of professionals qualified to use Brazelton's NBAS). However, even more perfected design of facilities for children, mothers, families, and any other person is necessary, together with behavior, practices, scheduling, and the design of facilities that can stimulate the emergence of the whole range of skills in young children while reassuring and giving roles to the mother, the family and the other habitual or potential partners. I have chosen to describe here two examples of strategies and facilities that we have designed to meet these requirements. They can help to make progress in the views, images, decisions, and practices of families, child-care professionals, and decision makers of all kinds (political, economic, social and cultural) for the benefit of children and their families and for society as a whole.

Meeting Room at the Maternity and Obstetrics Department, Bagnol-sur-Cèze (Gard Department, South of France).   The meeting room is separate from the hospital sector and rooms for mothers and their babies. It is designed for meetings between new mothers and their husbands, other children, family, and friends in an atmosphere of positive interaction. It has two parts. One consists of a structure 90 cm high with nests in which mothers can place their children. A bench runs around it so that every mother can be seated near her child and maintain bodily or visual contact with it, especially when the mother is talking to her husband and other children. The structure ensures permanent physical and affective security for the child and the affective security of the parents (the baby cannot fall).

The second part consists of a superstructure on which the elder child or children can develop their motor skills, interactive capacities, cognitive processes, and symbolic activities under the eyes of their parents (and also, on an imaginary scale, under the eyes of the baby, as is revealed by their speech) (cf. earlier in this chapter, "The complex behaviors which appear to become established during the first 3 years on the basis of the core skills of the first year").

The children who visit their mother and the baby are not, and do not feel, ignored, left out, pushed about, or subjected to aggression, in contrast with conditions in most maternity hospital rooms where the birth of a baby obliges the elder children to share the interactions and attachment links with their mother. By using the superstructure, they can demonstrate the whole range of their skills and simultaneously initiate diversified interactions with their mother, their father, their other partners, and the baby itself, without competition with the latter. The atmosphere is one of calls, exchange of looks, gestures, utterances and language, and happiness. Triangular relations develop between the elder child or children, the mother, the father, and the baby, and also interactions between four or five people. Roles and functions can be conserved and shared. Each person keeps his or her position and his or her status with regard to the others "in spite of" the arrival of the new baby and thanks to this arrival. A positive view of each by the other can become established because the design of the area does not force anybody into a conventional role. The mother can leave her proximal position in relation to the baby (who cannot slide out of the "nest") without worrying and have play exchanges with the elder child or children on certain parts of the superstructure. The father can set aside his role of father favoring the newborn child by playing with the elder child or children while his wife watches. The elder child or children can escape the conventional role expected of them in relation to the baby and display stress or demonstrate all their skills, without there being negative perception (in many other settings and situations, adults often talk of the behavior of elder children toward babies in terms such as "he's jealous, egotistical, unbearable, or nasty").

Grandparents, friends, and neighbors are astonished when they see the skills and reasonable behavior of the elder child or children and when they themselves experience their visit to the mother and child as a discovery of the adaptive capacities of everybody and as a moment of mutual confidence, friendliness, and reassurance with regard to their own difficulties.

All these phenomena can be "sublimated" when participants are accompanied in their discoveries by attentive but unobtrusive professionals who demonstrate in their attitudes "people skills" and capacities of attachment to each other. This is why the training of professional staff is considered indissociable from the design and fitting of such settings.

These phenomena are consolidated and acquire their full meaning when the family assembles in the same place on subsequent days or in subsequent weeks, at its own initiative or at that of the medical and educational team when mother and child have left the hospital. New references are then discovered or better understood by everybody in a place in which the baby can be enfolded in their interactions, putting real, imaginary, or fantasy difficulties in their place.

The innovation at Bagnols-sur-Cèze Maternity Hospital has led to a new research project involving obstetricians, pediatricians, psychologists, and researchers. The project concerns the regulation that can be demonstrated in this new site, which has not a priori a definite function and is thus not likely to be perceived as a location for medical, social, or other judgment. It is a meeting place for people to identify and be identified by others.

I believe that in the twenty-first century, while the insecurity of human life is liable to increase because of the increasing complexity of societies and because of the loss of many family and social references, it will be indispensable to design strategies and meeting places like those found at the meeting room in Bagnols-sur-Cèze. It seems useful and perhaps necessary that the high point formed by a birth should be followed by an intense period during which each participant both conserves his or her links and references in relation to his or her attachment partners and sees them under fresh light and with integration of the "newcomer" (the baby) in his or her image and interactions. Strategies must be designed for this, and settings should be organized to enable family members to meet in a "play" atmosphere outside the conventional structures of medicine and education. The presence of other families and the availability of child and family specialists help to intensify the positive atmosphere (and the resulting feeling of security), leading to laughter and jubilation on the part of the older children, the fathers, and other children, when they use superstructures comparable to that at Bagnols-sur-Cèze or other superstructures better suited to the cultural, ethnic, and ecological features of the geographical site.

The Mother and Child Sector of the Centre Médical National de la Mutuelle Générale de l'Education Nationale at Trois-Epis (Vosges Region, Eastern France).

Intended principally for teachers, the department mainly handles depressive, depressed, or convalescent mothers with their child or children and husband when the couple so wishes. We designed a room where the mothers meet their children every day at 3 p.m. (the time being fixed by the medical center, as the morning is reserved for medical treatment for the mothers and the personalized handling of the children in their sleep–wake rhythm, meals, and the hygiene and medical care required by their somatic state) and entrust them to the staff of the center at 5 p.m. The mothers thus spend only 2 hours with their children per day.

When the mothers meet their child or children at 3 p.m., they can see that the children climb, slide, and use the superstructures in complete security and with no signs of anxiety or distress. They smile, laugh, and communicate like the other children of the same age through looks, laughter, smiles, gestures, touching, and speech. They call out and have fun. They "escape" the apprehension, worry, distress, and/or feeling of guilt of a depressive, depressed, or convalescent mother and have an opportunity to explore, display, and stress the whole range of their core skills and simultaneously build up with their peers the complex behaviors described and quantified earlier in this chapter. The depressive, depressed or convalescent mothers can thus shift their positions with regard to their psychic, behavioral, psychophysiological, and physiological difficulties. They are in a situation that enables them to rediscover the skills that their child/children possess. When they accompany their child or children in the superstructures, they live their emotions positively and "come out of" their insecurity when in contact with the assurance and security shown by their child or children. They learn to smile, laugh, and listen again and to no longer feel guilty. Interactive loops are established or reestablished between mothers and children, enabling each to recover emotional, affective, and cognitive references with the subject of their initial attachment and to build up, strengthen, or rebuild attachment links that could not be established or that became distorted.

The mothers' behavior and reports show that they enjoy coming to this meeting place. Positive changes are noted at the end of the first week of stays of depressive, depressed, or convalescent mothers (Montagner et al., unpublished observations), both in their mental state and behavior and in their psychophysiological variables. Their views and images have changed with regard to both themselves and their child or children and their family, and their everyday environment in general.

I think that at the beginning of the twenty-first century, the placing of a mother or a father in a hospital establishment—and also in other establishments (work, culture, etc.)—will be accompanied by the reception of their children in settings designed for the reassurance, security and mutual esteem of all.

In parallel, it should be planned that child-care specialists can visit family environments, especially when the latter are socially and intellectually underprivileged and/or when the mother or the family cannot or does not know how to take steps to "show" their baby to others (and to learn to know their baby) without experiencing such visits as distressing, destabilizing, or guilt-forming. Regular information campaigns and displays in places frequented by families, such as supermarkets, grocery stores, squares, and village centers, might encourage mothers to visit a specialized center after gaining the assurance that they will not be judged, bothered, or dispossessed of the role as mother or simply as a person. Buses, caravans, or other kinds of vehicles could be fitted out as meeting places for mothers and child-care specialists. Here again, these could be sited in places frequented by families. Finally, because images have strong emotional force, attractive, easily accessible, functional libraries of video and printed material should be formed, where mothers and families could borrow all types of work in their language, providing information in a form that can be understood by everybody.

A network of perinatal and child-care specialists could organize and coordinate all these initiatives at the town or district level.

Proposal 2.   This is the possibility for mothers and families to entrust their young child for a few hours to an appropriate center, providing physical and affective security for all.

As is shown in the example described earlier of the hypertonic boy who "did not look at" his mother, some babies only fully reveal the diversity and complexity of their skills in situations in which they interact with partners other than their mother, especially when they have had painful experiences with her. It is as if these children display a defensive drive with regard to a mother in psychological and social difficulty. They seem to avoid responding to her behavior and perhaps perceive it as generating insecurity. In any case, no adjusted interactions are observed between such 4- to 8-month-old children and their mothers.

Monitoring these mother–child dyads shows that it may be essential to enable a child to be in the company of other children of the same age with roughly the same skills and thus likely to give meaning to its behaviors and utterances and simultaneously enable it to understand their various activities. This contact must last for a sufficient length of time. However, this time must be spent in the presence of specialists who know how to recognize the child's skills and show them to its mother without her feeling guilty.

This is why it is important to design new reception structures, which could be called "life and development itineraries." They would enable each child—even disabled children—to reveal, show, and stress its skills to its mother and its family without attendance of such facilities being a source of worry, distress, or guilt for the latter or—obviously—a source of worry or distress for the child. Children could attend for a number of hours, for a day, or for several days, according to the wishes of their parents and, in the case of disabled children, according to a combined request from parents and child-care specialists according to the type and severity of the difficulties experienced by the child and its family. This does not mean establishing day-care-type centers but more flexible, open centers organized for both children and their families and adapted to each individual case without judgment or rejection.

I feel that such centers should be based on three major principles: (a) They should enable mutually consented separation of a child and its mother or a child and its parents; (b) the rhythms of each child should be respected (Montagner, 1983, 1993; Montagner, de Roquefeuil, & Djakovic, 1992; Montagner et al., 1993a, 1993b); and (c) facilities should be organized so that children truly have the possibility of discovering the full range of their skills and showing them to the other children, to the center team, and to the parents (when the latter are discreetly present and especially when they can watch their child active among others).

The child's "demonstration" of unsuspected motor skills (which cannot emerge in the family niche for lack of suitable facilities and of affective security from the mother and the family), a great variety of already complex interactive and relational capacities, new cognitive processes, and unexpected symbolic activities changes the view of the various partners. This in return enhances the emergence of new skills and the process then continues. For this reason, it is important to design reception facilities for babies and young children not as "child-minding" centers to which a child is entrusted in exceptional cases because of an unexpected event or regularly because of its two parents' scheduled work, but as essential settings that enable a child to get to know him- or herself as fully as possible in an atmosphere of physical and affective security after separation agreed mutually with the parents and viewed in positive terms by all the other partners.

☐ Conclusions

I believe that the future of the family is closely linked with the development of three broad fields:

1. The establishment and intensification of multidisciplinary research by clinicians and workers involved in fundamental research (physiologists, psychophysiologists, psychologists, developmental specialists, etc.) whose main objective is to better understand the continuities and discontinuities between the characteristics of early development (from birth and during fetal life when this is possible and desirable) and development during the first 3 years of a child's life. It is essential to better understand how babies and young children can use their skills as resources either

to establish, consolidate, and diversify their interactions and attachment links with their various partners (and especially with their mother) or to protect or defend themselves when they cannot establish adjusted, attuned interactions with the person with whom they form their initial attachment, and thus conserve their skills, especially their core skills as defined in this chapter, or other skills in the light of comparison of data from various studies. It is necessary at the same time to clearly define the conditions required so that a child in difficulty can reveal, show, and stress its skills, especially when its family is itself in difficulty. Progress in research requires clinical and fundamental work on the temporal evolution of the mechanisms and processes through which young children establish, reestablish, or avoid interaction with their various partners and not only with their mother.

2. The development of strategies and the creation of settings enabling child-care specialists to modify the view, images, attitudes, and behaviors of the mother and the family toward babies and young children. The results of fundamental research back up the observations, experience, and conclusions of clinicians in stressing that significant changes can be achieved when mother and family become aware of a child's skills and especially its ability to establish and reestablish interaction with its various partners. If meetings can be arranged with child-care specialists in the family environment, it is also desirable that from birth onward, babies should—without any professional external support—be part of relational dynamics of the various members of families, especially with brothers and sisters because they may view a baby as a competitor. We have given an example with the installation at a maternity hospital of a room separate from the medical areas where mothers and babies can meet fathers, elder children, and other visitors in a recreational atmosphere and establish or reestablish their affective references with each other. Triangular interactions involving four people or more and that involve a baby and, around it, its mother, father, and one or more elder children already give the baby the status of person and participant. I find it important that neonatal officials and specialists develop strategies and locations to serve these meeting and discovery functions based on "the arrival of the newcomer" so that it can be awarded its position without feeling that it is taking someone else's place (father, brother, or sister). In special situations of mothers in the hospital when their child is only a few months old, it may be just as important for them to see their child at some time during the day in a nonmedical setting where they can observe the child's joie de vivre and vitality in an atmosphere that enhances interaction for interaction's sake and that "shifts" the mother away from her worry, distress, and guilt.

The example of a facility for meetings between mothers and their children in a specialized medical center taking depressive, depressed, or convalescent mothers for a few weeks was mentioned. The positive consequences are twofold. The mother suffers less worry, distress, and guilt during hospitalization (it is also possible that there are beneficial effects on the illness and on convalescence). The child or children benefit as they only experience temporary separation from their mother and they are among other children and other people with whom they can discover and show their skills in a gratifying context where they then meet their mothers.

Hospitals should also install places where sick, postoperative, or convalescent children can be at one moment or another in a recreational atmosphere in which they can live like children and use all their skills, moving out of the focus of their illness, operation, or convalescence. The place would be for meeting not only other hospitalized children but also their parents, brothers, sisters, and friends. We undertook this at Hopital Arnaud de Villeneuve in Montpellier (in the south of France) by designing settings in which children "in a terminal stage" (who may die in a few days or weeks of cancer, AIDS, etc.) can climb up and down, straddle, slide, hide alone or with another child, and develop diversified interactions on each side of walls with windows and apertures while laughing, gesticulating, soliciting, cooperating, and inventing new games and new uses of the objects. These children who rediscover themselves as children and who no longer live continuously as suffering beings can thus modify their perception of themselves and also the views, images, and practices of their parents and the medical team. Making hospitals a center of life for children and parents should be a major objective for the twenty-first century.

3. The development of strategies and the creation of reception structures outside the family environment for children of all ages for an hour or several hours or for a day or several days. The objectives are to enable children to reveal and demonstrate skills that they have been unable to bring out in the family environment and to display these skills to their mothers and their families, especially when the latter are in difficulty. It is necessary to be aware that many capacities and regulation features can only emerge in a child when it can behave at its own rhythm among other children, that is to say in the company of other humans who possess broadly the same skills and can thus give them meaning, or at least a different meaning from that in the family environment. "Life and development itineraries" for children of all ages should be set up not to replace the family but as facilities to complement, enhance, and shed light on the development of children by helping to enhance a positive view of their children by parents, whatever their somatic, psychological, and social difficulties. Such places also enable meetings between families with different habits and cultures. Children and parents thus learn to know new modes of behaviors, images and thought.

However, innovations of this kind are only possible with two major evolutions (or possibly "revolutions"?).

1. Awareness by political, economic, social, and cultural decision makers that a child must be considered as a separate entity and distinct from the family entity in the same way that the mother, father, and other members of the family are entities that must not be confused either with the child entity or the family entity, even though there are obviously reciprocal influences between these people. It is important for a baby to establish a secure attachment to its mother, and it is equally important that it should bring out its skills and use them as resources in interactions with its various partners at home and in any other place. The child can thus participate in its own development and not be merely the result of maternal or family modeling. A children's policy for the sake of children and, if possible, for the sake of each child must be designed for this and not merely a "childhood" policy. Decision makers must no longer shelter behind the institutional shields of the family, child, and/or family care systems and organizations, and medical and educational structures. The child as a person should also form part of considerations, projects and decisions. This is the price of a significant decrease in the frequency, duration, and seriousness of major developmental difficulties in a large number of children.

2. The multidisciplinary, nondogmatic training of child-care professionals and the setting up of interdisciplinary networks to develop strategies for helping children, moth-

ers and families and the construction and equipping of reception, care, education, and leisure facilities for young children and their families, especially when they display risk factors or are already in difficulty.

☐ Summary

This chapter shows how research can be used to develop new strategies and new facilities to enhance child development, avoid the emergence of difficulties, and simultaneously facilitate family life. The introductory section stresses the fundamental interest of Bowlby's attachment theory and Brazelton's NBAS in clinical and fundamental work aimed at understanding developmental processes in children or at forecasting the emergence of difficulties in a specific child. The obstacles to progress in knowledge are also examined. New research is described. This is aimed at achieving a more complete description of the range of potential and real skills in babies and young children, not only through their interactions with the mother but also with other partners and principally children of the same age.

The second section contains the main results of research on the capabilities displayed by children 4 to 7 months old when they are placed in an interaction situation with another child of the same age under conditions in which they can "escape" their tonico-postural immaturity. The work led to identification of five major capabilities that appear to be core skills essential to the normal development of children.

The main data gathered in longitudinal research on the complex behaviors that become established in the first 3 years of the life of children in certain human and spatial conditions are summarized in the third section of this chapter. The five core skills previously defined appear necessary for their emergence and development. Various developmental difficulties observed during the first year, especially with regard to attachment difficulties between mother and child and in the light of the five core skills, were then examined.

Finally, a longitudinal study of two mother/child-in-difficulty dyads during the first year was used to show how a mother's behavior and view can change while the child itself changes. This was followed by real examples of strategies and settings that, by enhancing the emergence of the skills of young children and enabling them to demonstrate them to their mothers and families, modify for the better their behaviors, views, and images, especially when the child, mother, or family displays risk factors or is already in difficulty. The examples consist of a meeting room in a maternity hospital and a meeting room in a medical center treating depressive, depressed, or convalescent mothers accompanied by their children. The future of young children and the family was then discussed on the basis of these strategies and facilities.

☐ References

Ainsworth, M. D. S. (1973). The development of mother-infant attachment. In B. M. Caldwell & H. N. Ricciuti (Eds.), *Review of child development research* (Vol. 3, pp. 1–94). Chicago: University of Chicago Press.

Ainsworth, M. D. S. (1974). *The secure base*. Baltimore, MD: Johns Hopkins University.

Ainsworth, M. D. S. (1979a). Attachment as related to mother–infant interaction. In J. S. Rosenblatt,

R. A. Hinde, C. Beer, & M. C. Busnel (Eds.), *Advances in the study of behavior* (p. 9). New York: Academic Press.

Ainsworth, M. D. S. (1979b). Infant–mother attachment. *American Psychologist, 34,* 932–937.

Ainsworth, M. D. S., & Bell, S. M. (1969). Some contemporary patterns of mother-infant interaction in the feeding situation. In A. Ambrose (Ed.), *Stimulation in early infancy* (pp. 133–170). New York: Academic Press.

Ainsworth, M. D. S., Bell, S. M., & Stayton, D. J. (1971). Individual differences in strange situation in one-year old. In H. R. Schaffer (Ed.), *The origins of human social relations* (pp. 17–58). New York: Academic Press.

Als, H., & Brazelton, T. B. (1975). Comprehensive neonatal assessment. *Birth and the Family Journal, 2,* 3–11.

Als, H., & Brazelton, T. B. (1981). A new model of assessing the behavioral organization in preterm and fullterm infants. *Journal of the American Academy of Child Psychiatry, 20,* 239–263.

Als, H., Lester, B., Tronick, E. Z., & Brazelton, T. B. (1982). Manual for the assessment of the preterm infant's behavior. In H. E. Fitzgerald & M. W. Yogman (Eds.), *Theory and research in behavioral pediatrics* (Vol. 1, pp. 35–63). New York: Plenum.

Als, H., Lester, B., Tronick, E. Z., & Brazelton, T. B. (1979). Specific neonatal measures: The Brazelton neonatal behavioral assessment scale. In J. Osofsky (Ed.), *The handbook of infant development* (pp. 185–215). New York: Wiley.

Als, H., Tronick, E. Z., & Brazelton, T. B. (1977). The Brazelton Neonatal Behavioral Assessment Scale. *Journal of Abnormal Psychology, 3,* 215–231.

Bowlby, J. (1958). The nature of a child's tie to his mother. *International Journal of Psychoanalysis, 39,* 350–373.

Bowlby, J. (1960). Separation anxiety. *International Journal of Psychoanalysis, 41,* 89–113.

Bowlby, J. (1969). *Attachment and loss. I: Attachment.* London: Hogarth Press and Institute of Psychoanalysis.

Bowlby, J. (1973). *Attachment and loss: II: Separation, anxiety and anger.* London: Tavistock.

Bowlby, J. (1980). *Attachment and loss: III: Loss, sadness and depression.* New York: Basic Books.

Brazelton, T. B. (1973a). Effect of maternal expectations on early infant behavior. *Early Child Development and Care, 2,* 259–273.

Brazelton, T. B. (1973b). Assessment of the infant at risk. *Clinical Obstetrics and Gynecology, 16,* 361–375.

Brazelton, T. B. (1979). Behavioral competence of the newborn infant. *Seminars in Perinatology, 3*(1), 35–43.

Brazelton, T. B. (1981). Clinical use of the Brazelton neonatal behavioral assessment scale. In M. Coleman (Ed.), *Neonatal neurology* (pp. 57–71). Baltimore, MD: University Park Press.

Brazelton, T. B., Kolowski, B., & Main, M. (1974). Origins of reciprocity: The early mother–infant interaction. In M. Lewis & L. Rosenblum (Eds.), *The effect of the infant on its caregiver* (pp. 49–75). New York: Wiley.

Brazelton, T. B., & Lester, B. M. (1983). *Infant at risk: Toward plasticity and intervention.* New York: Elsevier Press.

Brazelton, T. B., & Tronick, E. Z. (1980). Preverbal communication between mothers and infants. In D. Olson (Ed.), *The social foundations of language and thought* (pp. 229–315). New York: Norton.

Brazelton, T. B., Tronick, E. Z., Adamson, L., Als, H., & Wise, S. (1975). Early mother-infant reciprocity. In *Parent–infant interaction, CIBA Foundation Symposium* (Vol. 33, pp. 137–155). New York: Elsevier.

Brazelton, T. B., & Yogman, M. W. (1985). *Affective development in infancy* (Vol. 3). Norwood, NJ: Ablex.

Brazelton, T. B., Yogman, M. W., Als, H., & Tronick, E. Z. (1978). The infant as a focus for family reciprocity. In M. Lewis & L. A. Rosenblum (Eds.), *The social network of the developing child* (pp. 29–43). New York: Plenum Press.

Grenier, A. (1981). La motricité libérée par fixation manuelle de la nuque au cours des premières années de vie. *Archives Françaises de Pédiatrie, 38,* 557–561.

Lamb, M. E., Thompson, R. A., Gardner, W. P., Charnov, E. L., & Estes, D. (1984). Security of infantile attachment as assessed in the "strange situation": Its study and biological interpretation. *Behavioral and Brain Sciences, 7,* 127–171.

Montagner, H. (1983). *Les rhythmes de l'enfant et de l'adolescent.* Paris: Stock.

Montagner, H. (1988). *L'attachement, les débuts de la tendresse.* Paris: Ed. Odile Jacob.

Montagner, H. (1993). *L'enfant acteur de son développement.* Paris: Stock.

Montagner, H., de Roquefeuil, G., & Djakovic, M. (1992). Biological, behavioral and intellectual activity rhythms of the child during its development in different educational environments. In Y. Touitou & E. Haus (Eds.), *Biologic rhythms in clinical and laboratory medicine* (pp. 214–229). New York: Springer-Verlag.

Montagner, H., Epoulet, B., Gauffier, G., Goulevitch, R., Ramel, N., Wiaux, B., & Taule, M. (1994). The earliness and complexity of the interaction skills and social behavior of the child with its peers. In R. A. Gardner, A. B. Chiarelli, B. T. Gardner, & F. X. Plooj (Eds.), *The ethological roots of culture* (pp. 315–355). NATA Series D: Behavioral Sciences. Dordrecht: Kluwer.

Montagner, H., Gauffier, G., Epoulet, B., Restoin, A., Goulevitch, R., Taule, M., & Wiaux, B. (1993a). Alternative child care in France: Advances in the study of motor, interactive and social behaviors of young children in settings allowing them to move freely in a group of peers. *Pediatrics, 91,* 253–263.

Montagner, H., Restoin, A., Rodriguez, D., Ullmann, V., Viala, M., & Laurent, D. (1988a). Aspects fonctionnels et ontogénétiques des interactions de l'enfant avec ses pairs au cours des trois premières années. *Psychiatrie de l'enfant, 31,* 173–278.

Montagner, H., Restoin, A., Rodriguez, D., Ullmann, V., Viala, M., & Laurent, D. (1988b). Social interactions of young children and their modifications in relation to environmental factors. In M. R. A. Chance (Ed.), *Social fabrics of the mind* (pp. 237–259). Hillsdale, NJ: Lawrence Erlbaum Associates.

Montagner, H., Ruiz, V., Ramel, N., Restoin, A., Mertzianidou, V., & Gauffier, G. (1993b). Les capacités interactives d'enfant de 4 à 7 mois avec un enfant du même âge. *Psychiatrie de l'enfant, 36,* 489–536.

Montagner, H., Restoin, A., Ullmann, V., Rodriguez, D., Godard, D., & Viala, M. (1984). Development of early peer interaction. In W. Doise & A. Palmonari (Eds.), *Social interaction in individual development* (pp. 25–41). Cambridge: Cambridge University Press.

Nugent, J. K., Lydic, J., & Burke, P. (1986). *Newborn and infant assessment.* Boston: Little, Brown.

Stern, D. (1985). Affect attunement. In J. D. Call, E. Galenson, & R. L. Tyson (Eds.), *Frontiers in infant psychiatry* (p. 2). New York: Basic Books.

Stern, D. (1989). *Le monde interpersonnel du nourisson. Une perspective psychanalytique et développementale.* Paris: PUF.

Tronick, E. Z. (1982). *Affect, cognition and communication: The process of social interchange in infancy.* Baltimore: University Park Press.

Tronick, E. Z., Als, H., & Brazelton, T. B. (1977). The infant's capacity to regulate mutuality in face-to-face interaction. *Journal of Communication, 27,* 74–79.

Tronick, E. Z., Als, H., Adamson, L., Wise, S., & Brazelton, T. B. (1978). The infant's response to entrapment between contradictory messages in face-to-face interaction. *Journal of the American Academy of Child Psychiatry, 17,* 1–13.

Tronick, E. Z., Als, H., & Brazelton, T. B. (1979). Early development of neonatal and infant behavior. In F. Faulkner & J. M. Tanner (Eds.), *Human growth: A comprehensive treatise* (pp. 305–327). New York: Plenum.

Tronick, E. Z., Als, H., & Brazelton, T. B. (1980). Monadic phases: A structural descriptive analysis of infant-mother face-to-face interaction. *Merrill-Palmer Quarterly, 26,* 3–23.

Tronick, E. Z., Ricks, M., & Cohn, J. (1982). Maternal and infant affective exchanges: Patterns of adaptation. In T. Field & A. Vogel (Eds.), *Emotion and interaction: Normal and high risk children* (pp. 83–101). Hillsdale, NJ: Lawrence Erlbaum Associates.

Tronick, E. Z., Scanlon, K. B., & Scanlon, J. W. (1985). Behavioral organization in extremely ill preterm infants during the postpartum period. In *Advances in infancy research* (p. 5). Norwood, NJ: Ablex.

10
CHAPTER

Kathryn E. Barnard
Georgina A. Sumner

Promoting Awareness of the Infant's Behavioral Patterns: Elements of Anticipatory Guidance for Parents

☐ A Primer for Getting Acquainted

Infants are not the buzzing mass of confusion they were once thought to be. Understanding of infant neurological and behavioral organization has given us a road map of infant states, infant behavior, nonverbal cues, and cycles of attention/nonattention that prove to be very helpful to the infant's caregiver (Barnard, 1981; Brazelton, 1962, 1973; Brazelton, Koslowki, & Main, 1974; Parmelee, 1964). With this new understanding of infant behavior, parents can be equipped to care for their infant with an informed competency. Parental guidance incorporating the information that developmental and biological scientists have advanced in the past 25 to 30 years is a necessary part of the health professional's agenda of care. In this chapter we present a structure for providing guidance to parents that is highly supportive of parents, parenting, and parent–child interaction.

In the mid 1980s, our research group of nurses, psychologists, and a pediatrician tested a parent curriculum we developed to give parents information about their newborn and developing infant up to three months of age (Barnard et al., 1985; Barnard, Booth, Mitchell, & Telzrow, 1988). The Nursing Support for Infant Bio-Behavior program (NSIBB) was a structured, educational curriculum designed to facilitate the mutual adaptation process between the caregiver and the infant. The program was designed so that the content followed a specific progression during the first 12 weeks of the infant's life. Although the content and the goals remained the same for each family, the specific details were individualized to the personality and style of each mother and infant.

The NSIBB program's content and activities were developed or selected from the known biobehavioral changes occurring in all infants during their first three months of life. These biobehavioral changes and subsequent goals of anticipatory guidance were:

Week 1. Sleep–wake–feeding patterns and the baby's behavioral response patterns form the key issues the parents need to know about. During this period they will need to acquaint themselves with their baby and to understand their baby's unique characteristics. They begin to identify who their baby is and to develop ways of meeting the baby's needs. At this time the parents may express frustration about their infant's sleep-wake schedule, which will gradually increase in predictability.

The three goals of this visit were to help the parent become familiar with sleep–wake states, gain an understanding of sleep–wake state patterns and changes, and become aware of the baby's abilities and preferences.

Week 3. Anticipatory guidance about infant fussiness and crying was a primary focus. During this period babies may be quite fussy, because the infant's peak amount of crying begins at about 4 weeks (Brazelton, 1962). These crying periods are extremely frustrating and overwhelming for parents. Crying may interfere with pleasurable periods between parent and infant and may hinder any kind of positive communication they may have established.

The goals were to help the parent understand and develop an ability to cope with the infant's fussiness and crying; increase the awareness of the infant's emotional and security needs; become more aware of communication and infant cues; and facilitate contingent responding and appropriate infant stimulation.

Week 5. This is a transitional time for parents and infants. Parents are often more at ease with their role and feel more confident in caring for the baby. The infant's feeding and sleeping patterns may be more predictable. The parents begin to observe the infant smiling and establishing eye contact. On the other hand, the infant may still be fussy and the parents may be losing their patience with the baby.

The goals for this visit as well as the next two visits were to increase parental awareness of activities appropriate for the infant; to increase their feelings of parental competence; and to promote the infant's learning.

Week 8. During this period, infants consolidate their behaviors and give clearer cues. Parents observe sociable behaviors in their babies such as smiling, visual tracking, ceasing to cry when they have been picked up, and differentiating the parents from other people (Barnard, 1981; Murphy, 1973). These behaviors make the parents feel that the infant recognizes them as specific individuals.

The goals listed from week 5 continue to be emphasized.

Week 12. At this time, many parents have established routines in caring for their baby. The parent and infant usually have learned to read each other's cues and to respond appropriately. When the parent and infant are together they exhibit a "give-and-take" rhythm. This rhythm is usually evident in most interaction periods.

The goals of week 5 are emphasized, as well as the goal of preparing the parent for the wonderful period of social interaction that occurs beginning at about 3 months when the infant becomes a real social partner.

We next describe our experience of implementing this curriculum with mothers. In the NSIBB model the mothers were subjects in a research study comparing nursing approaches to working with mothers from the birth of the infant until the infant was 3 months old. The mothers were all referred from the local health department and in general were from low-income families.

We have subsequently used the principal components of this NSIBB model in new programs that we have developed concerning newborn care. One such program is a videotape instructional series for professionals called *Keys to CareGiving* (Nursing Child Assessment Satellite Training (NCAST), 1990). This series comes with a set of parent handouts for teaching parents about infant state, infant behaviors, infant nonverbal language, state modulation, and parent–infant interaction.

In this chapter we describe the successful elements of the NSIBB program. These elements represent both the process and content of appropriate early guidance to new parents. The content includes sleep–wake patterns, infant behavior, infant communication cues, and parent–infant interaction. Following the explanation of content, we describe the techniques we used to personalize the information about the content. The windows we set up for personalizing this guidance were the physical examination, sleep/activity records, behavioral observations, feeding observations, and various developmental activities. In thinking about anticipatory guidance, Winnicott's notion that every "mother sees her infant through her own window" is an appropriate metaphor for how the information should be framed. The presentation of information about her own baby's sleep/wake pattern or nonverbal behavioral cues provides that individual "window" the mother uses in learning to know and appreciate her baby. The same goes for fathers, although professionals have been slower to include men in this acquaintanceship process.

☐ Sleep–Wake and Feeding Patterns

All life within the family of a newborn revolves around the baby's periods of sleep and feeding. We have discovered that since the 1960s, when Parmelee (1964) began to report infant sleep durations, the amount of sleep parents report their infants having has decreased. In the 1960s sleep of the 1-month infant averaged 16 hours in 24, whereas in the 1980s it has decreased to 14 hours. Table 10.1 displays data about infants' sleep and feeding patterns during the first year of life. These data come from Nursing Child Assessment Sleep Activity records (NCASA). See Figure 1 for this 7-day record system completed by parents from across the United States and Australia during the late 1980s and early 1990s. The amount of sleep in 24 hours changes little during the first year of life; what does change is how it is organized. The baby begins with 2- to 3-hour sleep periods and by 3 months can put together six to eight 60-minute sleep cycles. Sometime after 2 months the infant generally begins consolidating sleep to occur more during the night. The duration-of-sleep data match well with physiological recording of

TABLE 10.1. Nursing Child Assessment Sleep Activity Data

	Age of child, months (number of subjects)			
	1 (255)	2 (180)	3–5 (178)	6–12 (160)
Hours of sleep[a]	13.8	13.3	13.1	12.8
Sleep segments	6.3	5.8	4.8	3.9
Feedings	7.6	7.3	6.4	5.5

[a] Significant difference. Hours of sleep between 1 month and all other times decrease.

sleep by Coons (1987). We recommend parents use the NCASA recording over a 7-day period. One 24-hour recall may not reflect a typical day; it is over several days that a pattern emerges.

In addition to noting the sleep and feeding episodes, it is useful to give parents an understanding of the components of sleep and how the sleep periods are organized. Table 10.2 gives the definitions of the common infant sleep states and their implications for caregiving. It is especially useful for parents to know how to recognize the states of sleep and drowsiness and to know when the infant will likely feed well. We have found parents occasionally mistake the active sleep state as a signal that the infant is waking. A lack of knowledge of sleep/wake states and their transitions makes it difficult to understand the basic organization of the infant's behavior in the early months.

We encourage the mother to feed the baby only when the infant is awake so the feeding will be successful. This is particularly true for early breast-feeding mothers. The baby sucks more consistently when awake, and this vigorous sucking helps establish adequate breast milk. We teach the mother techniques of state modulation, so that they can bring the baby to the appropriate state for feeding. Providing stimulation such as talking, touching, and moving the infant with irregular timing is often successful in arousing the infant to a more awake state. Table 10.2 also provides the average number of feedings, which is an important factor in making sure the infant has appropriate nutrition in the early weeks. We are concerned if infants in the first weeks of life have fewer than six feedings in a 24-hour period (Barnard, 1980; Blackburn, 1980). Another week's recording should be done if there are fewer than six feedings in a day, and the mother should be asked more about volume and content of the meals.

☐ Infant Behavior

Infant behavior provides a framework for understanding the newborn and observing the developing relationship between parents and infants. Although infant states occur automatically, infant behaviors are more complex. The complexity arises from the fact that infant behaviors are interactive, and therefore depend on certain dyadic conditions occurring simultaneously. The infant behaviors we have used come from the Brazelton Neonatal Behavioral Assessment Scale (NBAS) (Brazelton, 1973, 1984; Brazelton & Cramer, 1990; Cardone and Gilkerson, 1989). The behaviors we have found parents are very interested in include:

- Orientation to face and voice
- Orientation to face
- Orientation to voice
- Habituation
- Consolability
- Cuddliness
- Smiling
- Irritability
- Readability

Eliciting infant behaviors is an interactive process. It is helpful to show parents how to get the infant to respond to visual and auditory stimuli, demonstrating the ability their infant has to process information from the environment. When parents see for themselves this remarkable capacity, their approach to their baby incorporates a new understanding of the baby's capacity to see and hear. Showing the parent how to maximize the baby's response by positioning the baby in an upright position, making use of a natural quiet alert state, and pacing the voice or face so the infant can track, confirms

TABLE 10.2. The Six States of Consciousness

State Behaviors	Implications for Caregiving
Quiet sleep (non-REM) Lack of body activity Regular respiration Lack of eye or facial movements Bursts of sucking Occasional startles Generally unresponsive	Difficult to awaken Appropriate for activities requiring little infant activity, e.g., cutting nails Feeding will be unsuccessful
Active sleep More body activity Irregular respiration Movements of face, smile Movement of lidded eyes More responsive	Less difficult to awaken Parents may think baby is awakening Feeding will be unsuccessful
Drowsy Variable activity Irregular respiration Opens and closes eyes Eyes glazed or heavily lidded Delayed responsiveness	More easy to awaken Difficult to tell if awake or asleep If left alone, may go back to sleep Take time to fully awaken for feeding To awaken baby, give something to see, hear, or suck
Quiet alert Minimal body activity Regular respiration Face and eyes bright Most attentive to stimuli	Good time to feed or socialize Babies respond and learn best Most newborns have an intense period of this state shortly after birth
Active alert Much body activity Irregular respiration Facial movement Eyes open, not bright Fussy Sensitive to stimuli	State in which most babies begin feeding May signal a need for change, feeding, repositioning May be difficult to interact with baby If left alone, babies will often go into a lower state
Crying Irregular respiration Facial grimace Cries Color changes Variable sensitivity to stimuli	Babies' limits have been exceeded Signals need for a change May console self May need consoling by caregiver

Note. From NCAST Publications (1990, p. 9), with permission.

that the baby does see and hear them. When parents understand infant behavior, they respond more positively and tailor their responses to the needs of the infant. For instance, parents with irritable infants try more ways to console them. Where before they may have first fed their baby in response to crying, now they may try talking to the baby, holding both of the baby's arms close to the baby's body, swaddling, and/or rocking.

Another example of parents changing their behavior with the infant is, when they have learned that their infant can see and hear, they talk to the baby and provide more stimulating and interesting things for the baby to see. It is only logical that parents have this information about infant behavior; it makes parenting the infant much more fun and rewarding.

☐ Infant Communication Cues

Infants communicate very clearly by their body language (Eriks, 1979). We call these nonverbal forms of communication engaging and disengaging cues. Engaging cues communicate the needs and desires of the infant to interact. They say, "I want to interact," or "I'm interested." Some familiar engaging cues are smiling, looking at, and reaching out to another. Disengaging cues, on the other hand, signal the need for a break in the interaction. They communicate "I need a break" or "I've had enough." The cues we are most familiar with include crying, turning head away, and falling asleep. Cues that are obvious are termed *potent*; those that are less obvious are termed *subtle*. Subtle cues that are engaging include widening and brightening of the eyes, raising of the head, and brightening of the face. Subtle forms of disengaging cues include yawning, hand to ear, and turning eyes away. Subtle cues are thought to precede potent cues. Parents and caregivers who can read the subtle forms of their infant's cues are more sensitive in their interactions with babies.

Infants have the capacity to take in only so much stimulation before they need to take a break from the interaction. They engage for a period of time and then need to

---

TABLE 10.3. Clusters of Hunger and Satiation Cues

Subtle	Potent
Hunger	
Fussiness	Crying
Mouthing	Back arching
Clenched fingers and fists over chest	Mouthing
or tummy	Rooting
Hand to mouth	Hand to mouth
Sucking movements/sounds	Turning to caregiver
Turning to caregiver	Flexed arms and legs
	Feeding sounds
Satiation	
Falling asleep	Decreased sucking
Arms and legs extended	Back arching
Lack of facial movements	Extended and relaxed fingers
Extended and relaxed fingers	Arms straightened along sides
	Pushing away

Note. From NCAST Publications (1990, p. 32), with permission.

turn away before turning back to reengage. Caregivers who allow the baby to turn away and then wait for the infant to reengage have longer and more rhythmic interactions with their baby (Brazelton, 1974).

Cues become more meaningful when a combination of engaging and disengaging, potent and subtle cues occur around a specific situation such as feeding. Two types of cue clusters occur around feeding. The first is hunger cues and the second is satiation cues. All parents need to know these clusters. Hunger cues include clenched fingers and fists over the chest and tummy, flexed arms and legs, mouthing movements, and rooting behaviors. Satiation cues include arms and legs extended indicating a relaxed state, arms straightened along the sides, finger extension (fingers may be straightened, hyperextended, and can include one or all fingers), and pushing away with the arms. Table 10.3 lists hunger and satiation cues. We have found that these cues, especially satiation cues, are very useful to breast-feeding mothers. By watching the amount of mouthing and the position of the baby's arms, they can confidently know when the baby is full.

☐ Parent–Child Interaction

Critical to the success of any interaction is the ability of the parent and infant to adapt to one another. Parents and infants both have responsibility for this "fitting together." Barnard (1976) published a model of caregiver–child interaction that captures this process. A central concept embedded in the model is the reciprocity or contingent responding of the caregiver to the child and the child to the caregiver. It is important to establish this response pattern early in the relationship. This pattern of responsiveness gives the infant a sense of how the environment in general responds to her behavior. Through the responsiveness of the caregiver, the infant will learn either to trust or mistrust the world.

The Barnard model has four characteristics of the caregiver's behavior during the interaction and two for the infant/child. For the caregiver these are Sensitivity to Cues, Alleviation of Distress, Provision of Social Emotional Growth Fostering, and Provision of Cognitive Growth Fostering. For the child they are Clarity of Cues, and Responsiveness to the Caregiver. Scales have been developed to measure the characteristics of the dyadic interaction during both feeding and teaching tasks (Barnard, 1976; Barnard, Hammond, Booth, Mitchell, & Spieker, 1989; Sumner & Spietz, 1994a, 1994b).

The mother's interactive behavior is correlated with the child's later mental development (Barnard, 1994; Morisset, 1994).

Table 10.4 describes a listing of the caregiver and infant responsibilities during a feeding. These ideas can be used to give the parent feedback about their feeding interaction. The Barnard model of interaction was used to give the mothers feedback about the feeding interaction in the NSIBB program.

☐ "Windows" for Anticipatory Guidance

A physical examination of the infant was done for each mother during the first visit. During this exam the infant's reflexes were elicited and discussed. Some mothers who had seen, for example, the startle response were unsure of their infant's normalcy. By

---

TABLE 10.4. Parent's Interactive Roles and Responsibilities During Feeding

---

Sensitive to cues
1. Position the infant so they can see the infant's eyes and face and hold the infant in close contact with their body.
2. Recognize and respond contingently to the infant's cues.
3. Pace the amount and intensity of their responses to the needs of the infant.

Responsive to distress
1. Recognize and respond to the infant's potent disengagement cues by stopping the feeding, changing the infant's position, or touching or talking in a soothing manner.

Provide growth-fostering situation

  Social/emotional
  1. Make eye contact, say positive things, touch affectionately, laugh and smile during the feeding.
  2. Hold the infant in close contact with their body.
  3. Relax and enjoy the feeding.

  Cognitive
  1. Talk about sights, sounds and experiences.
  2. Allow and encourage exploration of them and the feeding equipment by the infant.

Note. Adapted from NCAST Publications (1990, p. 53), with permission.

conducting a thorough infant exam in front of the mother, the nurse was able to elicit areas of concern and to point out unique features of the infant. The nurse was also able to note potential attachment problems as he or she observed the mother's response and interest in the infant's examination. Most mothers watched the exam closely and tried to soothe their infants when they fussed. Other mothers displayed no interest in either the exam or their infant's response to it.

Physical care techniques were also demonstrated if the mother needed them. For example, umbilical-cord care was the area that caused many of the mothers the most concern and represented the skill in which the mothers were least experienced. The handling of the infant and demonstrating of physical care techniques, such as umbilical care and diapering, seemed to serve multiple purposes. First, the skill was taught by both modeling the steps involved and verbally explaining each step. The nurse also modeled the positioning of the infant as the nurse interacted with the baby in the "en face" position. This positioning enabled the infant to get a better view of the nurse's face, thus, increasing the likelihood of the interaction. Second, the nurse was able to assess the health of the infant as well as the infant's style of interaction and movement, that is, "cuddly," "slow to warm up," or "jittery," and thus could make her comments individualized. Finally, the mother's trust in the nurse was enhanced by her observation of the nurse's sensitive handling of the infant.

Demonstration of infant behavioral responses was also important in teaching the mother about her infant's abilities. A few items were selected from the NBAS to show the baby's visual and auditory responsiveness. Mothers were better able to understand and assimilate this information when it was demonstrated in a concrete fashion by the nurses.

For example, during a first visit with a 19-year-old unmarried primiparous mother, the Brazelton items were attempted without success due to the infant being asleep. However, information was shared with this mother about her infant's visual and auditory abilities. Objects in the room were pointed out as examples of good infant stimulation, and the mother was encouraged to show them to her infant. Two weeks later, at the 3-week visit, this mother asked the nurse, "When can Bonnie see?" It appeared that because the mother had missed the behavioral demonstration, the information had been too abstract for her to apply to her baby.

Another mother, in contrast, was shown the Brazelton demonstration. Her infant attended and followed briefly the red ball and red ring and turned to seek out the rattle. This mother, although a 30-year-old mother of four children, was amazed to discover that her baby could see and hear. She stated, "I had thought that they only slept and ate." During the next home visit with her, at 3 weeks, she reported that the baby had "watched and followed well a yellow ball but lost it if the ball moved too quickly." Thus, the demonstration of newborn behavior had helped her become fully aware of the infant's abilities and to incorporate some of the techniques she had observed into her own activities with her infant. Information regarding infant abilities would be thought to be a review for this mother of four children, but for her it first became real when she saw her infant's abilities demonstrated.

The NSIBB observation record basically asked the parents to observe their infant and to record what they saw. This was a technique selected to tune the parents into their infants between visits, to increase their knowledge of important behaviors, and to help parents become better assessors of their children. The parents' observations were used as the basis for discussion during which the nurse was able to provide the parents with reinforcement and validation of what they had seen and what they were doing with their baby. Often during these discussions the mother would mention behaviors that were confusing to her. The nurse was able to act as an interpreter of the infant's behavior and thus help the parents gain further knowledge about their child. The NSIBB observational record was a simple sheet of paper to put down reminders used to increase the parents' own awareness of what they knew about their infant and to validate them as the expert assessor of their infant.

The Sleep/Wake Behavior Record

Another information-giving strategy used in NSIBB was using the NCAST record for a sleep/wake, 24-hour recall (see Figure 10.1). The mothers were asked to recall their infants' behaviors during the previous 24 hours. During this recall, the nurse was able to get a sense of how things were progressing for the mother-infant pair. The nurse could detect from the recall how infant caretaking was perceived by the mother, that is, if it was "a lot of bother," or "taken in stride," and note specific trouble areas, such as feeding, spitting up, and fussiness. From this recall, the nurse could determine if the feeding and sleep/wake patterns were normal. By this assessment, teaching needs and areas for anticipatory guidance can be identified.

For example, in one of the cases a 28-year-old primiparous mother of a 5-pound, 5-ounce, small-for-gestational-age infant revealed on recall that in a 12-hour period she breast-fed the infant nine times (from midnight to noon). The infant's longest sleep period during these 12 hours was 1½ hours. Further exploration of the record showed that her infant was falling asleep soon after the feedings began and thus was never

NCAST

SLEEP/ACTIVITY RECORD

Date of Recording _____

Pregnant Woman / Parent / Caregiver	Infant / Child	Sleep Concerns of Parent/Child

Pregnant Woman / Parent / Caregiver

Name _____

Age _____

Expected date of delivery _____

Usual Bedtime _____

Usual Awakening _____

Infant / Child

Child's Name _____

Gestational Age at Birth _____

Child's Age (wks./mo.) _____

Child's Sex ☐ Male ☐ Female

Location of Child

During Day ☐ Home ☐ Child Care Other _____

During Night ☐ Home ☐ Child Care Other _____

Number of people sleeping in same room as baby _____

Sleep Concerns of Parent/Child

Do you have any concerns about your sleep or your baby's sleep? ☐ Yes ☐ No

If yes specify:

☐ Getting to Sleep ☐ Waking Up at Night

☐ Sleeping Too Much ☐ Sleeping Too Little

☐ Sleeping Wrong Time

☐ Other, specify: _____

DAY TIME (6AM to 6PM)

Day of Week	6 AM	7	8	9	10	11	NOON	1	2	3	4	5	6 PM	SUMMARY		

DAY TIME TOTALS

148

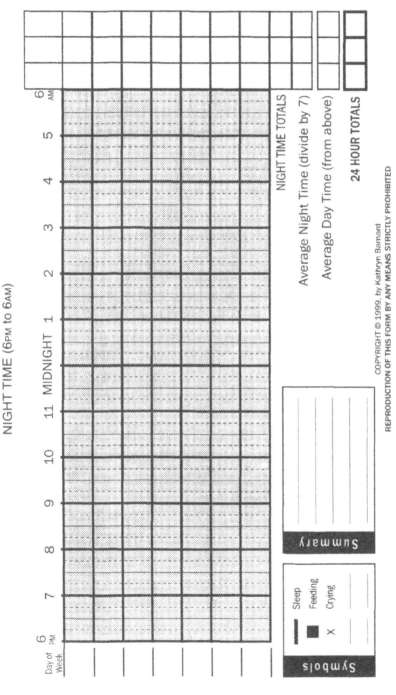

FIGURE 10.1. NCAST record for a sleep/wake, 24-hour recall.

149

receiving a full feeding. This mother profited from learning more about (a) infant states, (b) the best times for feeding, and (c) how to keep the infant awake in order to complete a feeding. The nurse shared information about the states of consciousness ranging from deep sleep to fussiness and crying. When parents were helped to tune into their infant's state, they were better able to assess the infant's needs and to select appropriate activities to do with the infant.

Trying to feed an infant when she drowsy or in a light sleep can be very frustrating for new parents. If they are prepared that their infant might make sucking noises or might cry during light sleep, they will be less likely to interpret these as hunger cues. The nurse suggested certain activities that are appropriate to specific states, such as showing objects to the infant during quiet, alert times; clipping fingernails during deep sleep; and baby exercises during active, alert periods. We teach parents about how the infant makes natural transitions from sleep to wake and then back to sleep after being awake. We discuss with them ways of helping the baby modulate his or her state when they have difficulty, which is common for infants born preterm. Crying and fussiness are to be expected, and we teach parents how to anticipate this behavior. We teach them that modifying the environment in specific ways can prevent fussiness, reduce the amount, or at least help parents not feel immobilized or responsible for it when it is not easy to console the baby. Parents understand better when they have an appreciation of the enormous brain development that is occurring and realize that the irritability is related to the infant learning how to handle all the stimuli coming into the developing central nervous system.

The parents' observations were used in the NSIBB program as much as possible in order to make these somewhat abstract ideas more concrete. By building on the use of their observations, parents' confidence was reinforced by the nurse, who showed them that they were the best source of information about their own baby. The nurse's role was to help the parents understand the behaviors, to interpret what the parents observed, and to validate what the parents reported.

In a visit with a 15-year-old primiparous mother and 17-year-old father, the nurse was able to involve both parents as they each reported on their infant's behaviors. They were able to pinpoint the infant's various states and behaviors that they had noticed during each state. For example, the parents reported that their infant made sucking noises and furrowed its brow during sleep. The nurse further confirmed this and identified this as being a period of light sleep.

By using what they had noticed, explaining what they had seen, and noting the practical implications, the nurse was able to help these parents understand and use the state information in their "window." Finally, using the 24-hour recall, the nurse was able to give anticipatory guidance as to what changes might occur in the infant's sleep/wake pattern. By being prepared for these occurrences the parents would not be caught off guard, and therefore there was less chance for them to become anxious about various behaviors. By letting the parents know what normally can be expected, such as that there are temporary changes that are signs of the infant's growth and development, a positive perception of some of these behaviors can be facilitated.

Feeding Interaction

It is recommended that for newborns you do your first feeding interaction observations shortly after the first 2 weeks. We recommend using the NCAST Feeding Scale

(Sumner & Spietz, 1994a). The Feeding Scale is a 76-item binary scale built around the model of parent–child interaction described previously (Barnard, 1994). In addition to the subscale structure of the parent and child characteristics, there are a number of concepts included in scale items. These include contingency, positioning, verbalness, sensitivity, affect, and engagement/disengagement cues of the infant. In the NSIBB program the feeding was observed at the second visit, at 3 weeks. If you are already concerned about the dyad at birth, you should try by all means to do an assessment as soon as possible and begin supportive feedback. You can use the episode to give the mother immediate help with whatever would improve the feeding interaction, such as positioning, waking the baby first, demonstrating how to respond contingently, and/ or talking to the baby. Because we know that infant behavior is not stable, you may want to do several observations and pool your observations to get a more representative picture of the infant's role as a social partner. Also, the mother's responsiveness might be influenced by her circumstances: We find mothers with low education and poverty conditions are less responsive, and mothers with depression are less active in the interaction. The dyadic dance is developing during these early weeks, and it is ideal to support the mother, father, and infant during this time.

☐ Parent Activities to Encourage the Infant's Development

When the infant was 5 weeks old, *vocal imitation* was discussed. This was taught as a fun activity for the parents and infant, as well as a time of learning for the infant. The role of imitation in early learning was presented, but the infant's developing awareness of his or her impact on the environment was stressed. As the infant is imitated, he or she gains awareness of effect on the world, and by hearing his or her own sounds the infant is encouraged to further vocalize.

Infant massage, infant exercises, and physical games were taught during both the 5-week and 8-week visits. To teach these techniques the mothers were given a picture booklet that showed each massage stroke or exercise along with a brief written description. The techniques were further taught by the nurse as she demonstrated and verbally explained the booklet contents (Booth, Johnson-Crowly, & Barnard, 1985). If possible, the nurse demonstrated the techniques on the baby. In teaching the massage, if the baby was unavailable, the nurse briefly demonstrated the main strokes on herself or on the mother. This was done so the mother would have as clear an understanding of the activity as possible without a live demonstration.

After presenting the activity, the nurse reviewed those areas that may have been confusing to the mother. She then encouraged the mother to try the activity each day, or as often as possible. The nurse suggested ways in which massage could be incorporated into the infant's bath time, or how the mother could do infant exercises while she watched TV. The nurse also encouraged each mother to share the booklet with her partner as an activity he might enjoy as well. One NSIBB mother shared both activity booklets with her babysitter and encouraged her to do them while she cared for the infant.

Baby exercises were introduced during the fourth NSIBB visit, when the infant was about 8 weeks old. If the infant was alert, the nurse demonstrated these while she and the mother sang a song such as "This Old Man." The exercises were introduced as an arousing activity, with a livelier beat and more vigorous movements than the massage. They were encouraged as a fun activity to do with the infant as well as providing some benefits for the infant's motor development.

In addition to the exercises, *physical games* were introduced and taught to the mothers during this visit. These games combined physical stimulation with singing. Although the exercises moved only one body part at a time, physical games moved the baby's whole body at once, thus creating a unique sense of space for the baby. Again, if the baby was in an appropriate state, the nurse would demonstrate the games for the mother so she could see how they were done.

Many mothers were already doing some of these games, which they would show to the nurse. These games were encouraged as a fun, non-task-oriented activity that they could do with their infants. Some of the NSIBB mothers who reported that they did not know what to do with children this young were excited to get these ideas. Success for the mothers pertaining to these activities depended on their ability to incorporate the infant communication information and state information into their activities with their infant. The mothers who were able to judge their infants' mood, activity level, and likes and dislikes were successful with these activities and enjoyed doing them. Generally, massage was best liked if the mother had selected a time when the infant was in a quiet-alert state, such as after a bath or early in the morning. The exercises were more often enjoyed in the afternoon and when the infant was in an active-alert state.

A case from the NSIBB sample is presented to show how this important content about infant behavior, parent–child interaction, and developmental activities is incorporated into the ongoing nurse–client relationship and the ongoing life of the family. The NSIBB aspects of the case are highlighted and some explanatory clinical notes are italicized. Mrs. N, a 25-year-old mother, had recently moved to the West Coast from New York City. She had 12 years of education. She lived with her husband and two children, ages 3 and 5, in a temporary shelter. She had begun prenatal care when she was 3 months pregnant, gaining 36 pounds during her pregnancy. The pregnancy was complicated by a seizure during the third month. She began seizure medications during the last month of pregnancy. She described the labor and delivery as "hard." She delivered a 7-pound, 11-ounce infant.

> It is helpful to have as much information about the pregnancy and birth as possible. These events are important to the parents and will be a point of conversation as you begin your acquaintance.

First contact with this mother was by phone while she was still in the hospital. She was friendly and interested in our future home visits. The first visit was scheduled for three days following discharge, when the infant would be 6 days old.

> With shorter hospital stays your first contact may require assessment of physical status of both the infant and mother.

The nurse made the first home visit at the temporary shelter home. The visit began with a review of the program. After telling Mrs. N what this first visit would involve, the physical assessments of both mother and baby were done. Areas of concern were discussed in more detail, such as breast-feeding problems, the mother's nutrition, contraception, and umbilical cord care.

During the infant's physical exam, the nurse verbally commented on what she observed, such as the infant's calm manner and ability to maintain a quiet-alert state without becoming upset by the physical manipulations of the exam. The sleep/wake recall was done and was used as a base from which to teach Mrs. N about infant states and possible changes to expect in the infant's schedule. The nurse first demonstrated the infant's visual abilities by using her face and then the red ball. The mother then took the ball and tried to elicit the infant's responses as well. Pictures were used to reemphasize the information about infant abilities, and examples of good stimuli were identified in the environment.

> The "windows" the nurse used were the physical and behavioral exams to bring the mother closer to the window of understanding her baby. Most parents find the recording of sleep and wake states to be very organizing. The actual recording makes them aware of patterns and the relationship of caregiving events and the infant's pattern of feeding or sleeping.

This mother was attentive and receptive to all the information given during this visit. At the end of the visit, Mr. N and their two other children arrived. Mrs. N. introduced the nurse to them. This father was clearly involved with their children and was supportive of his wife's participation with the nursing visits. He had a part-time job and was looking for additional work but until he found better employment, the family was applying for welfare assistance. The nurse directed them to the WIC (Women, Infants, and Children) program and provided them with the address and phone number of a nearby clinic that had a WIC office.

> During the first contact with a family it is important to get acquainted and develop the relationship. We try to restrict the program content of this initial visit and spend more time on developing the relationship.

The second visit was made 2 weeks later when the baby was 20 days old. The family had moved to a small single-family home by the time of this visit. All the physical problems or concerns noted during the first visit were monitored in this and in subsequent visits. Mr. N had filled in the sleep/wake records from the notes his wife had kept. They recorded the infant's sleep/wake activity for 10 days instead of the 7 requested. This mother had found the NCASA record helpful and interesting in that she was able to see her infant's pattern. Both parents had filled in the observation record, which had been left with them during the previous visit. These records were used by the nurse to guide the discussion about their infant's behaviors.

> This was an excellent way to involve the father in getting acquainted with their infant. We have found fathers react positively to such activities and read the parent handouts more eagerly than the mothers.

The fussy periods, noted on the NCASA, were not frustrating for this mother. She reported that these periods seemed to occur when the family was tired but that the father was especially helpful during these times. In going through the crying booklet, the nurse reinforced and supported much of what the parents had been doing for their infant.

The consistency of their caregiving was emphasized as the infant's developing trust was discussed. Infant communication and cue information was received with enthusiasm and was further clarified by using photos. The mother was excited and proud of her infant's development and was eager to tell the nurse that the infant was already looking at his hands. She also reported that she thought she heard the infant "coo," but added that her husband said he was too young. After reassuring the mother that the infant might be making cooing sounds, the nurse encouraged her to begin imitating his sounds. When her husband came home, his wife greeted him saying, "He is cooing, he's not too young."

When infants give responses the parent can relate to, such as looking at his hands and cooing, and you can validate that they are real behaviors, you can help parents better understand their baby's behavior.

The mother began this visit by complaining of headaches and dizziness, and she said she wanted to stop breast-feeding and return to work. The nurse asked about the physical symptoms, exploring possible reasons for them and some possible remedies before she moved into the NSIBB program content. Mrs. N brought out the observation and NCASA records she had kept. The observation record was only partially completed, so the rest of the record was finished together with the nurse as the nurse and mother discussed the infant's behaviors and the mother's observations. Infant cues were further reviewed as this record was completed. Mrs. N had no difficulty tuning into her baby's cues. She felt that his cues were very clear when he wanted to play, eat, or rest, or when he was full.

> It is important to realize the heavy demands on a new parent; therefore, when they haven't completed a task, such as the behavioral observation record, accept where they are and take them a little further in their window of understanding their baby.

The mother, as the expert observer, was reinforced when her observations were validated and encouraged. She again completed more sleep records than the nurse requested. She continued to find them helpful in learning about her baby and in organizing her own day. Massage was introduced. The nurse demonstrated the massage strokes as the mother watched and followed along in the written booklet.

The last topic to be discussed in this visit was Mrs. N's feelings about her infant's responsiveness. She felt that he knew her voice and that he responded especially to her. She noted that he was better able to follow her movements as she moved across the room than he was during the first week at home. The nurse ended the visit by giving her some anticipatory guidance as to what might occur in the next 3 weeks of their baby's development.

The week 8 visit was made when the infant was 8½ weeks old. The nurse noticed, on arrival, a change in Mrs. N's mood. She was grumpy and short-tempered with her 3-year-old daughter. As the visit began she reported that she was tired and had painful cysts on her ovaries. She was receiving appropriate medical care for her condition, so the NSIBB nurse listened and gave her support.

Regarding her fatigue, an evaluation of the NCASA identified specific problems. From this assessment the nurse was able to suggest some alternatives the mother could try. These records were compared to earlier records, which clearly showed the infant's maturing as evidenced by more prolonged alert periods and longer stretches of night sleep. The mother's experience with the massage was explored. She liked doing it and reported that her husband was doing it as well. She reported that the infant "will laugh and get excited, then will stay quiet and alert afterwards just looking around and entertaining himself." She demonstrated the massage. She had modified the techniques to her style, using her fingertips rather than the palms of her hands. She added that she usually used oil which she warmed, and discovered that the massage strokes were useful for burping.

> Feedback for the parent's observations and activities is important. The infant at this stage is only beginning to be a good social partner and doesn't always make it clear that his mother is doing great. It is music to the mother's ear to hear praises from "experts."

Infant exercises were introduced. The nurse was only able to demonstrate some of the techniques because the infant was hungry. The exercise picture booklet was relied on for the rest of the exercise discussion. Vocal imitation was actively being done by these parents. The mother reported that when the father did it, he and the baby got a mini-conversation going back and forth.

The infant's development was further discussed as the mother reported that "he has become a real member of the family. He accepts the other children and responds to each one of them." During this visit, the nurse observed interactions between the mother and infant that were full of mutual gazing and smiling. These observations were noted and the mother was given positive reinforcement and encouragement.

Mr. N had been laid off from his two part-time jobs, so the financial situation of the family was shaky. Both parents were optimistic about his returning to work after the holidays. At the end of the visit, this mother again asked for extra NCASA records because she found them helpful in her daily planning.

The last NSIBB visit was made 4 weeks later, when the infant was about 12 weeks old. First the sleep/wake records were reviewed. Mrs. N noted how her infant's schedule had become more predictable. Her observation record was done and her observations were discussed with the nurse. Her observations were astute, indicating that she was sensitive to her infant. These observations were complimented and the nurse provided her with validation and reinforcement.

Mrs. N gave a return demonstration of the exercises. She reported that she did not like them as well as the massage, but she found the infant liked them after his bath. The father enjoyed doing them and was doing them daily. The nurse discussed with her the benefits of "tuning in" to the infant. Mrs. N noted that it seems to make her interactions more satisfying. She also commented that her husband often "plays beyond the early cues till the baby fusses and cries." The nurse gave her support for her interest in, enjoyment of, and pride in her infant. She also encouraged Mrs. N to share what she had learned with her husband.

In concluding this visit, the nurse gave the mother some pamphlets regarding accident prevention, growth, and development, and suggested activities for babies up to 1 year. Further community resources were suggested that the family could use. Mrs. N was given back all the records she had completed in the NSIBB program, which she planned to keep with her infant's baby book.

> This case was very appropriate for the focused, NSIBB educational program. The activities were well received by the family, especially the massage and vocal imitations. The father, who learned the NSIBB activities from the instruction booklets and from Mrs. N, also enjoyed these activities. Mrs. N was able to maintain the records which were part of this program. In fact, she consistently requested additional ones. This mother was able to focus her attention on her baby and was receptive to new information and ideas.

Many communities have a nurse or lay home visitor going to the home for the first weeks after birth. Sharing information that will foster the acquaintance between the parents and infants will intensify and enhance the parent–infant relationship. This approach can be integrated into the health-care professional's agenda.

☐ Conclusion

In this chapter we have presented the elements of what should be included in anticipatory guidance for all new parents. This includes information about infant sleep/wake patterns, infant behavioral responses, which include the infant's ability to see and hear and learn from the environment, infant nonverbal communication cues, parent–child interaction skills, and techniques for engaging the parent and infant in rich interaction during the early months of life. It is our belief that all parents deserve at least this limited exposure to what developmental scientists have discovered about the infant's enormous capacity to interact with the environment. Developing the parent–infant partnership must be a top priority of any professional who interacts with the parents and infant during the first 3 months of life. We have described a curriculum we used in the NSIBB program and highlighted the elements of content and process that we feel were critical to the program's success. We presented the process of this curriculum with one family and showed how the program is tailored to the needs and interests of the parents and infant. To not give parents this type of anticipatory guidance and support is unacceptable for any society that treasures children, families, and our future. It is in the establishment of this early social partnership that the infant has the foundations for later learning and behavior. Parent–child interaction is the rich cloth from which the child is crafted into a developing child and a mature and caring adult. Opening the parental "windows" of understanding with each infant is one of the important opportunities in this world (Barnard, 1992; Barnard, Morisset, & Spieker, 1993).

☐ References

Barnard, K. E. (1976). *NCAST II learners resource manual.* Seattle: NCAST Publications, University of Washington.

Barnard, K. E. (1980). Sleep behavior of infants—Is it important? In K. E. Barnard (Ed.), *Nursing child assessment sleep/activity manual.* Seattle: NCAST Publications, University of Washington..

Barnard, K. E. (1981). General issues in parent-infant interaction during the first years of life. In D. L. Yeung (Ed.), *Essays on pediatric nutrition* (pp. 161–182). Ottawa, Ontario: Canadian Science Committee on Food and Nutrition, Canadian Public Health Association.

Barnard, K. E., (1992) Prenatal and infancy programs. In J. D. Hawkins, R. F. Catalano, & Associates (Eds.), *Communities that care.* San Francisco: Jossey-Bass.

Barnard, K. E. (1994). What the feeding scale measures. In G. Sumner & A. Spietz (Eds.), *NCAST caregiver/parent–child interaction feeding manual.* Seattle: NCAST Publications, University of Washington.

Barnard, K. E., Booth, C. L., Mitchell, S. K., & Telzrow, R. W. (1988). Newborn nursing models: A test of early intervention to high risk infants and families. In E. Hibbs (Ed.), *Children and families: Studies in prevention and intervention.* Madison, CT: International Universities Press.

Barnard, K. E., Hammond, M. A., Booth, C. L., Mitchell, S. K., & Spieker, S. J. (1989). Measurement and meaning of parent–child interaction. In F. J. Morrison, C. E. Lord, & D. P. Keating (Eds.), *Applied development psychology* (Vol. III). New York: Academic Press.

Barnard, K. E., Hammond, M. A., Mitchell, S. K., Booth, C. L., Spietz, A., Snyder, C., & Elsas, T. (1985). Caring for high-risk infants and their families. In M. Green (Ed.), *The psychosocial aspects of the family.* Lexington, MA: Lexington Books.

Barnard, K. E., Morisset, C. E., & Spieker, S. J. (1993). Preventive interventions: Enhancing parent–infant relationship. In C. Zeanah (Ed.), *Handbook on infant mental health.* New York: Guilford Press.

Blackburn, S. (1980). State organization in the newborn: Implications for caregiving. In K. E. Barnard (Ed.), *NCAST I learner manual.* Seattle: NCAST Publications. University of Washington.

Booth, C. L., Johnson-Crowley, N., & Barnard, K. (1985). Infant massage and exercise: Worth the effort? *American Journal of Maternal–Child Nursing,* 10, 184–189.

Brazelton, T. B. (1962, April). Crying in infancy. *Pediatrics, 29,* 579–588.

Brazelton, T. B. (1973). *Neonatal behavioral assessment scale.* Philadelphia: J. B. Lippincott.

Brazelton, T. B. (1974). *Toddlers and parents.* New York: Delacorte Press.

Brazelton, T. B. (1984). Neonatal behavioral assessment scale, 2nd ed. Clinics in developmental medicine, #88. London: Spastics International Medical Publications. Philadelphia: Lippincott.

Brazelton, T. B., & Cramer, B. G. (1990). *The earliest relationship: Parents, infants and the drama of early attachment.* New York: Addison-Wesley.

Brazelton, T. B., & Nugent, J. K. (1995). *Neonatal behavioral assessment scale* (3rd ed.). London: MacKeith Press.

Brazelton, T. B., Koslowki, B., & Main, M. (1974). The origins of reciprocity: The early mother-infant interaction. In M. Lewis & I. Rosenbaum (Eds.), *The effect of the infant on its caregiver* (pp. 123–129). New York: John Wiley & Sons.

Cardone, I. A., & Gilkerson, L. (1989). Family administered neonatal activities: An innovative component of family centered care. *Zero to Three, X*(1), 23–28.

Coons, S. (1987). Development of sleep and wakefulness during the first six months of life. In C. Gulleminault (Ed.), *Sleep and its disorders in children* (pp. 17–27). New York: Raven Press.

Eriks, J. (1979). Infant talk. In K. E. Barnard (Ed.), *NCAST II. Learner manual.* Seattle: NCAST Publications, University of Washington

Morisset, C. (1994). What the Teaching Scale measures. In G. Sumner & A. Spietz (Eds.), *NCAST caregiver/parent–child interaction teaching manual.* Seattle: NCAST Publications, University of Washington.

Murphy, L. B. (1973). Development in the 1st year of life: Ego and drive development in relation to the mother–infant tie. In L. J. Stone, T. Smith, & L. B. Murphy (Eds.), *The competent infant.* New York: Basic Books.

NCAST. (1990). *Keys to caregiving manual.* Seattle: NCAST Publications, University of Washington.

Parmelee, A. H. (1964). Infant sleep patterns. *Journal of Pediatrics, 64.*

Parmelee, A. H., Wenner, W. H., & Schulz, H. R. Infant sleep patterns: From birth to 16 weeks of age. *Journal of Pediatrics, 65,* 576–582.

Sumner, G., & Spietz, A. (1994a). *NCAST caregiver/parent–child interaction. Feeding manual.* Seattle: NCAST Publications, University of Washington.

Sumner, G., & Spietz, A. (1994b). *NCAST caregiver/parent–child interaction. Feeding manual.* Seattle: NCAST Publications, University of Washington.

INTERVENTION PRIORITIES FOR THE TWENTY-FIRST CENTURY

CHAPTER 11

Aidan Macfarlane

Total Population Pediatrics for the Child of the Twenty-First Century

How will the child health services of the twenty-first century grow to meet the health needs of the child of the twenty-first century?

The two major threats to the health of all children into the twenty-first century will remain the same as they are today. These threats are poverty and ignorance, with the added threat in some countries of war and violence. Any approach to the future of child health has to take this into account.

The new perspective for those working in the field of child health is therefore that of *total population pediatrics*—a pediatric specialty that is concerned with maintaining the optimal health and well-being of every child within a population. It promotes an integrated approach combining the health attitudes and behaviors of children themselves, the care given by parents, the primary health care team (family doctors and nurses), community/social pediatrics, public health medicine, secondary and tertiary care hospital pediatrics, and the socioeconomic and political environment. Thus, hospital pediatrics becomes just one of many facilities in helping to maintain the health of a whole population of children in the best state available given current knowledge. It is also a concept that puts increasing emphasis on (a) recognizing children's attitudes and behaviors as being vital to their own health, (b) the parents as the primary health care givers to their children, and (c) the importance of health promotion and prevention of illness.

☐ Developing Total Population Pediatrics

The future development of total population pediatrics is based on a logical approach to the overall delivery of health services for children that sets out to:

1. Define, by epidemiological studies, what health problems affect the population of children. A less sophisticated and more practical approach is to question those working in the field of child health as to what they see are the major health priorities and to take the common problems that are identified.
2. Review available research and carry out new research (if possible using specific controlled trials) to find the optimal forms of intervention available in order to improve outcomes (these forms of intervention can be social, environmental, political, medical, etc.).
3. Define the most appropriate personnel (parents, politicians, teachers, social workers, community nurses, and doctors) to carry out the interventions.
4. Set priorities for the interventions in light of (a) the severity of the health problem because of mortality and morbidity it causes, (b) the prevalence of the problem, (c) the effectiveness of the intervention, and (d) the resources available.
5. Set strategic objectives to include measurable targets, for example, reducing the rate of death of children from accidents by 5% per year.
6. Monitor whether the interventions are being implemented and monitor the cost and quality of the interventions.
7. Develop outcome measures by which to judge whether the prioritized interventions are effective if applied to whole populations.

The main measures involved in this scenario are therefore concerned with the health needs of a population, the effectiveness of the interventions, monitoring the implementation of outputs (interventions), and the inputs needed to achieve the outputs and the outcomes. Applying these strategies will ensure that the future services for the care of children within a population are increasingly flexible in order to maximize the use of what will always be limited resources.

☐ Developing Child Health Services

This broad-based approach leads to a wide range of possible interventions covering many different fields, including political, socioeconomic, public health, and primary, secondary, and tertiary medical care. However, in the future it is essential to try to be absolutely clear about what are the most effective (and cost-effective) ways of intervening, and which services are best at delivering the intervention.

For example, attempting to prevent children from smoking—via governmental intervention in raising the price of cigarettes, enforcing laws banning the sales of cigarettes to children, and banning cigarette advertising—is a far more effective intervention than having those involved in health education tell children that cigarette smoking is dangerous to their health.

Alternatively, providing an effective immunization program needs a combination of effort between government in their provision of resources and overall organization of services: the primary health care teams to give the vaccine, parents to bring their children, and research workers to develop effective vaccines.

☐ The Challenges of Total Population Pediatrics

Children and Parents

Child health services will need to continue to acknowledge that parents are the principal providers of child care and are ultimately responsible for the health of themselves and their children. In providing health services to the whole population of children and families with the aim of maintaining all children's health and development in an optimal state, it is becoming essential to ensure that the format and location of services allow for true partnership between parents and health professionals.

This philosophy is based on the research showing that parents deal with 80% of illness in their children without referring to a medical professional (Spencer, 1984). Before consulting a medical professional, the average parent consults at least three other nonmedical professionals, usually a relative, friend, or neighbor. It is therefore essential that parents are provided, via the media, books, magazines, and leaflets, information that helps them make informed decisions about the appropriate action they should take when their child becomes ill.

One major move toward this objective in the United Kingdom has been the development of a national, parent-held "personal child health record" (British Pediatric Society, 1993b). This record is now given to almost every mother having a baby. It is deliberately loose-leaved, with the aim that it will start with information about antenatal care and follow the child through the preschool and school years into adulthood. It is designed to be used not only by health professionals but by all those concerned with the care of the child. It contains extensive sections for the parent's own observations of the child's health and development, and sections for the child's preschool teachers, and pages can be added for therapists and others who may be involved in the child's care. Having the parents hold the record not only acknowledges the parents' essential role in the care of their child, but makes the appropriate information available at whatever point the parents seek help for their child, whether this be at home, at an accident and emergency department, at a hospital outpatient center, or at a doctor's office.

Perhaps in the future not only will parents universally have full access to all other medical records kept on their child, but everyone of any age will either have full access to their own medical records or actually keep them themselves.

The "personal child health record" is also used to provide health education messages, particularly concerned with "accident prevention." However, if there is one well-learned lesson over the years, it is that health education and prevention are not simple. One cannot decide on a method of preventing a health problem one day and expect it to work the next day. Changing people's behaviors requires a highly complex mix of influences, perhaps the most effective of which is legislation (at least in the United Kingdom, where there is a tradition of most people abiding by laws). Nevertheless, because in general the UK population is so law-abiding, government has been slow to use this route, preferring instead the more ethical approach of the provision of information from multiple sources, on which to base an informed decision. As a result, there frequently remains a gap between the knowledge of health hazards and changes of behavior.

Thus in a survey of school children (Macfarlane et al., 1987) although 98% knew that smoking was harmful to their health, 21% still smoked. We are only beginning to understand just how complex are the issues that guide people's decision making and risk taking and how dangerous it may be to interfere with people's own individual informed decisions. However, certain general principles based on careful research have emerged, two of which are (a) that feeding back specific information about a person's health, such as the serum cholesterol level, is more likely to be effective in changing behavior than providing general information, and (b) that where information is provided via the media, such as a television program about preventing injury to children, follow-up with a direct professional input—for example, a visit from a health visitor to discuss the program—is much more likely to be effective.

Over the last decade, there has also been a huge increase in basic knowledge about child health and child rearing. This knowledge is now cognizant of recent research, and the findings are gradually being translated into forms that are of practical use to parents and children. Thus increasingly, articles in magazines, television programs, and books contain information about child health relating to day-to-day child activities such as "sleeping," "eating," "behaviors," and so on, that is consistent, sound, and research based. The result has been an ever-increasing sophistication of knowledge among parents about child health and development matters, and this will continue.

In the future, information about child health will therefore be transferred directly to parents without the intermediary of the medical profession. Technologies such as interactive software programs for use at home and in public places, such as libraries, will allow future parents and children to have access to medical information, and will allow them to make their own information-based decisions on health matters by moving through carefully developed "decision-tree" technology. These technologies will not preclude the need for medical practitioners and nurses, but will help to ensure that their advice and services are used with greater appropriateness by a more sophisticated and informed clientele. This trend will continue with the children themselves. Research indicates that by adolescence, that is, 10–18 years (Macfarlane et al., 1987), the majority of children (a) see themselves as being responsible for their own health, (b) understand that their behaviors will influence their health outcomes, and (c) show increasing concern about environmental issues influencing their future health. However, while children remain without political power (even in the most democratic countries they have no vote), they will continue to have little influence over environmental problems created today that will influence their health and their children's health into the next century.

The role of total population pediatrics within this trend will therefore be to continue to encourage and carry out research on basic child health problems as perceived by parents and children, to act as advocates on behalf of children and families, and to ensure that information is provided to children and parents in appropriate forms.

Developing Future Services for the Sick Child

There are two extremes of services for children. At one end are services that have high volume and low unit cost, for example, treatment of sore throats, rashes, mild gastrointestinal symptoms, and otitis media, which is mainly delivered by parents and the primary health care system within a local community setting. At the other end of the spectrum is low-volume, high-technology, very-high-cost care, mainly delivered via hospitals but now increasingly also being adapted to provide "hospital at home" facilities, such as the giving of factor VIII to hemophiliacs at home and the care of oxygen-dependent children at home.

Spanning the spectrum of care is medium-technology, medium-cost care by health professionals, delivered either in the home or as close to the home as possible on an ambulatory basis. Ambulatory care services can be defined simply as all health and illness care provided that does not involve overnight admission to hospital facilities (British Pediatric Society, 1993a). Included in this are emergency department pediatric care, pediatric day care (either medical or surgical), all outpatient care, acute ward assessments, home care, child health surveillance, specialist clinics, "hospital at home" schemes, primary care pediatrics, community pediatrics, child development and disability care, child protection, social pediatrics, health promotion, and pediatric community nursing services

Two compatible options to cover ambulatory care are (a) the provision of care in the community by an "outreach" from the hospital by health professionals whose main employment is in hospitals and (b) provision by doctors, nurses, and therapists whose main work is in the community and who are employed by community services, with "inreach" to cover some ambulatory functions that take place in hospital.

"Outreach" services from the hospital are usually for acute and chronically sick children who have been in the hospital and are subsequently, with adequate community support, then cared for earlier and better in the community, either by permitting earlier discharge from the hospital or even by preventing initial admission. The medical, nursing, and therapeutic care in these cases is normally provided by "specialist" pediatric doctors, nurses, and therapists based in a hospital and caring for children with relatively rare diseases such as diabetes, cystic fibrosis, and leukemias, and who are willing and able to help support the children and their families as close to their home as possible. This model will increase into the twenty-first century, with more and more pathology in children, such as diabetes and oncology, being treated entirely on an ambulatory basis, with no hospital admissions at all.

The "inreach" into the hospital from community services centers around the care provided in hospital emergency rooms and acute assessment units. In many hospitals in many countries, hospital emergency rooms are used as the primary health care facility (this is unlike the UK model where the family doctor and primary health care nurses act as "gatekeepers" to the hospital services, including, to a large extent, the use of emergency rooms). Having the most experienced doctors working at the "front doors" of the emergency rooms of these hospitals is most essential to the "inreach" concept. These doctors need to be experienced pediatricians with an intimate knowledge of community facilities or experienced family physicians. Either way, the emphasis in the twenty-first century will be on ensuring that whenever feasibly safe, children with acute medical problems are either sent back into the community to be treated at home, or treated in a short-stay (less than 12 hours) acute assessment or observation facility attached to the emergency room, rather than being admitted to a hospital.

A huge amount of the workload of emergency departments involved with children can be carried out with such a simple short-stay observation facility, which can be run by nurses, using parents as the observers. The commonest problems that could be managed in this way include much traumatology, including head injuries, ingestions and poisons, asthma, diarrhea and vomiting, and respiratory infections. Depending on the pediatric workload of the emergency room, such an observation facility could be run on an 8-hour, 12-hour, 16-hour, or 24-hour basis.

The cost of such a facility (which already exists in some hospitals) is relatively low compared with the costs of full inpatient admission, with its long "turnaround" time–

the time between admission and discharge, inevitably lengthened by paperwork, routine workups, dependency on the timing of senior doctor ward rounds, and loss of immediate contact with parents who may have returned home.

Also within this equation of preventing hospital admission are the emotional needs of the children not to be separated from their parents, not to have to be admitted to a strange and frightening environment for longer than necessary, and the far from negligible dangers of children picking up infections while in the hospital.

The Care of Chronically Ill Children with Complex Medical Problems

One of the most challenging aspects of child health in the twenty-first century is our increasing technological ability to keep alive severely ill children with highly complex medical problems (oxygen-dependent children, children with tracheostomies or gastrostomies, children with parenteral feeding needs, etc.) who would previously have died. Society's willingness and financial ability to provide full support to the families of these children, with 24-hour-a-day nursing needs, lags far behind its willingness to provide the technology that only ensures immediate survival. A challenge of the twenty-first century will therefore be to ensure that these short-term technologies are only financed if the finances are also available to bear the enormous financial cost of supporting the families in their long-term care of these children. The resources required for one form of treatment should never be separated from the other, as they are at the moment.

Clarification of Child Health Services in the Community

Within total population pediatrics, the future roles of social/community pediatrics need clarification. At the present time these include:

1. Provision of parental support, clinical cover, health promotion, immunizations, surveillance, and management and treatment of health problems for all preschool and school children.
2. Responsibility for the early identification, assessment, management, and treatment of all children with impairments, disabilities, and handicaps.
3. Provision of clinical care in the community for children with acute and chronic illnesses on an ambulatory basis.
4. Provision of specialized health services to all families who may have difficulties accessing medical services (e.g., children from homeless families, migrant families, ethnic minority families).
5. Provision of diagnostic, assessment, support, and management services to all children who have been subjected to physical and sexual abuse.
6. Provision of initial medical assessment and continuing medical supervision to all children who are adopted, fostered, or taken into care.
7. Liaison with all the acute hospital services concerned with the care of children, with the primary health care teams, with the local education authorities, with the local county council, and with social services.
8. Planning, monitoring, managing, administering, and auditing all these services.
9. Provision of training for staff working in all these services.

Development of Appropriate Information Technologies

Crucial to the developing concept of the child health services in the community has been taking on responsibility for the health of every child within a population—a concept as already stated of total population pediatrics, with concern for every child, whether that child is at home, in care, in a hospital, or at school. A major movement report (Steering Group on Health Services Information, 1984) in the United Kingdom said of health services information systems in England that:

> Screening and surveillance of children, as well as immunization, require a level of administration and co-ordination which cannot be undertaken effectively without a computer-based system. As most programs directed towards children are intended for every child, there is agreement on the need to develop a single integrated administrative system in each district designed to schedule appointments and ensure an accurate record of immunization, surveillance, screening tests and action in relation to special educational needs.

The result in the United Kingdom has been a proliferation of child health computer systems run on anything from personal computers used by individual child health doctors to "mainframe" computers running a national child health software system at the national level. In most UK health districts, some health information is being collected on computer on every child. At the time of writing, 80% to 90% of 90 English health districts are using the national system for their immunization date data, 40% are using it for preschool child development data, and 20% are using it to record school health information. Increasingly, the systems are "real-time" with access to information on visual display units in the community, in health centers and in hospitals. In the not too distant future, all computer systems at the health district level will be compatible so that family doctors, community doctors, community nurses, and hospital doctors and nurses will all be able to get the same basic information on every child from any terminal. With children in the community with handicapping conditions who need help from services supplied from health, education, and social services, detailed computer information about the child will need to be shared among all three services. Concerns about the confidentiality issues for such information appear ill founded. When parents understand that such sharing of information brings more and better resources to meet their child's needs, they are more than happy, research shows.

Other invaluable information for the community child health services has been provided by national surveys carried out by epidemiologists. For example, details of 13,135 children born in 1970 and followed up in the Child Health and Education Study have been reported in the book *From Birth to Five* (Butler & Golding, 1986). This provides a wealth of information concerning correlations between the children's social and environmental circumstances within the community and their health. Future studies along the same line are an integral part of the concept of total population pediatrics.

Future Integration of Community and Hospital Pediatrics

Integration between hospital and community pediatrics in the United Kingdom has been most rapid in the field of nursing. Specialist clinical pediatric nurses working with children with diabetes, asthma, epilepsy, and cancers are now appearing in increasing numbers. Their main roles are in the community, either directly supporting the children and their families or helping teach and support other members of the primary health care team, including the family doctor. The benefits of such nursing support in the community are clear. For instance, in the Oxford Health District in 1981 there were 44 acute admissions of children with diabetes due to poor control of their blood sugars. The diabetic nurse began work in 1985 and, in spite of an increasing prevalence of children with diabetes both locally and nationally, the number of admissions of children with diabetes fell to 14 in 1989. The estimated cost benefits in saving of hospital admissions not only covers the salary of the nurse, but saves a further £29,000.

Future specialist pediatric nurses in the community are most needed for children with asthma, cancer, intensive neonatal care, and cystic fibrosis. Such nurses will be responsible for not only the care of individual children in the community but also the transfer of care of these children to the primary health services, such as family doctors and primary health care nurses.

Children will therefore, in the future, be able to grow up in the community with the knowledge that they will receive maximum support from an integrated community/ hospital service. There will be widespread benefits for the children and their families and for the hospital, which can redirect scarce resources at more needy areas, by ensuring that unnecessary hospital admissions are avoided.

The main developments between community and hospital pediatric care include:

- Developing day care for a wide variety of surgical and medical pediatric problems with the resulting cost benefits for the services and emotional benefits for parents and child.
- Working to achieve the aim that no child should be admitted to hospital unnecessarily.
- Developing joint protocols for the care of specific conditions in the community and in the accident and emergency departments.
- Monitoring of accident and emergency department statistics.
- Monitoring hospital admissions.
- Monitoring referrals from primary health care teams.
- Developing a clinical pediatric community nursing service for children with chronic clinical problems.
- Developing an integrated service for the care of handicapped children.

Future Integration of Pediatrics and Public Health Medicine

This will be mainly in the following areas (Faculty of Public Health Medicine and the British Pediatric Association, 1990):

- Monitoring screening programs.
- Organization of immunization programs.
- Liaison with social services and education services.
- Organization of health promotion programs.
- Health advocacy (especially political).
- Community approaches to prevention.
- Training other health professionals.
- Planning and developing children's services.
- Developing outcome measures for child health.

Primary Prevention

Primary prevention—through political intervention, advocacy with industry, forming alliances, and health education—is perhaps one of the fastest developing and rewarding areas of total population pediatrics. Much of the work demands careful research, data collection, and data use. It is impossible here to touch on more than two specific areas. Immunization is, of all the work of community pediatrics, perhaps the most important and in many countries the most successful. This has also demonstrated the benefits of a central organization and administration. A senior medical officer at the Department of Health in the United Kingdom manages the immunization service nationally by having established a designated immunization coordination in each district with overall responsibility for the immunization rates. These immunization officers meet regularly to discuss, among other things, methods of increasing immunization rates, new immunizations, and new schedules. It would be difficult to single out anything specific as having so effectively increased immunization rates nationally; nevertheless, there has been a dramatic increase. Further, the use of triple vaccines has been demonstrated to have a 14:1 cost-benefit ratio—that is, it is 14 times cheaper to immunize children than to bear the medical costs of the diseases themselves.

As well as greatly improved immunization rates, we have information showing that outcomes, measured as the actual prevalence of the diseases that we are seeking to prevent, have also fallen dramatically.

The aim of the World Health Organization's Health for All 2000 program includes countries being able to manage at least a 90% uptake rate for all basic immunizations, and this has already been achieved by the United Kingdom. For the future, international child health organizations are working to move manufacturers toward the next goal of developing vaccines that are even more polyvalent so that a single injection might protect a child against six or eight infectious diseases. The other goal is that such vaccines should be thermostable so that the cold chain will no longer be the vital and vulnerable link that it is at present.

Prevention of Injury

A further example of both primary prevention and liaison between various services is in the field of injury prevention. In Oxford we are using a community liaison nurse to collect statistics at the accident and emergency department. From January 1988 to December 1989 out of a total of 2273 visits to the emergency department at Oxford's John Radcliffe Hospital in children aged 0–16 years for treatment for accidents, 808 (36%) were due to head injuries, and of 303 admissions because of accidents, 140 (46%) were due to head injuries. Information was also collected on other types of accidents. Subsequently a health education program via community nurses was implemented, and we are continuing to monitor visits at the accident and emergency department and admissions to judge the outcome of the intervention. This is an example of hospital community liaison, the value of information and information systems, and having an outcome against which to judge an intervention design to prevent injuries to children.

Injuries remain the single commonest cause of death in children aged 1 to 19 years, and American data show that for each child death due to injury there are 45 children who need admission to a hospital and 1300 who require some form of medical treatment (Guyer & Ellers, 1990).

Twenty-nine percent of deaths in children could be prevented by instituting 12 preventative measures at present available, according to estimates (Gallagher, Messenger, & Guyer, 1987). The major causes of severe injuries and death are motor vehicle accidents, both as car occupants and as pedestrians, drowning and near drowning, and burns. Injuries to children require special consideration because children depend on society to protect them from harm and to minimize their vulnerability from injury. Most injuries result from complex interactions of the environment, the host, and the energy source. No single intervention will normally be wholly effective, but opportunities for accident prevention certainly exist but are frequently not implemented.

The roles therefore of those involved in total population pediatrics in preventing injury are many—but the first is undoubtedly obtaining information concerning accidents in children in the local district. This can be achieved from many sources: local accident and emergency departments, the police, and the road safety officer of the local country council, to name but three. Many health districts in the United Kingdom are setting up joint planning committees on injury prevention between health, local country council, education, and the police.

☐ Conclusion

For the child of the twenty-first century to grow up healthy, we need to learn from one another and not try to reinvent the wheel. Many data about child health, effective interventions, and ways to best help children are already available in different countries, but in many cases we do not know about them, or if we do know about the data, we do not use them.

Careful reviews of already available national and international research are our most important and immediate priority for the future. Having identified effective means of intervention, we then need to implement them and monitor them against standard criteria.

It will be of enormous benefit to children worldwide if we can manage to swallow national pride and realize that we have a vast amount to learn from one another. We should begin to gather our information together and, as in this book, share it and make it available to all.

☐ References

British Pediatric Association. (1993a). *Flexible options for pediatric care*. London: Author.

British Pediatric Association. (1993b). *Parent held and professional records used in child health surveillance*. London: Author.

Butler, N., & Golding, J. (1986). *From birth to five*. New York: Pergamon Press.

Faculty of Public Health Medicine and the British Pediatric Association. (1990). *Together for tomorrow's children*. Report of joint working party.

Gallagher, S. S., Messenger, K. P., & Guyer, B. (1987). State and local responses to children's injuries: The Massachusetts Statewide Childhood Injury Prevention Program. *Journal of Social Issues, 43*, 149–162.

Guyer, B., & Ellers, B. (1990). Childhood injuries in the United States. *American Journal of the Diseases of Children, 144,* 649–652.

Macfarlane, A., McPherson, A., McPherson, K., & Ahmed, L. (1987). Teenagers and their health. *Archives of Disease in Childhood, 62*(11), 1125–1129.

Spencer, N. (1984). Parent's recognition of the ill child. In A. Macfarlane (Ed.), *Progress in child health* (Vol. 1, pp. 100–112). London: Churchill Livingstone.

Steering Group on Health Services Information. (1984). *Fifth report to the Secretary of State.* London: Her Majesty's Stationery Office.

Sheila Greene

Child Development:
Old Themes and New Directions

Developmentalists have a ready metaphor to describe the history of their own discipline. Thus one might be tempted to pinpoint the date when developmental psychology was born, to view developmental psychology at the turn of the century as being in its infancy, and to ask whether or not it has now, after traveling on through its childhood and youth, arrived at its maturity or whether it is still suffering from the *sturm und drang* of adolescence. I have resisted this temptation. Using the metaphor of steady, progressive development through predictable stages may always have been glib, but from the standpoint of the 1990s to write in this way would be to invite embarrassment. We have reached a different vantage point in terms of our general understanding of science and in particular of our understanding of the history of child psychology

It could be argued, and indeed has been argued most persuasively by Kessen (1986), that for most of this century, developmental psychologists shared the Western conviction that the march of science and civilization was leading us onward and upward. As a discipline, developmental psychology may well have been more prone than other branches of psychology to this belief in progress, because it is intrinsic to the concept of development itself. In reality, some of the more hopeful recent developments are rediscoveries of insights that were lost or are variations on very old themes.

The notion of science as a linear, unified enterprise advancing toward the truth or truths that could be expressed in universal laws or quantified in theorems was challenged fundamentally by Kuhn's book *The Structure of Scientific Revolutions* (1962), which argued that the history of science could be seen as the struggle for ascendancy between competing scientific paradigms. Kuhn was but one of many theorists who attacked fondly held nineteenth- and early-twentieth-century beliefs in absolutist notions such as progress and universal truth. The cherished idols of the modern era have been subject to the skeptical analysis of those writers who have been influenced by the postmodern shift in consciousness.

Inevitably this postmodern sensibility has become evident in the work of developmental psychologists. Its influence can be detected in a number of changes in contemporary preoccupations and practice. A self-critical stance has been brought to histories of the discipline (e.g., Bradley, 1989; Bronfenbrenner, Kessel, Kessen, & White, 1986). There is a new willingness to unpick the previous self-congratulatory discourse, to deconstruct and reinterpret. In this process a tangled story has emerged, or rather numerous tangled stories have emerged. Just as literary history, when reexamined through a feminist lens, permits the rediscovery of buried women writers, the new histories of developmental psychology have disinterred psychologists whose place in the history of the discipline deserves reappraisal. Accordingly, the work of early writers like Baldwin and Dewey has been reread and reevaluated (Cahan, 1992; Cairns, 1992). What is of particular interest now is that the work of these rediscovered writers, given its quality and undoubted resonance for psychologists of our time, was relatively neglected in its own time and certainly did not become part of the received history of the discipline. Despite the fact that this century has seen very distinctive phases in terms of the dominant perspectives on child development in Europe and North America, some underlying assumptions about the nature of development and the nature of childhood have been constant, as have underlying assumptions about the appropriate methodology for the discipline. The mood of skepticism and doubt that is emblematic of our time—though not necessarily common to all—has led in recent years to a radical reexamination of the foundational assumptions of the discipline.

☐ What Is Development?

One mark of the new critical reflectiveness is the attack on *developmentalism*, which could be defined as the imposition of an unwarranted uniformity of structure and directionality onto the changes associated with the ageing process. For most of this century the notion of unidirectional and natural progression lurked at the heart of the word *development* and at the heart of developmental psychology.

Morss (1990) traces the naturalistic assumptions behind the traditional developmental paradigm back to the romantic notions of social progress and human perfectibility that emerged in the nineteenth century. Theories about evolution proliferated at this time, and the views that were taken up by influential figures like Herbert Spencer and G. Stanley Hall were in many ways pre-Darwinian. Early developmentalists were certainly more concerned with notions to do with recapitulation and evolutionary hierarchies than with natural selection. As Morss noted:

> Perhaps the most fundamental assumption concerning an overall picture of individual development is that of *progress*. Derived from, or at least legitimated by biological sources, the notion that the individual gets better and better as time passes has been central to most developmental thinking. (Morss, 1990, p. 173)

The most obvious consequence of this commitment to ontogenetic progression can be seen in the proliferation of stage theories of development; Freud, Piaget, Erikson, and Kohlberg are examples of the most well-known stage theories in relation to child development. They all see development as moving toward what Labouvie-Vief and Chandler (1978) have called an idealistic endpoint, different in each case. Erikson (1953) encapsulated the biological thinking and the prescriptiveness behind these stage theories when he wrote, "the healthy child, if halfway properly guided, merely obeys and on the whole can be trusted to obey inner laws of development" (p. 61).

To the extent to which psychologists adhere to an unexamined and outdated form of biological thinking, there is undoubtedly a place for the critique offered by radical critics like Broughton (1987), Morss (1990, 1996), Burman (1994) and Bradley (1989). However, they are not alone in their dissatisfaction with the conceptualizations of development that have dominated this century to date, and there are definite signs of change. Some contemporary definitions of developmental psychology do not emphasize progression alone—they also emphasize regression. For example, Magnusson stated, "Development of living organisms refers to progressive or regressive changes in size, shape and function during the lifetime" (Magnusson, 1995, p. 20), and Baltes similarly referred to development as characterized by gains and losses (Baltes, 1989). There is much more awareness in contemporary thinking of the erratic and variable nature of psychological change and the extent to which change is a product of exchanges with the external environment rather than a matter of the unfolding of inherent potential. This realization begs the question of whether the terms *development* and *developmental* are the appropriate defining terms for this discipline because the emerging usage of these terms in psychology does not correspond to any dictionary definition.

Despite the fact that adherence to a nineteenth-century form of biological thinking can be seen to have produced a developmental psychology that was unduly prescriptive and universalistic, it is essential that the study of child development come to terms with the nature of the biological contribution to psychological development and change. In relation to child psychology, it is inescapably the case that many psychological changes are prompted by, or associated with, changes brought about by the growth and maturation of the body. Flavell (1970) went further and claimed that "it is the underlying presence of a biological growth process that lends to childhood changes their inevitability, magnitude, directionality, within-species uniformity and irreversibility" (p. 248).

No one would wish to deny the importance of physical maturation to childhood. However, what is questionable is the commitment on the part of child psychologists this century to the view that psychological change has the same characteristics and dynamic as physical change. Thus, just as the development of dentition occurs in a predictable, universal sequence in all healthy children, so, it has been assumed, does cognition, or attachment, or the self-concept, or moral reasoning. What such a perspective leaves out of account is the fact that although many of the psychological phenomena of interest are subject to change, the nature of that change may not be identical to or even comparable with genetically prompted physiological changes. Some psychological "developments" result from a process that can only be understood by reference to the active, constructive role of the person or the meaning-infused interactions of that person with others. Psychological phenomena are to a greater extent socially and historically contingent, and many of the important changes that occur in childhood are—to contradict Flavell—not inevitable, unidirectional and uniform.

As doors were opened to awareness of the complex nature of biological influences, the central role of social and cultural influences, and the active role of the person in shaping her or his own development, it became clear that human psychological change across time defies neat characterizations and that the old meaning of development has proved inadequate. The restricted developmental paradigm has operated like a straitjacket in this century, and it is time for it to be discarded.

In recent decades, the study of child development has been strongly influenced by many other disciplines, and many developmentalists have their roots in disciplines other than psychology. Within psychology the widening of the developmental focus to cover the life span has had an important influence on the conceptualization of child psychology and the nature of developmental processes. Of course, life-span psychology can be seen to subsume child psychology, but for a long time developmental psychology was confined to the study of children and adolescents. Examining psychological development from the life-span perspective casts a very different light on childhood. Much of the challenge to long-lived assumptions about development in childhood arrived with the extension of theory and research into adulthood. Thus the tendency to see childhood as a world apart psychologically has diminished, and the inadequacies of reductive accounts of psychological development become strikingly evident when they are applied to adults, to ourselves. Issues to do with continuity and discontinuity, constancy and change are highlighted by a life-span perspective in which recognition of the relative open-endedness and unpredictability of developmental processes has become unavoidable. The life-span developmental approach has helped to highlight the multiple mechanisms involved in the process of developmental change and to indicate the way in which childhood experiences may or may not be carried forward into adulthood (Baltes, 1987; Rutter, 1989).

At this point in time most developmental researchers would see themselves as only just beginning to understand the causes of development. The starting point for early developmentalists was to decide on *where* to look for the explanation—the biology of the organism or the environment.

☐ Nature and Nurture

Most child development textbooks start off with a history of the struggle between the empiricists—neatly epitomized by Locke and his *tabula rasa*—and the nativists, championed by Rousseau and his "noble savage." The resolution of the conflict, which was seen to continue in child development with the opposing views of the behaviorists like Watson and the maturationists like Gesell, was the civilized compromise of interactionism. Anastasi's paper "Heredity, Environment and the Question, How?" (Anastasi, 1958) marked a new way forward and supposedly put an end to the question, "How much?" As we have seen in recent years, with publications such as *The Bell Curve*, this question has still not gone away (Murray & Hernstein, 1994). In their rational moments the vast majority of child psychologists would reject extreme environmentalism and extreme hereditarian views. However, when it comes to the crunch, most developmental psychologists and scientists seem to lean in one direction or the other, and the old dichotomy can be seen in the emphasis on either genetic determinants or environmental/social determinants. The persistence of this split could be seen recently in the dispute that took place in the pages of *Child Development* between Scarr and Baumrind (Scarr, 1992; Baumrind, 1993). Baumrind took exception to Scarr's view that "genotypes drive experiences" and argued that "the details of socialization patterns are crucial to an understanding of normal and deviant development." Although the vocabulary and the data are different, the essentials of the old debate remain.

In relation to the origins of individual differences, one way forward might be seen in the work of those behavioral geneticists, such as Plomin, who do not diminish the role of environment but assert quite convincingly that the data that provide evidence of the strength of hereditary influence on individual development "provide the best available evidence for the importance of environmental influence" (Plomin, 1989, p. 105). On the other side, environmentalists find it increasingly difficult to disregard findings on the contribution of genetic factors to individual differences in ability or temperament or on the role of biological preparedness in determining the character of children's activities and experiences. Bronfenbrenner, for example, has taken the biological into fuller account in recent modifications of his ecological systems theory (Bronfenbrenner & Ceci, 1994). Plomin considered that "modern theory and research in both nature and nurture are converging on the interface between them" (Plomin, 1994, p. 20). New concepts, such as niche-picking, active, passive, and evocative genotype–environment effects, and proximal processes, are emerging as researchers struggle more assiduously to answer the question "How?" by identifying the mechanisms involved in the interplay between genes and environment (Bronfenbrenner & Ceci, 1994; Scarr & McCartney, 1983). But not all developmentalists would see this approach as representing the way forward. Gottlieb, for example, thought it was time to abandon entirely the nature–nurture dichotomy because it is an unfortunate hangover from "a pre-formation like predeterministic view of human development that has persisted to the present day . . . one that holds that traits are caused by genes in a staightforward unidirectional manner" (Gottlieb, 1992, p. 8). Instead, Gottlieb called for recognition of the "non-linear, emergent, coactional nature of individual development" (Gottlieb, 1992, p. 171).

At a species level, the importance of biologically based propensities and competencies cannot be denied, although the resurgence of interest among developmentalists in evolutionary theory as a grand explanatory framework (e.g., Belsky, 1995) is surprising, given its inability to account for complex psychological phenomena and its reliance on circular reasoning (see, e.g., Lerner & von Eye, 1992).

☐ What Develops?

For most of this century, the focus of interest in relation to the psychological development of the child has been very restricted. Even the so-called "grand theories" that have dominated child psychology in this century can be seen as focusing on an aspect of children and their psychology rather than the full picture. Thus we have "the child as conditionable organism" of the behaviorists, the "instinctual child" of Freud, "the child as logical thinker" of Piaget. More recently we have the child as information processor and the social child.

There are interesting signs of attempts to break down the long-standing barriers between the realms of cognition, emotion, and social development, which can be seen, for example, in recent work on social cognition (e.g., work on the theory of mind and person perception) and on the social-regulatory function of emotions (e.g., work on emotional self-regulation and social referencing). A consequence of the adoption of the supposed natural science method by mainstream child psychology has been the fragmentation of "the child." As Magnusson (1995) noted, we have concentrated on variables rather than persons. In recent years there has been a welcome renewal of discussion of the need for a holistic model of development, and models have been offered by a number of theorists such as Magnusson himself (1995) and Bronfenbrenner (1995).

Adopting a particular perspective on what it is that develops can all too readily lead to a very narrow vision. There are undoubtedly many examples of this kind of narrowed perspective and its consequences from the early days of the discipline onward, but I will take just one example from the study of infancy.

According to Piaget, the development of the concept of object permanence is an essential step on the road to rationality. Piaget observed that if a toy is hidden underneath a cloth in front of the infant's eyes, the infant will fail to search for the toy. Others have replicated his observations. Piaget claimed that the infant has not yet understood that objects are permanent and that they cannot disappear in this manner. The achievement of object permanence occurs with the development of the child's capacity to represent the world mentally, thus freeing the child from the here-and-now intelligence that is the hallmark of the sensorimotor period. Although critics of Piaget abound, his interpretation of his observations and the conclusions he drew about the crucial importance of the child's arrival at an understanding of the permanence of objects have been uncontested.

In a recent article, Greenberg (1996) pointed out that an alternative light can be cast on the child's understanding of the existence of objects. He said, "Piaget and his intellectual heirs have forgotten that the 'permanent' object is in principle and a priori impermanent and incapable of existing forever" (p. 118). Greenberg took, as an example of Piaget's bias, the preoperational child's failure to understand the conservation of matter. He reexamined one of Piaget's examples to do with the children's responses to the dissolving of a sugar cube. Piaget stated:

> The conservation of matter does not seem necessary to the child three to six years old in cases of changes of state or even changes of form. Sugar melting in water is believed to be returning to the void. . . . Just as the baby begins by believing that objects return to the void when they are no longer perceived and emerge from it when they re-enter the perceptual field, so also the six year old child still thinks that a substance which dissolves completely is annihilated. (Piaget, 1954, pp. 417–418)

As Greenberg pointed out, children are correct in thinking that the cube has been destroyed *qua* cube, although they have failed to understand that the matter that constituted the cube is still present in a different form.

Piaget's dismissive approach to the child's understanding of the impermanence of objects, arguably as important to their understanding of the world as an understanding of the possibility of conservation or of the relative permanence of some objects, is seen as a consequence of his emphasis on scientific, logico-mathematical thought. Rationality is thus equated with thinking of objects as permanent, invulnerable, and infinite, and irrationality with the failure to treat objects as though they had these properties. In fact, the infant must develop a rational understanding of the extent to which objects, including people, can be impermanent. Greenberg's article can be seen as representative of the current, deconstructive approach. It is notable that decades of criticism of Piaget have left untouched Piaget's assumptions about the nature of human rationality and its origins because these particular assumptions were cherished, one assumes, as much by his critics as by Piaget himself. Greenberg (1996) can also be seen as representative of the current interest in breaking down barriers between theoretical accounts of the child's cognitive, social, and emotional experiences. His dissatisfaction with the received interpretation originated in his interest in "that other form of reason that concerns itself with those impermanent objects of desire that are the focus of love and hate, hunger and revulsion, attachment and loss" (p. 130). It would seem that very often in the history of child development, the focus of theorists and researchers has been narrowed by an unduly restrictive, received wisdom about what aspects of the child are fit to be studied and what questions are permissible to be asked.

☐ Who Is the Child?

Putting the child back together again is not enough; we also have to recognize the richness and plurality that exist in the lives of children, the sources of their heterogeneous experiences, and the resultant constraints on the production of universalistic accounts of developmental processes.

The object of knowledge for mainstream child psychologists of the twentieth century has been "the child." This objectification of children has been the inevitable consequence of the emulation of the natural sciences and the associated quest for universal laws. Clearly there has had to be some recognition of individual difference, but the need to describe "the development of the child" and the underlying assumption that much of what develops represents an unfolding of natural propensities lead to a process that has been labeled the normalization of child development (Walkerdine, 1984). In the history of child development, normalization can be seen to go hand in hand with the biological view of development. The discipline has created norms against which all children's (and parents') behavior has been judged. Normalization constrains all children because it determines people's expectations of them and their own expectations of themselves. Children who do not conform to the natural developmental path are liable to be seen as deviant. In a circular process, children from the culture, class, or gender that is excluded from the definition of what is developmentally the norm are fated to be categorized as deviant, and therefore problematic.

In the latter part of this century, the civil rights movement and other social changes have led to a greater awareness of the extent of exclusion and of the role of science perpetuating a middle-class, Western, and male-centered view of the universe. The picture of ideal or "normal" development promoted by child psychologists was also permeated with these kinds of bias, although the delusion that science was a value-free enterprise kept people from a recognition of their own embeddedness in ideology.

Because, for most of this century, mainstream child psychology conceptualized the child in much the same way as a chemist conceptualizes an interesting compound, it made absolute sense for the psychologist to take the child into a laboratory for closer inspection and testing. To use Kessen's term, the child was seen as "isolable" (Kessen, 1979). Bronfenbrenner's accusation that much of mainstream developmental psychology could be summarized as "the science of the strange behaviour of children in strange situations with strange adults for the briefest possible periods of time" (Bronfenbrenner, 1979, p. 19) heralded a welcome awakening of concern for the ecological validity of child development research. The recognition of the problem of lack of ecological validity was part of a movement within developmental psychology to reconceptualize the nature and significance of the child's social context. This reconceptualization has had a perceptible impact on the focus of research, with an increased interest on the part of psychologists in observing children in their home, play, or school settings and in understanding how they negotiate and understand their social world. With the recognition of context and a renewed appreciation of the importance of culture come recognition of the plurality of children's experiences and an acknowledgment of the narrow cultural focus of much of the child development work carried out this century.

The questioning of traditional assumptions underpinning norms and prescribed sequences has led to an increased recognition and understanding of the heterogeneity that exists in children's lives and experiences. It is only comparatively recently that developmental psychologists have taken on board a view of culture as intrinsic to the child's psychology and not just an add-on that could be pared away to reveal the true child underneath. Contemporary child development is thus more about children in their cultures than about the child in isolation.

A further basic dichotomy that has been played out in this century is between the view of the child as passively responding to the forces operating on him or her versus the view of the child as an active agent in his or her own development. This is a struggle that has reached a resolution. The view of the child as active would appear now to be dominant—which is not to say that the child's behaviors and experiences are not constrained, because inevitably they are, but that children play an active role in shaping their own environments and in making sense of them.

☐ Reinstating Meaning

It could be argued that, in child psychology, as in other branches of psychology, a great deal has been lost by the neglect of the role of personal meaning in human life. Again, one can see evidence of a forgetting of earlier insights. For example, Dewey (1899) saw psychology as centrally involved with understanding issues concerned with meaning and issues concerned with values. He said, "Psychology, after all, simply states the mechanisms through which conscious value and meaning are introduced into human experience" (Dewey, 1899, p. 150).

Piaget had a great interest in the child's understanding of the world but he saw that world primarily in physical terms. Vygotsky has reminded psychologists of the extent to which the child's understanding of the world, whether it be the world of objects or of people, is socially mediated. As Bruner pointed out in his book *Acts of Meaning* (1990), "the child does not enter the life of his or her group as a private and autistic sport of primary processes, but rather as a participant in a larger public process in which public meanings are negotiated" (p. 13). The larger public process is culture which is permeated with meaning.

Bruner (1990) argued that "psychology stop trying to be 'meaning free' in its system of explanation. The very people and cultures that are its subject are governed by shared meanings and values" (Bruner, 1990, p. 20). He is not alone in his appeal. It is somewhat reassuring to hear a similar view being expressed most forcibly by Sperry, one of the major figures in neuropsychology and a winner of the Nobel Prize, who, shortly before his death, saw a sea-change, not only in psychology but in science, on the horizon. He saw a time approaching when "The former stark, strictly physical, value-empty, and mindless cosmos previously upheld by science becomes infused with cognitive and subjective values and rich emergent macrophenomena of all kinds" (Sperry, 1995, p. 506).

☐ The Child's Perspective

In line with their outdated natural science model of their relationship to their subject matter, for too long psychologists have seen as objects the people who were the focus of their observations or experiments—although in a strange inversion of meaning they have referred to them as "subjects." In child development, as in other areas of psychology, there is a new appreciation of the necessity to take "the subject's" perspective into account. There are increasing numbers of studies that involve the observation and recording of meaningful chunks of children's behavior and in which children's own, naturally occurring activities and narratives are given pride of place. There are many examples. One is Furth and Kane's recording and analysis of the spontaneous, pretend play of three 4- to 5-year-old girls who are planning and enacting a "royal ball" (Furth & Kane, 1990), and another is Dunn's account of the social interactions of young children in their home settings in which she "observed the children within the drama and excitement of family life" (Dunn, 1988, p. vii).

Qualitative methodologies, which had been part of the psychologist's armamentarium earlier this century but had been all but forgotten in the misguided insistence on quantification and nothing else, have been rediscovered and elaborated. An example of the insights to be gained from the application of qualitative methods can be found in the research of Gilligan and her colleagues with adolescent girls. In *Meeting at the Crossroads*, Brown and Gilligan (1993) described the development of a method of recording, listening to, and attempting to understand girls' voices. They were concerned to find an approach that would let the girls speak to them in their own words. They call their method the "Listener's Guide," and through it they have obtained new insights into the girls' experiences as they travel from late childhood into adolescence. It is interesting to recall that Bühler as far back as 1927 collected and analyzed information from the diaries of teenage girls but that this kind of qualitative work fell into disfavor in mainstream developmental psychology for the following half-century (Bühler, 1927, cited by Cairns, 1983).

Bruner (1990) and others have called for an approach to children's psychology that is interpretative and hermeneutic. Such an approach, which recognizes the importance of meaning in human psychology and of the need to address the existence of subjectivities and intersubjectivities, may permit a scholarly understanding that is more consonant with the dynamic of children's lives as they are experienced and constructed. An interpretative approach does not mean the abandonment of objectivity; it simply takes account of and respects the role of meaning and subjectivity. It can complement other approaches and methodologies; it does not necessarily supplant them. To use Kagan's terminology, there is a need for both the objective and the subjective frames in developmental psychology (Kagan, 1984). The discipline is impoverished if it fails to find a way for them to coexist.

☐ Applying the Science

Despite early concerns on the part of some child psychologists about "the perils of popularization," histories of the discipline show that the work of developmental psychologists has never stayed in the laboratory, nor was it insulated from the political concerns and ideological commitments of the time, despite its pretensions to being value free. As Schlossman (1985) and Smuts (1985) pointed out, from a very early stage the pressure to apply new theories and supposedly "pure" research was strong and some psychologists were themselves strong advocates of the view that the redemption of society lay in the proper management of children and that psychology had a major role to play in that process. Schlossman referred to the "gospel of child development" in the United States, and similarly the Newsons in the United Kingdom referred to "the cult of child development" (Schlossman, 1985, p. 65; Newson & Newson, 1974).

Through their interventions in advising parents and teachers and policymakers, psychologists and other developmentalists have had an impact on the upbringing, education, and management of generations of children and also played their part in shaping society's notions about the nature of the child, thus playing a central role in "the social construction of childhood."

Child psychology has been involved in a circular process by which it is both directing and directed by the prevalent political and historical circumstances. The way in which child psychology can lend itself to prop up the status quo, or the status that is politically desired, is well illustrated by Riley's analysis of the role of child psychology in the glorification of motherhood in post–World War II Britain (Riley, 1983). At the end of the war, state-funded nurseries, previously needed to enable mothers to join the workforce and support the war effort, were closed overnight and mothers were secluded in their homes. Thus the jobs were left to the returning soldiers and mothers were free to concentrate on producing and raising the next, well-adjusted, generation, who, Bowlby's early work assured them, required their constant presence and devotion.

Advice to parents, or, more often than not, to mothers, on child rearing provides a salutary reminder of the faddishness of child psychology and the problems involved in applying developmental research. Advice to mothers from experts has had a much longer history than that of the formal discipline of child development, but the early experts were also in the habit of leaning on access to specialized knowledge or "science" for the justification of their views.

Hardyment (1983) started her history of three centuries of advice on child care by quoting the words of a British physician:

> It is with great Pleasure I see the preservation of Children become the Care of Men of Sense. In my opinion this Business has been too long fatally left to the management of Women, who cannot be supposed to have a proper knowledge to fit them for the Task. (William Cadogan, 1748, cited by Hardyment, 1983, p. 10)

Nearly two hundred years later, the view of "Men of Sense" was still that mothers are not capable of rearing children properly and that science will provide the answers. Although Watson (1928) considered that "the world would be considerably better off if we were to stop having children for twenty years (except for experimental purposes) and were then to start again with enough facts to do the job with some degree of skill and accuracy," he swallowed his principles and gave mothers the benefit of his advice and his science.

In magazine articles and in his best-selling book *Psychological Care of Infant and Child,* Watson promoted a new and scientific approach to child rearing based on behaviorism (Watson, 1928). Watson's pronouncements on child rearing, in which parents were admonished for hugging and kissing their children and in which the main aim seemed to be to produce little self-contained automatons who bothered their parents as little as possible, seem bizarre and unacceptable from our vantage point today.

The influence of Freud, Bowlby, and Piaget on child-rearing manuals can also be traced. Hardyment (1984) gave an example of a Freudian, Buxbaum, author of *Your Child Makes Sense, A Guidebook for Parents* (1951), who advised patents that "from birth onwards children feel the pressures of urgent bodily needs and powerful instinctive urges (such as hunger, sex and aggression) which clamour for satisfaction."

Toilet training created particular difficulties in the household devoted to rearing children according to the Freudian way. According to Fraiberg (1959), the child who produces a bowel movement "comes to regard this act in the same way that an older child regards a loved person" and to flush it down the toilet was "a strange way to accept an offering of such value."

The favored theories changed in due course. By the 1960s and 1970s the influence of Piaget was more apparent. Leach, the psychologist author of the very popular child-care manual *Baby and Child* (1977), showed her Piagetian leanings when she told her readers:

> If you provide the space, equipment and time for your child's play, she will see to the development of her thinking for herself. She is the scientist and inventor: your job is merely to provide the laboratories, the facilities and a research assistant—you—when she needs one. (Leach, 1977, p. 351)

Twenty years later, this view of the young child as independent scientist does not chime with the current Vygotskian emphasis on socially supported learning.

In the last few decades, child developmentalists, fed on cognitive developmental and attachment theories, tell the modern mother that she should always be alert to her child's needs, ready to interact, to provide the right kind of stimulation combined with plenty of warmth and sensitivity. She is expected to be well informed and actively involved. As Urwin pointed out, the current emphasis on the need for quality maternal involvement has led to "the idea that the normal mother can function as a tutor or pedagogue" and that children need lots of "one-to-one attention" (Urwin, 1985). Urwin's study suggests this expectation creates a burden of obligation that many mothers feel guilty about because they invariably fail to give sensitive, loving stimulation and attention at all times. It is not hard to imagine the feelings of harassed mothers as they read, "housework can seem like pleasant play all over the house if you are prepared to take the baby with you and bounce her on the bed you are making, play peep-bo around the furniture and give her a duster to wave" (Leach, 1977, p. 270).

A review of the numerous ways in which the findings of developmental psychology have been applied is well beyond the scope of this short chapter. Some of the hailed contributions of the discipline to the welfare of children can be seen, with hindsight, to have been less than helpful. For example, the IQ test has often been used oppressively as a way of labeling and excluding rather than a way of understanding and assisting children. Binet himself opposed the view of intelligence as a fixed attribute and said, "We must protest and react against this brutal pessimism. With practice, enthusiasm and especially with method one can succeed in increasing one's attention, memory and judgment and in becoming literally more intelligent than one was before" (Binet, 1909, p. 126). He would probably have been horrified at what happened to his invention. There are plenty of cautionary tales but there is also considerable evidence of success

Some developmental psychologists today argue that the need for careful analysis, well-informed advice, and tried-and-tested interventions has never been greater. From different sides of the Atlantic, leading developmentalists have expressed their concerns about the circumstances in which young people are growing up. Rutter commented on "the substantial body of literature indicating that . . . there has been a considerable rise in the level of psychosocial disturbances in young people over the last half century" (Rutter et al., 1995, p. 62). Bronfenbrenner also sounded a pessimistic note, warning of "a progressive decline in American society of conditions that research increasingly indicates may be critical for developing and sustaining human competence throughout the life course" (Bronfenbrenner, 1995, p. 643).

It is clearly necessary to be cautious about such pronouncements, and the criteria for judging whether things are getting better or worse must be subject to the closest scrutiny. Even if there is little change, there are far too many children who are leading lives that are less happy and less fulfilled than they could be. As Erikson said in 1950, "human childhood provides the most fundamental basis for human exploitation." At best this exploitation consists of children being used as the repository of the desires and expectations of their parents and their society. At worst, children are neglected and abused or trapped in distressing situations not of their own making. Many children are caught up in the wars and conflicts created by the adults around them, and there are, sadly, few signs of change in that direction. Psychologists have a role to play in understanding and helping all of these children. As Scarr noted in 1979,

> Unlike some academic fields of psychology where swings away from application have been pronounced, child psychology has not strayed too far into abstraction. There have always been real children whose welfare could be served by new knowledge and new applications. (Scarr 1979, p. 810)

It is clear that if the psychologist is to act in the service of children, he or she does so from a particular value base and that it is incumbent on us to at least make our values clear, open to challenge and revision. Sarason called for applied psychologists to be "advocates of social change" rather than "willing agents of social policy" (Sarason, 1981, p. 176). Whatever the standpoint one takes, intervening in the lives of children is a political act and should be recognized as such.

☐ Alternative Visions of the Future

Predicting the future is always a risky occupation. If I had to make a prediction about the major theoretical thrust in the immediate future, I would say that it would be in the elaboration of the social and cultural perspective on child development and in the exploration of the child's own phenomenal and subjective world. Lerner and Dixon noted the beginning of this shift, commenting that "the growing interest in contextualism during the 1970s and 1980s was associated with the recession of the other major models to the backburner of theoretical and empirical activity" (Dixon & Lerner, 1992). As Morss (1996) pointed out, the reincorporation of the social into the developmental perspective on the child takes a number of different forms, ranging from the examination of the child plus his or her social influences, to radical social constructivism, to the Marxist critical psychology of development espoused by Morss himself. Once again it must be recognized that an appreciation of the extent to which the child's psychology is socially constructed is not new. One hundred years ago, James Mark Baldwin said, "The development of the child's personality could not go on at all without the modification of his sense of himself by suggestions from others. So he himself, at every stage, is really in part someone else, even in his own thought of himself" (Baldwin, 1897, p. 30). Implicit in this way of thinking is a systemic view of development which should be capable of successfully incorporating the biological, the social and the personal as inextricably enmeshed, reciprocally influential elements.

Other people's predictions will be quite different. I was interested to see in the recent textbook by the British psychologists Butterworth and Harris (1994) that, in a section called "Developmental Psychology in the Twenty-First Century," their first prediction is "an ever closer link between developmental psychology and developmental biology. . . . Advances in evolutionary theory, in genetics and in the biology of the developing nervous system are beginning to give evidence that converges with the behavioural and cognitive measures typical of developmental psychology." Their second prediction concerns closer links between developmental psychology and new theoretical models in biology such as "selectionism" or "neural Darwinism" (Butterworth & Harris, 1994, p. 229). This would not be the future as I see it or, perhaps more to the point, as I would like to see it, because it appears to place an emphasis on biologically deterministic explanations to the detriment of the other forms of explanation. But these eminent British psychologists are probably correct. The future will be built on many different, sometimes compatible and sometimes incompatible visions.

In his examination of the future of developmental psychology, Kessen concluded, "whatever style of reasoning we adopt, the evidence of past decades, from different cultures and from different groups in the United States, supports a strong case against the Grand Simplicities of theory or of method" (Kessen, 1990). His view applies equally to Europe. Whatever the future holds, it will not be neat an simple. If it is, we can be sure that we have gone seriously awry. Our examination of the past should tell us that in human psychology the simple formulation is usually an inadequate formulation. The time of Grand Theories in psychology has gone, notwithstanding the claims of evolutionary psychology. Child development has had more than its share of these grand theories, and despite their importance in the history of the discipline, each has toppled in its turn. But the need for Grand Thinkers has not gone. It would seem from the data-driven and, at best, microtheoretical nature of much of the research in child development—the kind of work that can be methodologically meticulous but terminally uninteresting—that large-scale theorizing is to be avoided. Thankfully, there are many developmentalists who, despite impeccable credentials as empiricists, are also interested in the big issues. I have in mind people like Bronfenbrenner, Rutter, Baltes, Kagan, and Bruner. These writers synthesize and systematize and generate fresh hypotheses. To a greater or lesser extent, they are also willing to stand back and ask what it all means and whether it could be done any better. People with the capacity to act and think in this way are always going to be essential in a discipline like developmental psychology, where a self-critical stance may help to guard against answers that may be not only wrong, but also dangerous.

☐ Conclusion

In the past century we have explored a multiplicity of methodologies and tried out a multiplicity of theories. The history of the discipline is the history of the assembly and dismantling of theoretical frameworks. The overturning of old ways of viewing the child and the search for the best way to conceptualize his or her development continues but the interest in examining the basic assumptions of the discipline is currently particularly intense, as befits this era of skepticism and deconstruction.

As we enter the years of the new century, there are many recent signs of an increased willingness to confront the complexities involved in understanding children's development and also of willingness to construct conceptual frameworks and methods that will enable the study of these complexities. It is to be hoped that we can use this changed consciousness and the experience accumulated over the past decades to advance to an understanding of children that does better justice to their complex, changing, and multiple ways of being in and with their worlds.

☐ References

Anastasi, A. (1958). Heredity, environment and the question "How?" *Psychological Review, 65,* 197–208.

Baltes, P. B. (1987). Theoretical propositions of life-span developmental psychology: On the dynamics between growth and decline. *Developmental Psychology, 23,* 611–626.

Baltes, W. (1989). *Lebensmittelchemie.* Berlin, Hamburg: Springer-Verlag.

Baumrind, D. (1993). The average expectable environment is not enough: A response to Scarr. *Child Development, 64,* 1299–1317.

Belsky, J. (1995). Expanding the ecology of human development: An evolutionary perspective. In P. Moen, G. H. Elder, & K. Luscher (Eds.), *Examining lives in context: Perspectives on the ecology of human development* (pp. 352–355). Washington, DC: American Psychological Association.

Binet, A. (1909). *Les idées modernes sur les infants.* Paris: Ernest Flammarion.

Bradley, B. S. (1989). *Visions of infancy: A critical introduction to child psychology.* Cambridge: Polity Press.

Bronfenbrenner, U. (1979). *The ecology of human development: Experiments by* nature and design. Cambridge, MA: Harvard University Press.

Bronfenbrenner, U. (1995). Developmental ecology through space time: A future perspective. In P. Moen, G. M. Elder, & K. Luscher (Eds.), *Examining lives in context: Perspectives on the ecology of human development* (pp. 619–647). Washington, DC: American Psychological Association.

Bronfenbrenner, U., & Ceci, S. J. (1994). Nature–nurture reconceptualized in developmental perspective: A bioecological model. *Psychological Review, 101,* 568–586.

Bronfenbrenner, U., Kessel, F., Kessen, W., & White, S. (1986). Toward a critical social history of developmental psychology: A propaedeutic discussion. *American Psychologist, 41,* 1218–1230.

Broughton, J. M. (1987). *Critical theories of psychological development.* London: Plenum Press.

Brown, L. M., & Gilligan, C. (1992). *Meeting at the crossroads: Women's psychology and girls' development.* Cambridge, MA: Harvard University Press.

Bruner, J. (1990). *Acts of meaning.* Cambridge, MA: Harvard University Press.

Bühler, C. (1927). Die ersten sozialen Verhaltensweisen der Kindes. In C. Bühler, H. Hetzer, & B. Tudor-Hart (Eds.), *Soziologische und psychologische: Studien über das Erste Lebensjahr* (pp. S.1–102). Jena: Fischer.

Burman, B. (1994). *Deconstructing developmental psychology.* London: Routledge.

Butterworth, G., & Harris, P. L. (1994). *Principles of developmental psychology.* Hove: Lawrence Erlbaum Associates.

Buxbaum, E. (1951). *Your child makes sense: A guidebook for parents.* London: Allen and Unwin.

Cadogan, W. (1978). *Essay on the nursing and management of children.* London: John Knapton.

Cahan, E. D. (1992). John Dewey and human development. *Developmental Psychology, 28,* 205–214.

Cairns, R. B. (1983). The emergence of developmental psychology. In P. H. Mussen (Ed.), *Hand-*

book of child psychology. Volume 1: History, theory and methods (pp. 41–102). New York: John Wiley & Sons.

Cairns, R. B. (1992). The making of a developmental science: The contributions and intellectual heritage of James Mark Baldwin. *Developmental Psychology, 28,* 17–24.

Dewey, J. (1899). Psychology and social practice. In J. A. Boydston (Ed.), *The middle works of John Dewey* (pp. 105–124). Carbondale, IL: Southern Illinois University Press.

Dixon, R. A., & Lerner, R. M. (1992). History of systems in developmental psychology. In M. H. Bornstein & M. E. Lamb (Eds.), *Developmental psychology: An advanced textbook* (pp. 3–46). Hove: Lawrence Erlbaum Associates.

Dunn, J. (1988). *The beginnings of social understanding.* Oxford: Blackwell.

Erikson, E. (1953). *Childhood and society.* New York: Norton.

Flavell, J. H. (1970). Cognitive changes in adulthood. In L. R. Goulet & P. Baltes (Eds.), *Life-span developmental psychology: Research and theory.* London: Academic Press.

Fraiberg, S. (1959). *The magic years: Understanding and handling the problems of early childhood.* New York: Scribner.

Furth, H. G., & Kane, S. R. (1992). Children constructing society: A new perspective on children at play. In H. M. Gurk (Ed.), *Childhood social development: Contemporary perspectives.* Hillsdale, NJ: Lawrence Erlbaum Associates.

Gottlieb, G. (1992). *Individual development and evolution: The genesis of novel behaviour.* Oxford: Oxford University Press.

Greenberg, D. E. (1996). The object permanence fallacy. *Human Development, 39,* 171–131.

Hardyment, C. (1983). *Dream babies: Three centuries of good advice on child care.* New York: Harper and Row.

Hardyment, C. (1984). *Dream babies: Childcare from Locke to Spock.* Oxford: Oxford University Press.

Kagan, J. (1984). *The nature of the child.* New York: Basic Books.

Kessen, W. (1979). The American child and other cultural inventions. *American Psychologist, 34,* 815–820.

Kessen, W. (1986). Towards a critical social history of developmental psychology. *American Psychology, 41*(11), 1218–1230.

Kessen, W. (1990). *The rise and fall of development.* Worchester, MA: Clark University Press.

Kuhn, T. S. (1962). *The structure of scientific revolutions.* London: University of Chicago Press.

Labouvie-Vief, G., & Chandler, M. (1978). Cognitive development and life-span developmental theories: Idealistic versus contextual perspectives. In P. Baltes (Ed.), *Life-span development and behaviour* (Vol. 1, pp. 181–210). New York: Academic Press.

Leach, P. (1977). *Baby and child.* London: Michael Joseph.

Lerner, R. M., & von Eye, A. (1992). Sociobiology and human development: Arguments and evidence. *Human Development, 35,* 12–33.

Magnusson, D. (1995). Individual development: A holistic integrated model. In P. Moen, G. H. Elder, & K. Luscher (Eds.), *Examining lives in context: Perspectives on the ecology of human development* (pp. 19–60). Washington, DC: American Psychological Association.

Morss, J. R. (1990). *The biologising of childhood: Developmental psychology and the Darwinian myth.* Hillsdale, NJ: Lawrence Erlbaum Associates.

Morss, R. (1996). *Growing critical: Alternatives to developmental psychology.* London: Routledge.

Murray, C. M., & Hernstein, R. J. (1994). *The bell curve: Intelligence, class and structure in American life.* New York: Free Press.

Newson, J., & Newson, E. (1974). Cultural aspects of childrearing in the English speaking world. In M. Richards (Ed.), *The integration of the child into a social world.* London: Cambridge University Press.

Piaget, J. (1954). *The construction of reality in the child.* New York: Ballantine Books.

Plomin, R. (1989). Environment and genes: Determinants of behaviour. *American Psychologist, 44,* 105–111.

Plomin, R. (1994). *Genes and experience: The interplay between nature and nurture.* London: Sage.

Riley, D. (1983). *War in the nursery: Theories of the child and mother.* London: Virago.

Rutter, M. (1989). Pathways from childhood to adult life. *Journal of Child Psychology and Psychiatry, 30,* 23–51.

Rutter, D., Champion, L., Quinton, D., Maughan, B., & Pickles, A. (1995). Understanding individual differences in environmental-risk exposure. In P. Moen, G. H. Elder, Jr., & K. Luscher (Eds.), *Examining lives in context* (pp. 61–89). Washington, DC: American Psychiatric Association.

Sarason, S. B. (1981). *Psychology misdirected.* New York: Free Press.

Scarr, S. (1979). Psychology and children: Current research and practice. *American Psychologist, 34,* 809–811.

Scarr, S. (1992). Developmental theories for the 1990s: Development and individual differences. *Child Development, 63,* 631–649.

Scarr, S., & McCartney, K. (1983). How people make their own environments: A theory of genotype–environment effects. *Child Development, 54,* 424–435.

Schlossman, S. (1985). Perils of popularisation: The founding of *Parents' Magazine.* In A. B. Smuts & J. W. Hagen (Eds.), *History and research in child development* [Monographs of the Society for Research in Child Development, Vol. 50] (pp. 65–77). Chicago: University of Chicago Press.

Smuts, B. B. (1985). *Sex and friendship in baboons.* Hawthorne, NY: Aldine.

Sperry, R. S. (1995). The future of psychology. *American Psychologist, 50,* 505–506.

Urwin, C. (1985). Constructing motherhood: The persuasion of normal development. In C. Steedman, C. Urwin, & V. Walkerdine (Eds.), *Language, gender and childhood.* London: Routledge and Kegan Paul.

Walkerdine, V. (1984). Developmental psychology and the child-centred pedagogy. In J. Henriques, W. Hollway, C. Urwin, C. Venn, & V. Walkerdine (Eds.), *Changing the subject: Psychology, social regulation and subjectivity* (pp. 153–202). London: Methuen.

Watson, J. B. (1928). *Psychological care of infant and child.* New York: Norton.

CHAPTER

Bettye Caldwell

The Educare of Children
in the Twenty-First Century

Whenever a dramatic and cataclysmic event occurs, like the devastating Lisbon earthquake of November 1, 1755, the unaffected or minimally affected portion of the population instantly swings into action to deal with the emergency. This immediacy of response is not reserved solely for destructive events. Thus when gold was discovered in California in 1849, thousands of prospectors, merchants, bankers, outfitters, and adventurous ladies immediately began the long trek west to take advantage of the situation.

Rarely does such an immediate response occur when an "event" is gradual and happens over a long period of time, with increments that are barely noticeable from day to day or even year to year. Instead, in such situations, the public response is often tentative, perhaps confused and conflicted. Services that are offered to meet whatever needs are associated with the now-recognized situation tend to assume many forms and to vary widely in quality.

Such has been the situation, worldwide, with respect to the development of a network of services for young children who need some degree of supplementary care in addition to that provided by their families. This need has been with us for a long time—ever since we have had family life, in fact—but we somehow remained unaware of it. As most of us can only think in time units that fit a single life span, it was easy to overlook this need as it escalated gradually rather than suddenly. And with only a gradual increase rather than a sudden eruption, it failed to affect public consciousness to such a degree that informed action occurred.

But now we are acutely aware of this need. Whenever such awareness develops, it is as though we begin to look at events through the compressed time units that characterize the thinking of a historian. And, when that happens, we perceive a crisis, an emergency. That is precisely what has happened in most parts of the world with respect to the need to develop a comprehensive system of supplementary care for young children. All over the world we read about "the child-care crisis"—a crisis that, at subcrisis

189

levels, has been trying to generate an informed response for at least the last quarter of our now-departed century. As most countries can mobilize the public will to take needed action more successfully when there is an emergency, perhaps the current crisis orientation is a good thing.

☐ Alternate Care: A Necessary Service for Children and Families

For the participants in Baby XXI, I do not need to do much documentation of the importance of the development of national systems of supplementary care. However, agreement on the importance of doing so rarely coincides with agreement as to the possible consequences of such experiences—or, for that matter, with consensus as to the type of service that should be developed and become part of public policy.

In America, I am now often called a "child-care pioneer," and I sometimes find the need to confess that I got into the field by the back door—perhaps the only door through which anyone who wanted to retain professional respectability could enter a quarter of a century ago. My colleague Dr. Julius B. Richmond and I launched an infant day-care project in order to provide through such care health services, cognitive enrichment, and social support to poor children and their families (Caldwell & Richmond, 1964). Anticipating an enthusiastic endorsement from various professional groups of the wisdom of our venture, we were soon to learn that most mental health professionals and large segments of the general population did not agree with us. From pediatrics, in spite of Dr. Richmond's status in the field, there was not general acceptance. From developmental psychology there was indifference, from child psychiatry restrained opposition, and from child welfare overt hostility.

Since that time, however, there has been a steady accretion of research evidence demonstrating that such a service does indeed benefit disadvantaged children cognitively, can be offered without creating major health crises, and need not impair social and emotional development (Caldwell & Freyer, 1982; McCartney, 1990). The research also has identified enough questions (Belsky, 1986) to keep eyebrows raised and to drive continuing research into aspects of care that may be beneficial and that may be potentially harmful.

☐ Extent of Alternate Care Utilization

In spite of the great value of such research for answering the questions that trouble scientists and parents alike, utilization of such services does not wait for definitive answers. A brief examination of some of the recent data (Bureau of the Census, 1992) on child care utilization in America will illustrate that point:

- One-half of mothers with children under 1 year work.
- Two-thirds of mothers with children under 6 years work.
- Three-fourths of mothers of children under 18 years work.

However, we still do not seem to have good data describing the situation globally; different countries use slightly different reporting systems, making cross-cultural comparison difficult.

Such care is going to increase regardless of what our research might show. It is as though young parents of today have said to those of us in the older generation: "Look. This is the way we are going to raise our children. We're going to do most of it, but we're also going to have help. Now if you want to do something useful, don't keep scaring us by saying that it might harm our children. If you want to help, find out how to do it right." It is now a way of life, like urban living. With this in mind, energy needs to be directed to improving the service. In this chapter a plea is made to give the field a new name that better communicates the nature and importance of its service and to take the steps necessary to upgrade the quality of service provided.

☐ Needed: A New Label for the Field

One of the most important things we need to do for the early childhood field is rechristen it, give it a new name. The name I am proposing is the first one in my title: *educare*. I have several reasons for endorsing—actually carrying on a one-woman campaign for—the term.

The first and main reason is simply that we have a tower of Babel with respect to terminology that refers to early childhood programs. Is the correct name for the field early childhood education? Day care? Child care? And what is the difference between day care and child care? Are we talking about preschool? Nursery school? Kindergarten? Prekindergarten? Post-preschool? And on and on.

When multiple labels are used, the logical assumption is that you are referring to more than one type of program. My contention is that we are basically referring to one type of program and therefore need one label that will embrace all that we offer. Not only does this semantic variety confuse the general public, but it prevents the internal assimilation of a clear concept of the essential nature of the service we offer.

This multiplicity of labels would not be so bad if we did not justify our chosen words with formal definitions that presume to specify the services associated with different labels—most especially early childhood education and day care, terms that establish the polarities. Table 13.1 offers a summary of some of the common phrases that have been used over the years to communicate the presumed philosophy and service orientation connoted by these two terms.

Granted that these descriptors adapted from various professional articles describing the two presumably different services are to some extent caricatures and stereotypes, and granted that they are hopefully somewhat out of date, these artificial distinctions are still very real in the minds of many consumers, students, media representatives, and policymakers. Whatever else they indicate, they show that we do not convey a unified self concept describing a broad and inclusive pattern of human service.

By focusing on certain aspects (e.g., protection from harm versus providing developmental opportunities) of what we do and choosing a label based exclusively on one or the other set of program components, we have prevented the emergence of a concept broad enough to cover the full range of common services. With our devotion to labels that exclude rather than include, we have, quite literally, diminished ourselves conceptually. We have fostered the endorsement of a false dichotomy. Metaphorically it is as though we have said that, because their services are somewhat different, pediatrics and surgery and neurology are not all parts of medicine.

The words we use for any object or event profoundly influence the internal concept

TABLE 13.1. Labels Historically Used to Describe "Early Childhood Education" and "Day Care"

Early childhood education	Day care
	A social welfare program
For middle class/affluent	For lower class/poor
For successful families	For pathological families
A school	An institution
A service for children	A service for parents
Is supplementary care	Is institutional/custodial care
Is privately funded	Is publicly funded
Operates 2–3 hours/day	Operates for 8–10 hours/day
Provides education/enrichment	Provides care & protection
Is developmentally appropriate	Is inimical to development
Encourages value choice	Imposes values
Facilitates freedom and diversity	Fosters conformity
Is a family support	Weakens the family
Democratizes	"Sovietizes" children

that becomes assimilated. A historian described only as Vito, who worked in Naples in the early eighteenth century, offered a profound comment on the insight that linguistic study could shed on history. His words (from Collingwood, 1946) are beautiful and profound:

> Etymology can show what kind of life a people was leading while its language was coming into existence. The historian is aiming at a reconstruction of the mental life, the ideas, of the people he is studying; their stock of words shows what their stock of ideas was; and the way in which they use an old word metaphorically in a new sense, when they want to express a new idea, shows what their stock of ideas was before that new one came into existence. Thus Latin words like *intellegere* and *disserere* show how, when Romans needed words for understanding and discussing, they borrowed from an agricultural vocabulary the words for gleaning and sowing. (pp. 69–70)

When I encountered that quote I was entranced, for that is exactly what we have done in regard to a label for the field of early childhood. The chosen words reflect the stock of ideas we had when the labels were chosen. We now have new ideas, new awareness of what the service should be. And we need a new label.

In order to do a more effective job of communicating what we do both to ourselves and to the public at large, we need a term that is inclusive rather than exclusive, one that embraces a broader array of the services we provide. The term *educare* would accomplish this. By encompassing both of the major aspects of the early childhood field, the label would help demolish the false dichotomies outlined in Table 1. The word communicates, in three short syllables, that all early childhood programs must offer components of both of the services previously conceptualized as separate and distinct. One cannot educate without offering care and protection, and one cannot provide true care and protection during the precious early childhood years—or during any years, for that matter—without also educating.

But an even greater value associated with the adoption of a new name is the promise it offers that a new service has been created. This is not just a fancy new word for an old, not particularly valued service. This is a new service. It will be a good day for young children when no sort of early childhood program pretends to exist without providing components of both education and care, that is, integrated educare.

☐ Achieving Quality in Educare

If educare is to fulfill its responsibility to Baby XXI, it must be of high quality. In the United States, there is wide variability in the quality of programs in which different children are enrolled. There are at least four issues that must be dealt with internationally if quality of care is to improve: health, research, training, and funding. Each of these issues is here dealt with in turn.

Health Issues

If educare is to be a comprehensive service that is beneficial to children, it must include a major health-care component. This is especially important in programs for children younger than 2 years. In fact, many of the concerns and policy issues in this field center on the infant. Infants have frequent upper respiratory infections, put everything in their mouths, deposit their urine and saliva indiscriminately, occasionally bite others, contentedly pick up and eat food off the floor, and are reluctant to put their excrement in receptacles designed for that purpose. They are crawling/walking colonies of pathogens!

In the approximately 25 years that Western countries have had group care for infants, there have been several cyclical waves of research reassurance and alarmism. The earliest research (Glezen et al., 1971) tended to be reassuring, showing that infants in group care had about 1.5 more upper respiratory infections per year than controls, a nonsignificant difference. Following this early work came analyses alerting caregivers and parents to the increased possibility of haemophilus B influenza, of hepatitis A, of diarrhea associated with several pathogens, and of cytomegalovirus infection (of both infants and caregivers).

Perhaps the most powerful recent data offering reassurance are those from the multisite Infant Health and Development Program (IHDP, 1990) study of low-birth-weight premature babies, a group considered at high risk for susceptibility to morbidity. The children in the intervention group of that study, randomly assigned at birth, attended a high-quality educare program from the age of 1 year to 3 years. There were no major differences in health status between the intervention and the follow-up (control) groups. The only measure on which health differences were found (in the first analysis) was on a morbidity index based on the mothers' reports. The lighter babies (< 2000 g) enrolled in the intervention program were reported to have had a small but statistically significant increase in minor illnesses. There were no differences in serious health problems. Here it should be noted that sanitary procedures in the centers were undoubtedly exemplary, as there was continuous monitoring and supervision by health-care personnel throughout the duration of the intervention. Findings from this study need to be thought of not as what is typical in alternate care settings but as what is possible—even with a high-risk population—when the care offered is of high quality.

What is needed at this time is a set of enlightened policies and practices that can bring health maintenance routinely into educare. The multiple origins of educare, as chronicled earlier (mainly social service and education, plus a small mom-and-pop entrepreneurship), have militated against a consistent auspice for the service. It is fair to say that for all too many years, no one wanted the field. Now that it is coming to be recognized as an important human service, turf battles are common and are increasing. If the service is truly comprehensive, it needs all the disciplines represented under the broad umbrella of child development.

There is much to commend in the French system (Richardson & Marx, 1989), which places care for infants younger than 3 years under the Ministry of Health and programs for children in the age range of 3 to 6 years under the Ministry of Education. Training for the caregivers in this system is close to ideal—nurse's training first, followed by training in child development and early educational practices. All units for infants, whether centers (Crèche Collectives) or family day care arrangements (Crèche Familiales), are under the supervision of a pediatrician assigned to the Protection Maternelle et Infantile (PMI). The crèches are thought of as a vital part of preventive health care. Without a system comparable to the PMI, which reaches all children, it would be difficult to adopt this system without modification. Certainly there is no such system in the United States. Nonetheless, it offers an excellent model to be examined when considering ways to involve health professionals more extensively and more effectively in educare.

The American Public Health Association and the American Academy of Pediatrics (1992) recently developed National Health and Safety Performance Standards for Out-of-Home-Child Care programs. (Please note the committee's difficulty with what to call the field. Out-of-home child care was apparently a compromise that allowed them to avoid all the currently confusing terms.) The format adopted by the committee is incredibly detailed: First a standard is proposed, then a rationale for its inclusion is offered, and finally supportive comments and references are provided. These standards have already been reviewed by selected individuals and are now in the process of field review in several states. Hopefully, they will soon find their way into state regulations.

If adopted, these standards will have a major effect on the quality of educare in America, much as the accreditation system developed by the National Association for the Education of Young Children (Bredekamp, 1987) is having an impact on program quality. They will become the gold standard against which all health maintenance activities will be evaluated. When this is done, many will be found wanting. Then the task will be to set in motion a machinery for making the changes necessary to allow them to be implemented.

Research Issues

There is a pressing need for more and better research dealing with many aspects of the educare experience. Actually, in the United States within the past decade, there has been a flood of research dealing with either cognitive or social effects of alternate care (see the summary edited by McCartney, 1990). Of particular interest has been the question of whether maternal employment during the first year of the infant's life, and consequent utilization of alternate care, impairs the child's attachment to the mother and possibly to other important individuals to whom the child must relate. Controversy surrounding this issue has arisen repeatedly over the past quarter-century in roughly 5-year cycles—that is, reassurance (Caldwell, Wright, Honig, & Tannenbaum, 1970), alert (Blehar, 1974), renewed reassurance (Rutter, 1981), and then the sounding of a powerful alarm (Belsky, 1986).

The Belsky (1986) article generated as much controversy as the issue itself and led to charges of selective review of research and acceptance of inconclusive findings (Phillips, McCartney, Scarr, & Howe, 1987) and to reliance on a method (the Strange Situation test) considered by many to be inappropriate for children who have been in alternative care (Clarke-Stewart, 1988; Richters & Zahn-Waxler, 1988). People who had worked for years to help "day care" gain public acceptance resented the attention the scientific debate received in the media, thereby damaging the hard-won recognition of alternative care as a vital family support. However, regardless of one's interpretation of the "facts" in the debate, the tocsin sounded by Belsky had a generally favorable effect: It helped to call attention to the need for more and better research on this important subject.

Much of the research has been simplistic and careless—for example, not bothering to pay attention to the alternative care experiences of those children not officially enrolled in "day care." Samples have been small and casually assembled. And rarely has it had what Bronfenbrenner (1977) called ecological validity. The debate relating to attachment security illustrates this point better than anything else. Much of the research fueling the debate has used a procedure called the Strange Situation test (Ainsworth & Wittig, 1969). This is a laboratory procedure in which an infant is separated from its mother several times, remaining in the room with a stranger during one separation and entirely alone in another. Attachment security or insecurity is determined primarily by the infant's avoidance of or ambivalence to the mother during the reunions. This procedure has much to commend it in terms of scientific elegance, and, to be sure, it has been widely accepted by researchers the world over. However, its ecological relevance is minimal, and it may well have a quite different psychological meaning for a child who has rarely been separated from the mother versus that of the child who, experienced in alternative care, has learned how to cope with such separations. The latter child may, during the reunion episodes, be exhibiting independence and autonomy rather than avoidance. Research using such precise laboratory methods is important, but it needs to be supplemented with procedures that involve stationing a researcher at the door of the educare setting when the child is left (separation) and picked up (reunion). Only when both types are used will the full picture become clear.

Even more than having ecological relevance, research that will most help Baby XXI will consider simultaneously family as well as alternative care variables. Likewise, no assumption will be made about the quality of the alternative care—that will be measured as meticulously as the outcome variables. Children enter educare (which may be good or bad) from homes (which may be good or bad from the standpoint of the child's development). Likewise, sturdy and robust children enter alternative care, just as fragile and vulnerable children do. There are individual differences in the homes, in the educare settings, and in the children, all of which must be dealt with in the research of the future. Although research that deals simultaneously with all these variables is difficult to carry out, it is not impossible. And it is essential that it be done.

The National Institute of Child Health and Human Development Study of Early Child Care (see Friedman, 1990) represents an attempt to bring this broader ecological perspective into educare research. In this large-scale, 10-site study, children were recruited at birth and followed longitudinally until age 3. Recruitment went through 1991 until 1,200 subjects were in the study, and the first wave of data collection continued until 1994. At five major assessment points—1, 6, 15, 24, and 36 months—where assessments made of family variables (e.g., stimulation for development within the home, available social supports, quality of adult relationships), of child-care variables (quantity, stability, and quality), and of individual child variables (temperament, developmental level). Outcome measures included both socioemotional variables appropriate at the different ages (attachment, compliance, independence, peer relations, etc.) and cognitive variables (attention, language development, problem solving, intelligence, etc.).

This study represents mega-research of the first order, at least in the social sciences, and working out the details of the common protocol was not easy. However, all participants unanimously felt that the effort has been worthwhile in relation to the anticipated value of the research. Only from such efforts will the kind of information needed to guide policies for the educare of Baby XXI emerge.

These research issues are important in relation to achieving high-quality alternative care for children, not merely in terms of strengthening the knowledge base in child development. Although new knowledge is important, there is a special need for policy-relevant research—research that will establish which characteristics of educare are associated with which types of child outcomes. When that type of knowledge is available, program design and operational patterns can emerge in ways that will benefit the children as well as serve their families.

Training Issues

Educare quality will not improve until programs are staffed with individuals who are qualified for such work through personal attributes and training. Child caregiver bashing is very popular in the United States, and I do not mean to be adding to that strident chorus. From personal experience I well know of hundreds, even thousands, of dedicated workers who put in long hours for minimal reward. However, I also know of large numbers who lack the training, the understanding of how children develop and what their needs are in such situations, to create growth-fostering conditions.

Not every person working in educare must be a fully trained professional worker. Role differentiation can be effective here just as in other human service areas. However, every worker needs some training, and in some locales even this bare minimum is not specified.

One explanation for the dearth of highly trained personnel in educare is that, in most countries, compensation for such work is abysmally low. Again, it is difficult to offer data with global relevance, but this is clearly the case in the United States. The Child Care Staffing Study (Whitebook, Howes, & Phillips, 1989) confirmed the dismal truth about low salaries for child care workers: This predominantly female work force earns an average hourly wage of $5.35. Furthermore, in the last decade, child-care staff wages, when adjusted for inflation, have decreased more than 20%. Child-care teaching staff earn less than half as much as comparably educated women and less than one-third as much as comparably educated men in the civilian labor force. Until nations recognize the importance of educare and remunerate workers proportionately to its value for development, it will be difficult to recruit into the field the kind of workers needed to meet the needs of the children. And until better economic advantages can be promised, individuals who choose this work will not be able to afford the training they need to enable them to do a good job.

Funding Issues

The double bind just identified in relation to training leads quite logically to the last major issue identified in this presentation—namely, funding or economic issues. There is no way to develop a high quality educare system without willingness to put money into the system. That recognition, of course, leads to the question of where the money will come from. Will it be necessary to dilute or eliminate some existing services in order to improve quality in educare?

Even though personnel are underpaid, the service is costly for many families. Rounding, and generalizing across the country, and ignoring standards or quality, care in the United States costs about $50 per week (Child Care Action Campaign, 1990). These costs do not hit families equally; this represents 25% of the income of poor families but only about 6% of the income of others.

Many people who see similar figures use them to buttress the argument that it does not really pay to have women work, when one considers the cost of transportation, food and clothing, educare, and so on. The same people would be horrified at the suggestion that they should have to pay directly (obviously they pay indirectly through taxes) to build the roads and bridges they traverse to go to work. They have become accustomed to depending on roads and bridges to be there for them. They are tangible aspects of the infrastructure on which the economic world depends. But so is educare. Without the provision of proper developmental opportunities for the next generation, no community can prosper. And without assurance that their economic contributions to family, community, and nation do not imperil their children, workers cannot function effectively. When this concept of educare as part of the infrastructure for a nation's economy becomes assimilated by a people, willingness to pay for the service will rise exponentially.

In this context, it is important to remember that quality educare is cost-effective. In recent years, substantial evidence has been forthcoming to demonstrate that. Frequently quoted is the formula that for every dollar spent, five are saved. Results that show that children who participated in high quality early childhood programs are less likely to repeat grades or be referred for more costly special education (Berrueta-Clement, Schweinhart, Barnett, Epstein, & Weikart, 1984; Lazar & Darlington, 1982) have been powerful persuaders of policy makers to provide funding for such programs. The positive effect of early childhood programs has invaded the public consciousness more thoroughly during the past decade than many of us would have dreamed possible. Awareness hopefully leads to action. When a country develops the political will to provide the service, funds to pay for it can generally be found.

☐ Summary

One thing that must be done for Baby XXI is to design and operate a network of programs that can supplement the care and education the adult Baby XXI will provide for his or her children. If we do not leave a legacy of a quality supplementary care system for all the babies of the twenty-first century, they will have to develop it themselves. And that would be like having to rediscover the route to the New World, which the Portuguese explorers did centuries ago.

A first step toward achieving this is to coin and use a term that will adequately describe the full scope of the service. A more accurate term (in use in many parts of the world today) is *educare*. Consistent use of such a term would help eradicate the notion that what is needed is a unidimensional service that provides only care and protection; of equal or greater importance is the educational and developmental component of the service.

A redefined and reconceptualized service must then ensure that all children have access to programs of high quality. In order to achieve high-quality educare, we must make certain that the programs include a major health component, that research into outcomes associated with different types of programs be intensified, that training for personnel be mandated, and that adequate levels of funding be achieved that will attract competent personnel and help ensure favorable outcomes for children.

It is my hope that from Baby XXI will come new charts—rutters, they were called—to help guide the first faltering steps of the babies of the new century. And from those babies to whom we can give navigational help, may there come families who give love and support to the children of the twenty-second century. May we offer them as part of our legacy the wisdom to plan and the willingness to create a network of services that will help them transcend being merely human and instead become truly humane.

☐ References

Ainsworth, M. D. S., & Wittig, B. (1969). Attachment and exploratory behavior of one-year-olds in a strange situation. In B. M. Foss (Ed.), *Determinants of infant behavior* (Vol. 4, pp. 111–136). London: Methuen.

American Public Health Association & American Academy of Pediatrics. (1992). *Caring for our children: National health and safety performance standards: Guidelines for out-of-home child care programs.* Ann Arbor, MI: Edwards Brothers.

Belsky, J. (1986). Infant day care: A cause for concern? *Zero to Three, 6,* 1–7.

Berrueta-Clement, J. R., Schweinhart, L. J., Barnett, W. S., Epstein, A. S., & Weikart, D. P. (1984). Changed lives: The effects of the Perry Preschool Program on youths through age 19. *Monographs of the High/Scope Educational Research Foundation, 8.*

Blehar, M. C. (1974). Anxious attachment and defensive reactions associated with day care. *Child Development, 45,* 683–692.

Bredekamp, S. (Ed.). (1987). *Developmentally appropriate practice in early childhood programs serving children from birth through age 8.* Washington, DC: National Association for the Education of Young Children.

Bronfenbrenner, U. (1977). Toward an experimental ecology of human development. *American Psychologist, 32,* 513–531.

Bureau of the Census. (1992). Demographic state of the nation: 1992. *Current Population Reports Special Studies Series P-23,* no. 177.

Caldwell, B. M., & Freyer, M. (1982). Day care and early education. In B. Spodek (Ed.), *Handbook of research in early childhood education* (pp. 341–374). New York: Free Press.

Caldwell, B. M., & Richmond, J. B. (1964). Programmed day care for the very young child—A preliminary report. *Journal of Marriage & the Family, 26,* 481–488.

Caldwell, B. M., Wright, C. M., Honig, A. S., & Tannenbaum, J. (1970). Infant day care and attachment. *American Journal of Orthopsychiatry, 40,* 397–412.

Child Care Action Campaign. (1990). *Child Care Action News 7.*

Clarke-Stewart, K. A. (1988). "The 'effects' of infant day care reconsidered" reconsidered: Risks for parents, children, and researchers. *Early Childhood Research Quarterly, 3,* 293–318.

Collingwood, R. G. (1946). *The idea of history.* Oxford: Clarendon Press.

Friedman, S. (1990). NICHD Infant child-care network: The national study of young children's lives. *Zero to Three, 10*(3), 21–23.

Glezen, W. P., Loda, F. A., Clyde, W. A., Jr., Senior, R. J., Schaeffer, C. I., Conley, W. G., & Denny, F. W. (1971). Epidemiologic patterns of acute lower respiratory diseases of children in a pediatric group practice. *Journal of Pediatrics, 78,* 397–406.

Infant Health and Development Program. (1990). Enhancing the outcomes of low-birth-weight, premature infants: A multisite, randomized trial. *Journal of the American Medical Association, 263*(22), 3035–3042.

Lazar, I., & Darlington, R. (1982). Lasting effects of early education: A report from the Consortium on Longitudinal Studies. *Monograph of the Society for Research in Child Development, 47*(2–3), serial no. 195.

McCartney, K. (Ed.). (1990). *Child care and maternal employment: A social ecology approach.* New directions for child development no. 49. San Francisco: Jossey-Bass.

Phillips, D., McCartney, K., Scarr, S., & Howes, C. (1987). Selective review of infant day care research: A cause for concern. *Zero to Three, 7,* 18–21.

Richardson, G., & Marx, E. (1989). *A welcome for every child.* New York: French-American Foundation.

Richters, J. E., & Zahn-Waxler, C. (1988). The infant day care controversy: Current status and future directions. *Early Childhood Research Quarterly, 3*(3), 319–336.

Rutter, M. (1981). Social-emotional consequences of day care for preschool children. *American Journal of Orthopsychiatry, 51,* 4–28.

Whitebook, M., Howes, C., & Phillips, D. (1989). *Who cares? Child care teachers and the quality of care in America.* Executive summary. Oakland, CA: Child Care Employee Project.

CULTURE, FAMILY, AND INFANT IN THE TWENTY-FIRST CENTURY: CONVERGING CLINICAL SCIENCE AND NEUROSCIENCE VIEWS OF DEVELOPING ADAPTIVE MECHANISMS

CHAPTER 14

J. Gerald Young

Neural Mechanisms Underlying Parent-Facilitated Adaptation in Infancy

☐ Clinical and Neuroscience Views of Adaptation in Infancy

> This—some say—confirms the hypothesis that each man bears in his mind a city made only of differences, a city without figures and without form, and the individual cities fill it up.
>
> Italo Calvino
> *Invisible Cities* (p. 34)

Faced with the myriad details that our sensory systems have encountered in the course of our lives, we, too, wonder how we came to make sense of them—or *if* we *ever* truly made sense of them. This curiosity motivates our quest, an impulse to examine how the infant begins making sense of the confusion of stimuli showering upon him or her. Calvino gives a remarkably intuitive supposition, that we build the city in our minds (not the actual city, of course) by ceaseless recognition of and adjustments to the differences observed among the individual cities we encounter in the journey of life. Our city is constructed only of differences from the first city observed, and from the dawning city that evolves with difference detection as we grow in our experience of cities. Memories, which are really comparisons of stimuli with memories, guide us. So we return to first memories and begin our questions about them and their origins.

Clinicians are often criticized for an unscientific approach to clinical care and theory building. Yet, clinicians are at the final, integrative, decision-making point in the trajectory of helping children and families, and it is their task to know as much as possible and to select from and integrate this material in a manner that will optimally aid the child. Regrettably, so many streams of information flow into this final estuary that much of the material is lost as the clinician struggles to understand diverse research data (e.g., Young et al., 1996) and apply it in the extraordinarily complex task of evaluating a child (e.g., see Young, Kaplan, Pascualvaca, & Brasic, 1995). In fact, most of the selection is accomplished by the "culture" of clinicians deciding what types of information are useful, and implying that other information streams can safely be neglected. This necessity is accepted, but it is essential to refresh our perspectives on clinical care periodically, even if it requires trials of hypotheses that will require further research. This chapter presents data that are to be the source of conceptual models, drawn from emerging neuroscience research, with the aim of illuminating our understanding of infancy and early childhood. The purpose is to suggest the neural mechanisms underlying clinical research observations and data and to encourage novel concepts for guiding clinical care in infancy and early childhood. Moreover, clinicians can also reflect on a contrasting reality: Many clinical observations were derided by skeptical scientists wary of concepts like *emotional influences* and *unconscious memories*, but which repeatedly have been validated by neuroscience research. We recall a comment during a discussion of another scientific field, cautioning us to respect each of the components—experimental data, theory, and practice—of any human science: "if you want to understand what a science is, you should look in the first instance not at its theories or its findings, and certainly not at what its apologists say about it; you should look at what the practitioners of it do" (Geertz, 1973, p. 5).

The focus of this chapter on the impact of experiences during infancy and early childhood should not imply neglect of the assuredly profound effects of later experiences and development during the course of life, for good or ill, nor the presence of any of the other potent pathological influences—genetic, infectious, metabolic, or other causes—leading to developmental disabilities such as mental retardation or autistic disorder and contributing to the psychiatric disorders of childhood and adolescence and the everyday challenges to the adaptation of the "normal" growing child.

The roots of infant and parental behaviors are each so complex and deep that descriptions of the former and prescriptions for the latter are forever surrounded by doubt among parents, professionals, and scientists. The momentous knowledge emerging over the past 50 years, and presented or touched on in the previous chapters, is in danger of being unreasonably neglected because of these doubts. However, illuminating the basic brain functions underlying these clinical observations and recommendations is one of the most convincing means for substantiating their veracity and utility.

The fundamental challenge when writing about infants and families is to determine what to recommend to parents as most likely to be maximally beneficial to the development of their child. Knowledge of brain function and development can aid this undertaking, but presents its own challenges. Theoreticians have moved beyond disputes about whether outcome is determined by genes or environment, but examining environmental influences on behavioral or emotional outcomes is difficult due to the subtlety of the effects. Examinations attempting to separate internal influences and external influences at every level are active (e.g., the levels of the entire body, the brain, a brain region, a neuronal group, or a single neuron) and our knowledge is vastly improved (Nowakowski & Hayes, 1999). However, an external influence can be difficult to detect. Compare the demonstrable alteration of brain tissue by an infectious agent to the subtle molecular effects brought about by a repetitive, traumatic interpersonal experience. The latter leaves few traces and is only now beginning to be more fully understood.

Nevertheless, prolific neuroscience research is generating data that suggest conceptual models responsive to fundamental clinical questions; from among these we will survey examples that are illustrative of specific themes. Of necessity, much of such research utilizes animal models, but this limitation has been accepted for several reasons, of which two stand out. First, genes in humans tend to be homologous to those active in the regulation of brain development in the animals examined. Second, using the cerebral cortex as an example of extensive interest and investigation related to infants, it can be said that, in spite of the remarkable expansion of the surface of the neocortex over the course of phylogeny—the human neocortical surface has expanded to become 10 times larger than the surface in a macaque monkey and 1000 times greater than in the rat—both its thickness and the fundamental cytoarchitectonic organizational pattern are little changed (Rakic, 2000).

☐ Experiences Guiding Adaptation in the Developing Infant and Molding Early Brain Development

Genes and Environments

Gene–environment interactions. New scientific discoveries inevitably suggest the possibility of less complex explanations of observed phenomena, but this hope is unlikely to be fulfilled for the regulatory effects of genes on behavior. Discrete, high-level, complex functions, such as memory, mathematical abilities, or musical talent are recognized to be the product of multiple genes in complex interactions with the environment. The search for "single gene" causes of psychiatric disorders over the past half-century has led to the identification of a very limited number of such genes, and a resulting shift to efforts to unravel polygenic contributions, even for many of the developmental disabilities hoped to be less genetically complex. This is not surprising, as we should no more expect that a gene will code for a specific component of cognition than we would anticipate that one gene would code for the exocrine functions and another gene code for the endocrine functions of the pancreas, a much less complex organ than the brain. Of course, this is not to say that single gene effects on brain development are not observable at the initial stages of brain development, such as their effects on guiding the patterns of regional brain development. Nevertheless, the effects of a gene at later stages of brain development are complex because they are interwoven with other influences—their functions at these stages derive from complex polygenic interactions as well as the additional interactions of genes with their protein products and many types of environmental influences.

Instead, neural genes code for the development of fundamental elements that bit by bit generate brain structure, not directly coding for a specific structure like the amygdala, but by providing the responsive guiding factors that cause initial elements to interact with the environment and surrounding components in a manner that spawns an increasingly elaborate and coherent functional structure (Johnson, 1997). Developmental regulatory genes provide the mechanisms and piloting rules enabling these tissues to respond in predetermined ways, gradually building cerebral structures—from the molecular level to organized regional neural structures—that are themselves subsequently sculpted as much by environmental influences on the responsive guiding factors as the genetic programs. The pathways from genes to observable functions of the infant is complex, winding through innumerable turns selected by environmental characteristics which, when repeated sufficiently, "tune" the development of neuronal connections, in this manner conferring the child's emerging capacities. The task of tracing the pathways of this neural development is daunting, usually leading to the decision that it is too difficult follow when attempting links to clinical observations. Nevertheless, the tools are now sufficiently developed, and the initial data sufficiently encouraging, to attest that a great deal can be gained in understanding: Examining brain science data together with clinical observations increasingly will confirm, guide, and extend the parental care and nurturance of infants in an obviously beneficial manner.

The Formation of Brain Structure: Shifting from Genetic Regulation to Shared Genetic and Environmental Regulation. In order to observe examples of brain development in which the genetic effect is relatively "isolated" or clearly dominant, we typically think of the earliest developmental processes. We find that even the earliest processes of brain development are highly complex, such as the regulation of the determination that a cell will become a neuron rather than another cell type. Determination of the neuronal phenotype has been shown to involve multiple regulatory genes (transcription factors) and extracellular signals, with different characteristics of the neuron indicated by specific, interrelated subprograms (Anderson & Jan, 1997)

Moving closer to the genetic control of specific brain functions, we consider later developmental stages, such as the formation of basic brain structures. Of particular interest has been the patterning of the cortex, dividing it into structurally and functionally distinct areas. This process begins with the story of a set of genes that has been extensively studied. They control the specification of each of the segments of the body of an animal as unique and different from each other, and are known as *homeobox (Hox)* genes. Thus, the presence of antennae, wings, or legs on any of the thoracic or abdominal segments (in *Drosophila*, where *Hox* genes have been extensively studied) is determined by the activity of specific *Hox* genes. These genes have been conserved to an exceptional degree across the phyla, encompassing all of the major classes of animals, including mammals. More recent work has demonstrated that other kinds of comparable genes are active in the specification of the structures making up the head and brain. The forebrain is of particular interest, and a prosomeric model of brain development has been proposed that describes identifiable patterns of gene expression that subdivide the neural tube into specific regions (Puelles & Rubenstein, 1993). The regional expression of transcription factors has been examined, and many examples of their functions determined; one of these is of special interest, the *Pax6* gene. Humans with a heterozygous mutation of this gene cannot form an iris in the eye (aniridia). Similar disruption of eye formation occurs in other species, but most fascinating is that the misexpression of this gene at the wrong positions in the *Drosophila* embryo leads to the induction of ectopic eyes, such as on an antenna (Halder, Callaerts, & Gehring, 1995). This is an example of a single gene determining the development of a complete sensory organ, and suggests that the *Pax* genes might function at the top of a hierarchy, as if coordinating the signals and genes required for organizing an embryonic "field" or region (Sanes, Reh, & Harris, 2000).

Following regionalization of the brain, brain areas associated with specific brain functions begin to be identifiable. Environmental effects are recognizable even at this early developmental phase. The initial genetic instructional set uses varying specific molecular factors to establish a preliminary structural map. This process then gives way to greater interaction of the initial cortical neurons with varying signals from newly arriving afferents from other brain structures to determine the borders and specific cellular and synaptic arrangements of specific functional brain areas. This is a process—known as arealization—that plays a cardinal role in early infant adaptive learning (Rakic, 2000). The basic structure of the brain is still in the process of formation, yet the environment surrounding the cortex is beginning its increasing interactional influences—extrinsic molecular factors associated with arriving afferent pathways, and activity patterns driven by spontaneous activity of other brain structures or by sensory inputs—with the specific genetic developmental programs and their associated intrinsic molecular factors, as well as the spontaneous intrinsic coordinated activity patterns of the cortex. This balance of intrinsic and extrinsic influences is at the center of substantial research and debate.

Current data suggest that gene families regulate the regionalization of the brain, while areal subdivisions are largely controlled by thalamocortical afferents. The latter are well suited to furnishing this molecular or activity-generated patterning guidance, as their association with sensory organs gives access to the external world and their projections provide a platform of specificity to the associated cortical areas. Research has demonstrated that classical auditory cortical areas can be experimentally influenced by providing *visual inputs to the auditory thalamus* so that presumed auditory cortex is transformed into visual cortex according to some major properties. Thus, the sensory cortex appears to develop a modular organization reflecting the nature of the sensory input and the pattern of its activity, which additionally contribute to the maintenance and plasticity of these neuronal circuits (Pallas, 2001). The importance of this cortical responsivity for development and evolution is evident, and one view indicates how this would have profound implications for clinical understanding. This view asserts that this plasticity in the final stage of cerebral cortex formation is essentially influenced by neural activity, as opposed to differential molecular markers. Moreover, it is a more prolonged process in humans, stretching into the postnatal period and permitting the infant's interactions with the environment to influence functional specialization of the cerebral cortex, whether for improved adaptation or for developmental disruptions (Johnson, 1999).

A First Example of Single Gene Regulation of a Complex Social Behavior. When studying brain functions, and "defining" the relationships between genes and environments, however, there are always caveats. For example, recent evidence suggests that a single gene regulates a complex social behavior in fire ants (Krieger & Ross, 2001). This major gene, rather than the anticipated multiple interacting genes (each with small effects), may control whether there will be one or many queens in an ant colony. The mediating mechanism appears to be the gene's regulation of how ants perceive pheromones indicating to them who is or is not a queen. The curious manner in which this occurs indicates the potential for rare major effects from a single gene on complex social behavior. Social organization among ants is related to the *Gp-9* gene, encoding a pheromone-binding protein apparently essential for the recognition of fellow fire ants. This recognition is essential to generating one or another of the two fundamental social structures of fire ants: an independent colony established by a monogyne queen, or a high-density network of interacting colonies built by polygyne queens with worker ants. Pretender queens intruding into a monogyne community with a queen present are killed, while polygyne colonies accept large numbers of queens for their interacting colonies. In the monogyne colony all of the fire ants have two copies of the *B* allele, while the mutant allele, *b*, is present in the 10% who are heterozygous in a polygyne colony. Whereas potential *BB* queens are killed in polygyne colonies, the *Bb* workers fail to recognize *Bb* queens and the *Bb* queens are accepted by the colony, possibly due to a defective protein that diminishes the capacity of the *Bb* workers to recognize the pheromones as readily as the *BB* workers do. This research indicates how the mutation of a single gene, affecting a specific behavioral characteristic, can have an unexpected major effect on complex social behavior because this characteristic acts at a branching point that affects downstream behaviors that are crucial to the social organization of the group (Holden, 2001; Krieger & Ross, 2001).

Much further research will be necessary to determine whether a single gene can ever have a very strong effect on complex social behaviors in humans, but we are warned that there might occasionally be a role to play. Nevertheless, the usual source of genetic influences would continue to be expected to be multiple genes interacting with the environment. One source of this expectation is that human decision making tends to rest upon multiple sources of information, making it less likely that a single gene could direct a complex social behavior in a manner similar to that of the fire ant.

Experience and the Development of Individual Differences

The Effects of Early Experience on Brain Structure and Function: Synaptogenesis, Plasticity, and Sensitive Periods.

If genetic effects on the child are to be forged, together with environmental influences, into the "experiences" that mold the brain, what is it in the brain that is changed in response to parental behaviors that clinical experts recommend or discourage? As might be expected, there is controversy about the answer to this question. One of the preferred concepts uses the "selectionist" view that active use is determinant, as a period of overproduction followed by relative inactivity of synapses leads to the selective pruning of these synapses and possibly neuron elimination. Among other views, "constructivist" approaches stand out, with neural activity guiding the construction of synaptic networks. To consider the most prominent example, we first recall that studies of adults indicate that the most conspicuous neural mechanism underlying the effects of experience on behavior and the brain is the modification of synaptic connections. But we wonder whether experience-induced brain changes are different during infancy and early childhood, when neural circuits are being constructed, or might they be similar throughout the life span? If these brain modifications are different, then we shall be interested in whether they might contribute to a "sensitive period" when environmental influences might have a unique and enduring effect. As one example of a potential developmental change in brain structure in infancy and early childhood, we ask yet another question: When do synapses appear, and does experience alter how they are constructed before the learning-related changes that might occur in mature synapses?

The greatest number of synapses is to be found in the cerebral cortex, where investigators are elucidating developmental characteristics of synapse formation. Synaptic connections are formed and maintained—or eliminated—through a prolonged, complex process that reaches into the adult decades of life. Five stages of synaptogenesis have been proposed in the macaque monkey (see Figures 14.1 and 14.2), and the first three of these stages advance together across at least the five major cytoarchitectonic areas in which the processes were investigated (Bourgeois, Goldman-Rakic, & Rakic, 2000). The fourth phase, initiated just after birth and extending until puberty, is characterized by high synaptic density and greater malleability: activity-dependent stabilization occurs, apparently accompanied by molecular alterations in synaptic strength. Following puberty, and extending into old age, the fifth phase is notable for a very slow decline in synaptic density and a lack of synaptogenesis. The absence or markedly reduced formation of synapses indicates stability of synaptic connections during adulthood, advantageous for the storage and conservation of acquired knowledge (Bourgeois et al., 2000). Learning and memory in adults appear to be accompanied by a remodeling of existing synapses rather than a formation of new synapses; the molecular changes associated with the strengthening and modification of existing synapses have been examined in detail.

Upon reflection, it is quickly apparent that concurrent synaptogenesis during infancy, across all of the cytoarchitectonic areas examined, has profound functional implications, particularly that the presence of all of the basic cortical functions within 2 or 3 months of life permits the coordinated emergence of these functions. The potential for the development of higher level functions, such as voice or face recognition, working memory, or initial social skills, requires that this cortical readiness be available for integration with the other cortical functions as they mature, producing both

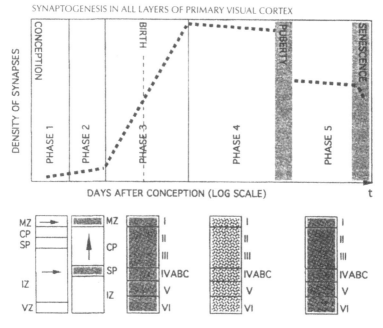

FIGURE 14.1. Changes in the relative density of synapses (dotted line in the upper frame) as a function of days after conception expressed on a log scale on the abscissa (t), in the primary visual cortex of the macaque monkey, during normal development. Five different phases of synaptogenesis are identified between conception and death. Each phase is superimposed above the density distribution of synapses in the cortical layers of the neocortex represented at the bottom of the figure. Abbreviations: CP, cortical plate; IZ, intermediate zone; MZ, marginal zone; SP, subplate. Bougeois, J. P., Goldman-Rakic, P. S., Rakic, P. (2000). Formation, elimination, and stabilization of synapses in the primate cerebral cortex. In M. S. Gazzaniga (Ed.), The new cognitive neurosciences (2nd ed., pp. 45–53). Reprinted with permission from MIT Press.

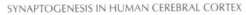

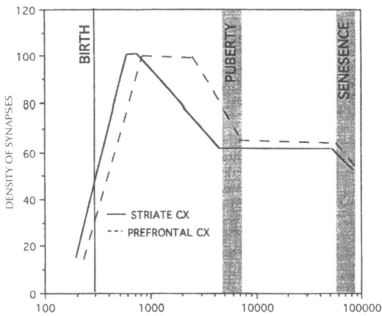

FIGURE 14.2. Changes in the relative density of synapses in the human cerebral cortex as a function of days after conception expressed on a log scale on the abscissa (*t*). Data are from Hutenlocher and Dabholkar (1997). Only phases 3, 4, and 5 are represented here. The same phases of synaptogenesis are observed in both the primary visual cortex (black line) and prefrontal cortex (dashed line). Note that phase 4 is longer in the prefrontal cortex than in the striate cortex. Huttenlocher, P. and Dabholkas, A. S. (1997). Regional differences in synaptogenesis in human cerebral cortex. Journal of Comparative Neurology, 387, 167–178. Reprinted with permission from John Wiley & Sons, Ltd.

unified structure and function—even though full maturation of cortical functions requires more than 10 years for the child. The first two phases of synaptogenesis, and the first half of the third phase, appear to be a genetically programmed, "experience-independent" process. However, by the time of the second half of phase 3, and during phase 4, the time of high synaptic density lasting from infancy to puberty, synaptogenesis takes on "experience-expectant" characteristics, as various sensory experiences spawn the necessary adjustments of the neuronal circuits of the cortex through their effects on synaptogenesis. As these events ebb, there is a transition to the molecular and cellular mechanisms typical of learning and memory in the adult (Bourgeois et al., 2000; Goldman-Rakic, Bourgeois, & Rakic, 1997).

This focus on synaptogenesis is not intended to indicate that it is the primary or sole mediator of experience-driven changes in the brain of the very young child. However, the pattern of synaptogenesis would appear to fit clinical observations about various important features of development during infancy (possibly conceptualized as a constructivist phase), such as the correspondence between emerging infant capacities and the rapid phase of synaptogenesis at the end of phase 3, and extending after birth. This rapid phase might occur for the first year or 18 months of the infant's life, depending on how we interpret the data describing synaptogenesis in humans (Huttenlocher & Dabholkar, 1997), as opposed to the information derived from analogous processes in the developing macaque monkey, as described. Other component activity patterns would also be active, such as selectionist activities in which the loss of synaptic connections at a somewhat later period contributes to the selective stabilization of these patterns of synaptic connections by the elimination of connections according to experience-guided activity patterns—in this way stabilizing the (apparent) "core" of the connections constructed earlier. This sequence of events suggests both the continuing plasticity of the brain during a substantial portion of early development, the orderly nature of the processes, and an apparent uniqueness characteristic of each developmental component which would make each a candidate for contributing to a sensitive period. Similarly, a "connectionist" perspective could play a role, inferring that statistical regularities of the environmental stimuli have a powerful formative influence on the developing brain; this view can be integrated comfortably with other components.

Are There Potential Clinical Applications of the Interacting Patterns of Brain Development and Early Experience?   We wonder again, however, how remote these brain-building events might be from the concerns of parents and professionals. Have we evidence suggesting any profound effects of experience during infancy that might be favorably managed through augmented research knowledge and parent counseling? Neuroscience and clinical investigators have unquestionably demonstrated that a child's experiences are accompanied by changes in the brain. From the perspective of later development—the older child, adolescent, or adult—there are clinical observations about specific early childhood experiences that have been accorded a central role in the genesis of adaptive or maladaptive behaviors. Have studies of the developing brain identified any brain–behavior relationships that indicate how these experiences might influence brain function in a manner suggesting neural mechanisms underlying the behavioral outcomes following repeated early childhood experiences of these kinds? There are such neural mechanisms, and we will briefly consider two mechanisms to make this point, and act as the rationale for pursuing an extended review of major elements of brain function in more detail preparatory to suggesting a conceptual model for use with families.

Two fundamental clinical problems, often encountered when caring for children and families, lead to discussions about the causes of a child's behavior, and that they presumably are related to experiences during infancy and early childhood. Often invoked as leading to "maladaptation" (from whose point of view?) they are as follows. First, differences in behaviors among children are often accompanied by highly compelling evidence that they reflect differences in the environments and experiences to which they were exposed, and special importance is given to the earliest repetitive experiences in infancy and early childhood. Here the idea is that unusual environments produce children behaving in unusual ways. But if the behavior looks less unusual, and more like simple "bad behavior," then there is diminished interest in examining the early childhood environment of the child. Second, children with significant emotional and behavioral problems are often reported to have had to accommodate to consistently contradictory cues from their caregivers, particularly aggressive behavior, while its presence or significance is disclaimed. In this instance, there is the theory that, not only is this likely to confuse the child, but that it can interfere with his or her adaptation. Yet, we wonder whether any brain mechanisms for resolving contradictory stimuli have developed. Research data now exist that provide instructive examples of interesting neural mechanisms related to each of these developmental experiences. We will not pursue here the question of whether the child's behavior in response to these phenomena should be described as "maladaptive," given that the behaviors are adaptive in relation to his own unique early childhood environment.

Sensory Mapping: A Model Neural Substrate for Individual Differences in Sensory Awareness. The creation of "social maps"—maps of a child's social space—and the tuning of the resulting "social coordinates" to the actual environment of the child, encompass complex processes utilizing the plastic properties of the developing brain. Components of these social maps, moreover, contain elements constructed during probable "sensitive periods" in early development, and not thereafter. Clinical observations have long suggested that an individual child, while adapting to a highly specific environment, subsequently "expects" and responds to specific multimodal environmental and social features and not others. Is it possible that this clinical observation is accurate, or is it a convenient explanatory mythology? What might be the physiological basis of this "expectation," or enhanced or diminished responsiveness to certain environmental features in preference to others—arising from the plasticity of response during infancy? Let us examine a simpler, though not simple, model, that of the development of sensory responses.

The tuning of the brain's response to the environment, in order to register significant sensory data, is a process that emerges in relation to, and dependent on, the data actually presented by the environment. This can be demonstrated by the brain's management of information derived from two different sensory systems. The brain needs to merge sensory maps of identical environmental phenomena that are registered by separate sensory systems. For the separate data to be adaptively useful (successful) the two must give corresponding "coordinates," so that the data can be merged; in other words, if used in isolation each will produce the same result. Cross-modal information must be in agreement, and the ranges of information in the modalities it is capable of sampling must conform to the ranges in the environment.

This principle has been demonstrated by Eric Knudsen and colleagues through studies of the merging of auditory and visual maps of space by young barn owls. Barn owls need to be able to localize sensory signals in space, including auditory and visual cues used to localize prey. Data from different sensory modalities, such as visual and auditory, must conform with great precision in the drafting of the spatial map. For example, using microsecond differences in the timing of sound reaching its two ears, the barn owl gives precise coordinates to the location of its prey, even in darkness, in the construction of its auditory map of space. Coordinates in a visual map drawn from viewing the prey are merged with auditory data in optic tectum neurons that respond to both visual and auditory signals from a specific location. Thus, the two sensory systems provide independent coordinates which are merged in the optic tectum (also known as the superior colliculus).

However, if there are alterations in these relationships in the experience of an individual during the sensitive period, adaptive adjustments are possible in order to maintain precise alignment. Knudsen altered the data obtained through the visual channel by placing prisms over their eyes (which are fixed in their sockets in owls), causing the owl to have visually responsive neurons tuned to an "off-center" location because of the displaced visual information; this meant that the visual and auditory maps were out of register and no longer associated. The auditory map had to be physiologically readjusted to compensate and again attain proper alignment between the two maps. Over about one month, the young owls adjusted so that the visual map was once again "tuned" and auditory and visual maps were again aligned (Barinaga, 1998; Knudsen, 1998).

While further research needs to be completed, it appears that the owls trained with prisms had developed additional neural connections as an adaptation to the prisms. While unused and inactive for a long period, such unusual functional connections formed during a sensitive period apparently can be reactivated at a later time during adulthood. Learning during the sensitive period permanently altered the brain, and the owl's capacities, so that it could relearn the task as an adult. The capacity for plasticity in response to experience during adulthood had been expanded and, in spite of disuse, had persisted. Owls lacking this prism training experience during the sensitive period were incapable of learning the needed response as adults. Is there reason to suspect that there is an actual change in neural connections? Knudsen's team earlier demonstrated that the young owls could adjust to various prism shifts applied, while the adults could not. They showed that a new pattern of connections—axonal projections—developed in these young owls, in addition to the original set of connections. Moreover, the original connections apparently were reactivated when the prism was removed and the young owls adjusted their sound localization.

While the later experiment demonstrated that the additional capacity for sound localization remained, it is important to recognize the limitation of this capacity in the adult: it cannot adjust to any prism shift presented, but only to the prism shift of the direction and magnitude identical to that used when the owl was young. This is a restricted, specific adaptive capacity, as compared to the broad adaptability of the young owl to shifts of varying directions and magnitudes. The adults appear to be limited to learning through the adaptation developed by the additional neuronal connections during the sensitive period, which remains available for relearning in adulthood. Knudsen's next research goal was to demonstrate that it is actually these specific additional neuronal connections that have persisted and have been utilized in the adult owls. This would indicate that experiences during the sensitive period would have their lasting effects through the development of axonal projections. Or is there some other mechanism that remains from early experience during the sensitive period, and is yet to be identified? Whatever the result, the experiments document the establishment of functional connections through experience during a sensitive period, leaving an enduring trace in the adult brain (Barinaga, 1998; Knudsen, 1998). Other examples of persisting effects of sensitive period experience in spite of disuse have been demonstrated in birds and mammals. An example in humans is language learning, discussed later (Kuhl, 1994; Tong, Busby, & Clark, 1988).

Social Mapping: A Hypothesized Model Neural Substrate for Individual Differences in Social Awareness in Infancy and Early Childhood. For the dependent child, most of adaptation means properly predicting the behavior of significant adult caregivers who provide the necessities of life to the child. Thus, there is a strong emphasis on the child's detailed study of interpersonal interactions and how they predict outcomes. These interpersonal interactions supply multiple indices of the adult's possible intentions as the child attempts predictions using increasingly familiar indices: language, facial expression, body posture, gestures, and the responses of other adults. All of these signs of possible intentions must be examined for their relations to outcomes. This involves the comparison of data from separate sensory modalities or separate information systems within a single modality and the merging of these data coordinates in a social map. Failure to build adaptive social maps that lead to reasonable levels of predictive and adaptive success cause confusion and the disruption of physiological and behavioral homeostasis, most prominently fragmented behavior, overactivity, and inattention in young children, or dysregulation of emotions and behavior in older children and adolescents.

Looking ahead to the vital role of attachment in development, discussed in the next chapter, one might conceptualize attachment as building physiological and behavioral systems, little by little, whose associated social map, and its subsequent tuning, is regulated by the mother. The initial emphasis is on the regulation of proper physiological and behavioral functioning, avoiding "escape" from the normal range of optimal function. Later, emphasis shifts to regulation of memory formation predictive of optimally adaptive outcomes. If physiological functioning is stable and the infant is able to enjoy a state of quiet alertness, then he is optimally prepared to learn. These ideas will be scrutinized in detail later.

Sensory Mapping: A Model Neural Substrate for Rapid, Intelligent Choice Responses to Conflicting Environmental Cues. One further example of brain function and early experience is useful, because it suggests both the diversity and fundamental significance of these early developmental events. The problem of dealing with conflicting information sources is not limited to a child attempting to decipher the varying indicators of an adult's sometimes contradictory cues indicating his or her emotions and intentions. It is a basic biological problem for a functional nervous system that begins at the level of responding to competing sensory cues. How do nervous systems manage the problem of utilizing multiple sensory cues when the sources of cue information presented might deliver internally contradictory information? And does this involve only memory and learning, or are genes somehow involved?

The problem of choice while responding to and merging sensory perceptual information exists for animals generally, and they use experience to select which of their available behaviors ought to be used. The rapid, rational choice reflects prior learning experience indicating the advantages and disadvantages of each. An example is the use of *Drosophila* to examine choice behavior, applying a visual learning paradigm in which individual flies are conditioned to select one of two flight paths in response to color and shape cues; following this training they are tested with two conflicting cues and their choice behavior is examined. The capacity to use multiple cues during visual learning creates a choice predicament for flies presented with contradictory information. However, it was found that wild-type flies can use small differences in the relative salience of competitive cues to make firm, stable choices, indicated by an observed distinct transition point in the flight behavior reflecting a choice that changed from one alternative to the other according to the changing visual cues. On the other hand, mutant flies (mbm^1) lacking brain structures known as mushroom bodies had a markedly reduced capacity for this choice behavior. Mushroom bodies are neural structures that appear to be involved in both multimodal sensory processing and context generalization, providing what has been described as "intelligent control" over instinctual behaviors. Thus, mushroom bodies appear to be an example of early neural structures that mediate intelligent responses to conflicting environmental stimuli (Liu, Wolf, Ernst, & Heisenberg, 1999; Strausfeld, Hansen, Li, Gomez, & Ito, 1998; Tang & Guo, 2001). This research indicates the existence of brain structures for generating responses to the environment that are substantially more complex—even in a much less complex animal than humans, and involving multimodal sensory processing, context generalization, and decision making in spite of contradictory information. The choice behavior utilizes previous learning, which is to say that there are brain structures responding in infancy that accomplish complex adaptive tasks.

Social Mapping: A Hypothesized Model Neural Substrate for Rapid, Intelligent Choice Responses to Conflicting Environmental Cues in Infancy and Early Childhood. This diversion into the behavioral challenges of the fruit fly is not meant to imply that we need mushroom bodies to cope with the often contradictory information confronting us. But it is to suggest that the nervous system has evolved in the context of a requirement for mechanisms for resolving conflicting sensory information, probably because it is so common. Similarly, it would seem judicious if adults were to assume that the social world of the infant or young child contains remarkable complexity, replete with internal contradictions. In spite of ample everyday evidence for this, parents typically seem little aware of or concerned with this problem for their babies. Judged at different levels of intensity and frequency of contradiction, these conflicting social data might be expected to interfere with learning after reaching a certain threshold; with ever greater exposure to contradiction, it would be expected to cause significant emotional distress according to the significance of the experiences and the persistence of the contradictions. This is the type of problem for which parent counseling can have a highly beneficial effect when applied. In addition, the complexity of these processes indicates that it is necessary for us to survey possible neural substrates for organizing perceptual information, even when contradictory, and for utilizing higher cognitive processes to adapt to these sometimes perplexing environmental cues.

☐ Conceptualizing Brain Function: Stimulus Evaluation and Adaptive Prediction Using Memory and Emotion

Brain Mechanisms for Adaptation

In the background of these discussions of genes, environments, and experiences lies a concept of the mind and the brain and how they function, and this will have to be articulated in detail if we are to consider the links between the developing brain and the infant's experiences. From the point of view of a neuroscientist studying the young child's emerging behavior, the essential question is, How does the brain extract from the environment the information necessary for it to adapt, survive, and reproduce?

The ultimate function of the brain is to predict the environment and its responses, in order to enable the animal to adapt optimally. The brain accomplishes this predictive activity, with more or less success, through *stimulus evaluation mechanisms* that utilize difference detection and significance detection. These evaluation mechanisms become more complex, functioning through successive levels of greater neuronal circuit complexity, molded by evolution, that utilize increasingly elaborate forms of memory—that themselves reflect added levels of complexity, such as categorization, relational data, and symbolization. All of these levels continue to function and interact with one another. Memories are the basis for *difference detection*, enabling comparison of the current stimulus with memories of prior environmental stimuli and responses to them. As these memories become more complex, by their inclusion of additional associated qualities, and even more so with elaborated data about the context of the stimulus and the relationships among memories, the animal is increasingly able to identify elements predictive of later environmental responses or conditions, favorable or unfavorable to its needs.

A second component of stimulus evaluation is *significance detection*, useful for boosting the rapidity of the animal's response (e.g., for survival purposes), for better identifying salient features of the environment demanding attention and specific adaptive responses, and for motivation. Significance detection utilizes (1) the reinforcement history of individual neurons to alter the strength of synaptic transmission (potentiation or depression) and (2) the elicitation of emotion, or, additionally, the memory of emotions, to guide behavior. Emotions continue to affect behavior even when the most complex memory systems are active.

In order to accomplish difference detection and significance detection, the brain also must continually form new memories in order to update data about environmental features that will guide subsequent adaptation. Memories increase in complexity both with reference to the complexity of stimuli to which they respond (e.g., a face activating a single amygdaloid cell as compared to a color activating a cortical cell) and in relation to the complexity of neuronal circuits and functions utilized to achieve difference or significance detection (e.g., recalling a lock combination, which lock it pertains to, its color, where it is, who has access to the lock, and what it protects—requiring working memory operating in tandem with long-term memory of different types in different neuronal circuits—versus recalling the smell of smoke, which requires long-term memory in a specific cortical area). Most important, however, is that the increasing complexity encompasses greater attention to both the details of context in the memories and the relationships among memories, permitting the person to identify repeated elements that tend to predict certain outcomes. It is this complexity that is so important in a learned behavior such as fearful avoidance, because the associations of anxiety with specific conditions in this person's earlier life, which had considerable predictive value, might no longer be associations with valid predictive utility. In spite of this, they could retain lingering, intense significance in the person's current life, and simultaneously appear unimportant to others, whose lives were radically different from his or hers, and who impatiently express their frustration with the person.

The increasing complexity of memories enables adaptive behaviors of increasing complexity, especially through a new capacity for strategies, such as enhanced attention to social and abstract factors, to aid in adaptive prediction. Moreover, this increasing complexity enables the replacement of some types of unconscious (implicit) memory and learning by conscious (explicit) memory, learning, and thinking when it is advantageous.

We do not mean to ignore in this discussion the ultimate need for action as a completion of the classical stimulus–response cycle view of brain function. The need for a behavioral response from the child is undisputed, but this is outside our immediate focus other than how memories and emotion influence the behavior. In this context, we will only say the obvious, that once stimulus evaluation is complete and a response strategy selects a behavioral goal, response systems are activated, including the basal ganglia, the cerebellum, and the premotor and motor cortices—all of which participate in utilizing this response selection to initiate and coordinate the selection of sequential patterns of movements to achieve the goals. In addition, modulatory neuronal systems have important interacting functions, regulating thresholds for perception, evaluation, memory formation, and response selection. They include the noradrenergic system (active during stress), the serotonergic system, and the cholinergic system, among others. Limbic and neuroendocrine systems also play significant roles in these responses.

Does this survey of adaptive brain functions aid us in our attempt to understand how anxiety, lack of awareness, or laughter could be a learned behavior favored by a child's environment, or could result from subtle disorders affecting these neural circuits? Does it illuminate the underlying neurobiological functions and participating structures? Let us see how neuroscience information describing various features of brain function might explicate the genesis and repetition of a specific behavior of a child through learning and memory formation, never neglecting the realization that interference with these functions by either lesions or genetic mutations might lead to a similar result.

Neural Coding of Environmental Information

First, a word about something that we will not pursue in detail, but cannot be ignored: How does environmental information get into the brain of the infant? The infant's adaptation begins with his or her detection of stimuli from the environment by sensory organs, initiating subsequent perceptual and cognitive processes that generate a response. Each of the multiple processing stages manipulates this information, which is coded and recoded during higher processing in the brain. The action potential, the prototypical "spike," acting as a signal of neural activity and communication of information, is only one element registering information; the coding elements within the central nervous system are diverse and extensive, much too complex to be described here. Yet, as the first and fundamental step of adaptation upon which all others depend, a brief mention of some examples of neural coding—neural signals, with a special emphasis on coding for learning and memory mechanisms—is useful.

The formation of a network of mental representations of the infant's environment depends upon her brain's capacity to detect and transform the sensory stimuli to a sensory–perceptual code that is available for discrimination, comparison with memory templates, significance determination, memory formation, and higher cognitive processing. This process would seem to encounter insuperable difficulties due to its inherent complexity, but the neural coding mechanisms and memory formation processes contain a similar diversity and complexity that enable the brain to accomplish these tasks. For example, information is coded variously as electrical signals, signals both from individual neurons and from pools of neurons (Reich, Mechler, & Victor, 2001; Richmond, 2001); influences on the strength of dendritic synapses by backpropagating action potentials (Magee & Johnston, 1997; Markram, Lübke, Frotscher, & Sakmann, 1997; Sejnowski, 1997); a marked increase in the sensitivity of a neuron—involving a dynamic gain–control mechanism—to subtle changes in the firing patterns of afferent inputs through short-term synaptic depression (Abbott, Varela, Sen, & Nelson, 1997);

networks of signaling pathways storing information for learned behavior within intracellular biochemical reactions (Bhalla & Iyengar, 1999; Lisman & Fallon, 1999); or optimizing stimulus representations within a sensory network through temporal patterning—the transformation, by neuronal assemblies, of stimulus representations over time within the same circuit, enabling distributed representations to reflect distinct features of a stimulus at different epochs of a response (Friedrich & Laurent, 2001).

Coding for learning and memory specifically has been examined for decades (Martin, Bartsch, Bailey, & Kandel, 2000). Multiple molecular and cellular methods for capturing and retaining information as memories are utilized; examples include learning mediated by long-term potentiation (LTP) secondary to activation of NMDA-related receptors (Bliss & Lomo, 1973; Johnston, 1997; Murphy & Glanzman, 1997); the influence of growth factors, even on adult neural plasticity (Zhang, Endo, Cleary, Eskin, & Byrne, 1997); reactivation of the NMDA receptor as a synaptic reinforcement process for memory consolidation (Shimizu, Tang, Rampon, & Tsien, 2000); coordinated, rapid changes in the distribution of clusters of proteins in both the presynaptic and postsynaptic neurons during long-lasting potentiation (Antonova, Arancio, Trillat, Wang, Zablow, Udo, Kandel, & Hawkins, 2001), and other mechanisms. We can be sure that there are many coding processes, quite sufficient for any level of complexity required for adaptation. What do we know about how and where this coding is transformed into memories, and how memory systems are organized?

☐ Brain Systems for Learning and Memory: Modular Neural Information and Distributed Neural Circuits

Anatomy and Functions of Memory: Mapping and Predicting the External World

The word *memory* connotes a single entity, with an intuitively understood function of storing replicas of past occurrences. Nevertheless, there are different types of memory (or, said differently, memory functions in different ways) and this complicates our study of the role of memory as experience molds behavior. A long history of research on "memory" has finally begun to produce a potentially accurate map of how memory functions in the brain. In spite of this, memory remains notably elusive as a concrete concept for research and as an activity to be identified within specific brain loci. This does not diminish its significance for behavior, because memory is the vehicle by which the brain retains the consequences of a current behavior or thought. As an example, this capacity is the foundation for a child's gradual learning, including learning through consequences, whether or not to choose violent behavior as a means toward an end.

In our discussions below, the types of memory are accepted as understood according to the general descriptions indicated, so as not to burden the flow of topics with controversies that do not directly affect it. Nevertheless, a brief description of types of memory, given below, will verify how complex and unfinished this topic is. Similarly, different physiological–anatomical "levels" of memory will be considered, but their radical differences will not be discussed. For example, differences in the firing pattern of a single neuron will be considered as if it were a simple representation of memory function, even though it is not intended to imply necessarily that a single neuron codes a memory—but, rather, that its firing pattern is an element utilized in the formation of memories. In this sense, the observation of concrete changes in the firing pattern of an amygdaloid neuron in response to patterns of environmental stimuli helps us recognize the reality of intangible memories influencing brain function toward or away from adaptive behavior. Finally, the organization of memory (or any brain function) in the brain is an evolving topic of research central to the neurosciences, and any comments here about localization in the brain do not imply that neural information is modular or localized in its "geography," or the extreme alternative, that it is inherently contained in neural circuits distributed broadly throughout the brain. Instead, it is assumed that memory and other brain functions have varying modular and distributed characteristics.

Memory is fundamental to adaptation, as the process by which a representational map of the world is formed, continually revised as it increasingly converges with external reality; it is used to predict environmental responses to events and behaviors. Its sensitivity to environmental events rests upon its capacity to generate altered representational maps in response to current experiences that update adaptive responses. This would, in turn, be a source of its vulnerability to producing representational maps that are so specific in time or space as to be "abnormal" outside the conditions generating them. The ease of alteration of these maps must be limited, so that confusing, ever-changing maps are not produced and it is possible to have long-term memories; yet, if revisions of representational maps require substantial intensity and frequent repetition of new stimuli, older, "abnormal" memories related to experience in the limited environment of early life can be quite persistent and, sometimes, maladaptive.

A Classification of Memory Systems

Understanding the neurobiology of memory mechanisms requires specification of the type of memory concerned, for there is good evidence for differing neuroanatomical circuits for specific types of memory. The term *explicit* or *declarative memory* refers to the conscious recollection of facts (verbal, spatial, etc.) and events—memory with content. In contrast, *implicit* or *nondeclarative memory* includes various unconscious recollections, such as motor memory, habits, skills, priming, and some types of classical conditioning (Zola-Morgan & Squire, 1993). Like everything else related to the brain, there is controversy about this division also (Butler & Berry, 2001; Tulving, 2000), but it stands as a very useful perspective that is employed by most investigators and clinicians.

The understanding of memory emerging from the cognitive neurosciences has changed rapidly since the early 1990s, and will continue to do so. A description of the definitions and classification of brain memory systems at the current time is useful, because it highlights both how much we have come to understand and the nature of controversies at this time. For example, one classification of memory systems is proposed by Tulving (2000):

1. *Procedural memory*: the learning and memory are expressed through behavior, by doing something or executing a procedure. It is also known as *nondeclarative, habit*, or *implicit memory* (incorrectly).

2. *Cognitive memory*: the learning and memory are expressed in thought and can be held in mind, such as being aware of thoughts or contemplating something. Also known as *declarative, propositional*, or *explicit memory* (incorrectly).

Four cognitive memory types or systems are described:

(a) *Working memory*: holds information "on line" for cognitive operations over brief time intervals.
(b) *The perceptual representation system*: memory-based enhancement of perceptual identification of objects.
(c) *Semantic memory*: the acquisition and use of general knowledge about the world.
(d) *Episodic memory*: conscious access to the personally experienced past (Tulving, 2000).

This is a working model, with imperfect separation among the categories, and some disagreement among investigators (e.g., some consider procedural memory and implicit memory to be identical). An alternative scheme that differs slightly is used by Squire and Knowlton and its relationships are diagramed in Figure 14.3 (Squire & Knowlton, 2000). Many investigators equate unconscious memory with procedural or implicit memory, and conscious memory with cognitive or explicit memory, as is done in this chapter, although they are not necessarily the same (Tulving, 2000). These distinctions are not trivial, as they focus progressive research efforts, but, until the questions are answered, it is most sensible to use the general sense of the terms that is current.

Anatomical, Cellular, and Molecular Perspectives on Memory

Modular and Distributed Neuroanatomy of Memories.   The localization of long-term memory within the brain is an essential goal for research because it will illuminate how the brain functions in highly meaningful respects; yet, it has been frustratingly refractory to continuing research efforts. In spite of the unruly challenges, there

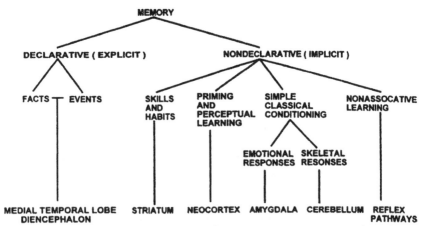

FIGURE 14.3. A taxonomy of mammalian long-term memory systems. The taxonomy lists the brain structures thought to be especially important for each form of declarative and nondeclarative memory. In addtion to its central role in emotional learning, the amygdala is able to modulate the strength of both declarative and nondeclarative memory. Source: Squire, L. R, Knowlton, B. J. (2000). The medial temporal lobe, the hippocampus, and the memory systems of the brain. In M. S. Gazzaniga (Ed.), The new cognitive neurosciences (2nd ed., pp. 765–779). Reprinted with permission from MIT Press.

are certain regions and processes that appear to function in a prototypical manner. For example, changes in firing patterns of neurons develop in response to stimuli, and result in long-term potentiation or depression of neuronal activity; they appear to be related to the memory encoding and consolidation processes. This acquisition process is likely to be related to morphological changes in the neuron, including synaptic enlargement, dendritic spine growth, expansion of the neuropil, and similar changes. This new memory formation process appears to occur particularly in the hippocampus and related structures (Figure 14.3), as indicated above. The locus of long-term memory storage is uncertain, but the neocortex is most often suggested, especially the association and polymodal regions. The amygdala and other areas play special roles in the formation of emotional memories, and working memory has a primary location in the prefrontal cortex.

At the molecular and synaptic levels it appears that the mechanisms underlying memory processes are essentially similar, while occurring in different anatomical locations. Similarly, it appears that common functional mechanisms are used, such as the temporal relations of stimuli, stimulus salience, massed versus spaced practice, and related factors (Rescorla, 1988a, 1988b). The structures underlying the formation of explicit memory have been studied in detail and are used as a model for the genesis of long-term memories. The formation of long-term explicit memory utilizes structures in the medial temporal lobe and the medial thalamus for a limited time after exposure to the stimuli, but these structures are not the locus of long-term memory. Instead, slowly developing, long-term explicit memory is built up elsewhere, particularly in various regions of the neocortex (Squire, 1992). Short-term, working memory is formed in another location, in the frontal region, and implicit memory formation appears to utilize interactions between the neocortex and structures in the neostriatum, cerebellum, and posterior cortical areas (Zola-Morgan & Squire, 1993).

Events underlying formation of long-term explicit memory in the medial temporal lobe and the medial thalamus have been delineated sufficiently to indicate that information from widespread regions of the neocortex arrive in the parahippocampal cortex and perirhinal cortex. Further processing takes place in the information flow to the entorhinal cortex and, subsequently, in the hippocampal formation (dentate gyrus, CA_3 and CA_1). Information is then dispatched through the entorhinal cortex and subiculum back to the neocortex, the apparent locus of long-term explicit memories. This information also goes to medial thalamic structures, including the anterior thalamic nucleus, the mediodorsal nucleus, and links to and from the medial thalamus within the internal medullary lamina. Moreover, projections to the frontal lobe (ventromedial frontal cortex and dorsolateral frontal cortex) make memories being formed available for guiding behavior through temporary influences on working memory, which is organizing behavior choices through comparisons of perceptual information with long-term memories. The formation of explicit memories in the medial temporal lobe and the medial thalamus thus influences working memory in the frontal cortex while revising long-term memories in broad regions of the neocortex (Zola-Morgan & Squire, 1993).

Multiple Mediating Mechanisms: From Experiences to Memories. How do cellular systems integrate sensory information and respond appropriately to the stimuli? The conventional molecular mechanisms of long-term memory formation that have been elucidated will be our focus, but an initial understanding is essential: There are multiple mechanisms for the formation of various types of memory. There can even be some difficulty when defining what constitutes a memory. Regulation of behavior in response to sensory information does not necessarily require the intervention of memory as usually conceived. For example, research has demonstrated that single afferent or efferent neurons can process information and initiate activities appropriate for maintaining the internal environment, such as monitoring and adjusting external osmolality and ion levels or blood sugar levels, or tuning the activity of multiple target organs in relation to the time or season. They are called "sensing effectors," cells that sense a single cue—the parameter they are regulating—and act to regulate the parameter. They can be a neuron (which is both sensory and neurosecretory) or an endocrine cell (equipped with smart detectors; Wenning, 1999). This concept cannot be overemphasized, because certain adaptive functions of the brain may use differing types of memory formation that need to be better understood, and have great significance for understanding learning and adaptation during infancy and childhood. Imitation is a notable example that will be discussed later.

Mechanisms of Long-Term Potentiation and Memory Consolidation.   Nevertheless, the multiple types of memory described above generally utilize more complex encoding, consolidation, and retrieval processes. These processes occur at molecular, cellular, circuit, and system levels, complicating our search for memory traces in the brain. However, cognitive neuroscientists have gained a solid foothold. The best studied model for the neurobiology of learning and memory at a molecular and cellular level is that of long-term potentiation (LTP) (Bliss & Lomo, 1973). LTP, described and studied in the hippocampus, is elicited by brief high-frequency stimulation; this engenders a long-lasting increase in the strength of synaptic transmission in this specific neuronal pathway. Correspondingly, long-term depression (LTD) occurs when low frequency, more prolonged (e.g., 10–15 minutes) stimulation is administered, and produces enduring decrements in the strength of synaptic transmission (Malenka, 1995). Most important for the functional understanding of these processes, and their clinical applications, is that the plasticity induced is bidirectional—meaning that a synapse can be potentiated or depressed according to the stimulus characteristics: LTP occurs after brief high frequency stimulation and LTD is produced by low frequency, sustained stimulation (Oliet, Malenka, & Nicoll, 1996). Specific molecular events in the intracellular second messenger cascades, producing altered gene expression, have been elucidated for each of these processes. The NMDA-type glutamate receptor is necessary for the production of LTP; while the AMPA-type glutamate receptor appears to be essential to its maintenance in one region of the hippocampus, other molecular mechanisms are utilized elsewhere, apparently reflecting the diversity of memory types and underlying mechanisms (Post et al., 1998).

Thus, if for many decades scientists have attempted to determine how memory is coded and where and in what form it is stored, the answers gradually are emerging. There is now agreement that memories are stored as altered synaptic plasticity in response to experience—an augmentation or decrement of synaptic strength, and sometimes in the synaptic structure (the pattern or number of synapses). The mechanisms differ according to the type of memory. Short term (working) memory is coded as the covalent modification of molecules already synthesized; the preexisting connections are then increased or decreased in strength. The mechanisms for long-term memory are more complex, and rely upon the synthesis of new messenger RNAs to form new proteins and the subsequent formation of new synaptic connections (Martin et al.,

2000). Long-term potentiation (LTP) is a process that most investigators believe to be a component of long-term memory consolidation, because the two processes parallel each other in so many respects. An interesting feature of LTP is that there is growing evidence that it is mediated by adhesion receptors, and that there appears to be an interaction of the two functions of the synapse—transmission and adhesion—in the LTP consolidation process. Junctional organization (through adhesion receptors) and trans-mitter receptors appear to be intimately linked, influencing one another (Lynch, 2000).

Classical and Extended Descriptions of Memory Pathology. Frank damage to specific brain structures causes multiple types of amnesia, varying according to the location of the lesion. However, the "pathology" of memory might include, in another sense, the maladaptive results of normally functioning memory systems in a trauma-filled environment.

The psychoanalytic concept that memories of traumatic events in childhood could significantly affect adult behavior has been validated and extended to include the marked effects of severe trauma during adulthood on later functioning; in both cases memory is the vehicle carrying these influences. Children who were abused at a young age are vulnerable not only to posttraumatic stress disorder (PTSD) but to other outcomes, such as unconscious identification with and repetition of aggressive behaviors of the abusing adult (identification with the aggressor), reflecting the activity of implicit memory in addition to conscious, explicit memory. Repeated exposure to aggressive violence can cause violent retaliation and preferential use of violence as a coping method; once encoded in memory, it guides behavior. Probably more common is the memory of childhood success at obtaining whatever one wanted by threats and aggressive behav-ior in the presence of an adult who failed to contain the aggression; this leaves memo-ries of unopposed, "successful" aggression as a preferred method of adaptation.

☐ Brain Systems for Learning and Memory Enabling Cognition and Planning

Motor Learning: Sensorimotor Transformations, Internal Models, Decoding the Actions of Others, and Governing Computational Processes

How do learning and memory become transformed into activities in the infant's world? All brain activities depend on movement for eventual interaction with the world, in-cluding communication and social interactions. This simple concept establishes the cardinal role of motor functions. Moreover, the transformation of sensory stimuli into purposeful action provides a guiding model for other activities of the brain. The con-stituent components of motor learning are being deciphered, and, while they cannot be reviewed in detail here, they are instructive when applied as a model for the under-standing of adaptive behavior generally, including social behaviors. Four principles stand out for our purposes. First, there are innate patterns of motor behavior, yet most motor behavior is learned, as it requires the flexibility to respond to novel needs. Sec-ond, motor outputs involve sensorimotor transformations, in that each command is affected by sensory feedback, consisting of sensory information from sense organs and also internal information in the form of an efference copy of the descending motor command. These transformations occur in both directions, "forward" (motor commands leading to sensory consequences) and "inverse" (a desired sensory consequence is transformed into the necessary motor commands for accomplishing it). This requires that both forward and inverse internal models be generated within the brain if we are to carry out skilled movements with complex goals (Wolpert, Ghahramani, & Flanagan, 2001).

Third, a principle related to the second, is that perceiving the action of others involves decoding their actions, at least partially, by activating one's own motor system at a subthreshold level; special neural mechanisms appear to be active during this decoding, as occurs during either observation or imitation, and can be demonstrated during neuroimaging. Fourth, motor activities can be considered as a computational system, and the same computation processes probably can be applied to social cognition and social interactions. For example, a forward social model would predict the reactions of other individuals to my own actions, and an inverse social model would guide my selection of appropriate actions in order to achieve a desired social outcome. This reflects the idea that, in spite of the increased complexity of social interactions, they are not intrinsically different computationally. It would appear that these computational processes are built up from fundamental units to highly complex units. While social cognition is more complex, examination of the extraordinary complexity of the motor system and its elaborate responses helps to form a basis for understanding how the brain can accomplish the complex computational processes governing the emotional and social functions necessary for the infant to develop optimally (Wolpert et al., 2001). Let us look in more detail at some of the essential brain functions that are occurring during this complex cascade of information processing.

Categorization: Complex Learning and Memories That Initiate Cognitive Functions

Categorization is a complex function, psychologically and neurobiologically. The basis of category structure can be complex and the range of neural circuits participating can be correspondingly broad (Ashby & Ell, 2001). Categorization is the grouping together of objects that share a specific feature or set of features, in spite of otherwise differing physical or functional characteristics. It is a vital brain function underlying survival and adaptive success—the purposeful utilization and organization of perceptual information—and is of great interest in the developing infant. However, its neural basis has evaded efforts to specify its components; the inferior temporal cortex and prefrontal cortex are considered likely participant sites due to their higher order processing of visual form and their important role in multiple visual behaviors.

Boundary differentiation is central to categorization, and it is a complex process because similarities have to be discarded as differences in relation to a particular category (e.g., motorboat), while seemingly distinct stimuli are determined to be similar (e.g., sailboat and plane). The search for underlying neural mediators must be attentive to distinguishing between processes indicating physical similarities as opposed to category membership. In an experiment using *cats* and *dogs* as categories to be distinguished by monkeys, accuracy was high even when the dissimilarity of a specific sample was substantially reduced by changing the form gradually toward the other category (using a "morphing" system). They found that neural activity in the prefrontal cortex (PFC) reflected category membership, and that the activity was similar regardless of the degree to which the sample reflected the category (e.g., *dogness*). Thus, neural firing rates followed stimulus category rather than a processing of physical characteristics making the sample increasingly like or unlike the prototype of *dog*. If the sample was judged to be within a category, the PFC neuron responds, whether the sample is a clear example of the category or is ambiguously close to the boundary. Moreover, these monkeys had not had prior experience with cats or dogs, and so they were learning these categories. When retrained with different, arbitrary categories, the monkeys performed at the same high level of accuracy in the novel category determination, and neurons at the same PFC locations were again responsive to categories, but now the new categories and *not* the original categories (Freedman, Riesenhuber, Poggio, & Miller, 2001).

Categorization links perception and cognition, and is an initial, vital step in cognitive processes. Thinking, and the resultant behavioral choices, use knowledge about the categories of things involved. Categories of emotions are likely to have more ambiguous boundaries than classical perceptual categories, so we would expect a more complex transition in neural firing rates. In order to categorize perceptual phenomena, combinations of features defining the category must be extracted. In this experiment, no instructions were given to the monkeys; instead, experiential training led to the formation of multivariate abstractions, and these perceptual categories were distinguished by more than a few simple characteristics. It can be anticipated that the sculpting of emotional categories and their boundaries will be accompanied by significant PFC neural activity, possibly related to attentional shifting while examining potential category-defining features. There are many possible complex methods through which neurons might code this information.

A core result of this research is that these PFC neurons are malleable, as they are capable of changing the category to which they respond. This suggests the capacity for rapid, flexible changes in the PFC neural circuits responding to categories as task requirements are altered. Other PFC neurons have been demonstrated to be responsive to experience by altering their sensitivity to stimuli or the learning of associations or rules. It is also anticipated that other brain areas might also have categorization functions, particularly inferior temporal cortex (ITC) neural circuits (Freedman et al., 2001). For example, earlier studies have indicated neural circuits in the lateral hypothalamus that are active with all stimuli considered as food by the monkey, providing a possible example of categorization within the hypothalamus (Thorpe & Fabre-Thorpe, 2001).

A significant feature of this research is the rapidity of response of PFC and ITC neural circuits, in spite of the number of processing stages occurring prior to the signal arrival. Category-specific neural activity has been observed in electrophysiological studies of humans also, but the latency to neural activity appears to be longer; the reason for this is unclear, but it might reflect the larger human brain and greater distance traversed. Whether the categorization methods in monkeys and humans are the same (e.g., single cell coding) and whether humans use additional brain areas for categorization functions (e.g., the fusiform gyrus) are among the questions remaining as subjects for research. One recent study in an epileptic patient showed selective neuronal responses in individual neurons of the human medial temporal lobe for animals, houses, natural scenes, faces, and famous people (Thorpe & Fabre-Thorpe, 2001).

The Prefrontal Cortex: Working Memory, Attention, Executive Functions, and Relational Representation

Descriptions of the functions of the prefrontal cortex became increasingly precise over the last two decades of the twentieth century. By the beginning of the 1990s, the functional components were less vague, and more readily permitted the distinction of functions from those in related brain regions and their application in clinical work. A representative description of the general cognitive functions of the prefrontal cortex was that it integrates information essential for planning and judgment, particularly through its role in the temporal structuring of behavior (using short-term memory, preparatory set, and suppression of internal and external influences), extracting sets of information, and integrating it into new information contributing to executive functions. Similarly, it enables sequencing of actions, attentional control based on mental representations of context, executive control, and the creation and use of abstract event knowledge. The information utilized is derived from the interior of the body, the external world, and the salience of stimuli in relation to prior experience. Moreover, these functions are particularly well suited for adapting to increasingly consequential and complex social interactions (Bear, 1991; Fuster, 1989; Stuss & Benson, 1986).

Further developments centered on elaborating links among these heterogeneous functional elements and constructing a foundation explaining how the prefrontal cortex accomplishes its cognitive tasks. This included special attention to ascertaining the common mechanisms that underlie their joint location, with an emphasis on the possible linking role of working memory. A compelling example of such a model for the mechanisms of cognitive function in the prefrontal cortex is that it creates and maintains explicit relational representations that guide thought and action (Robin & Holyoak, 1995). The work of many investigators is gradually unraveling the perplexing array of associated functional elements in research on the prefrontal cortex, sometimes using alternative terminology, such as *representational memory* (Goldman-Rakic, 1987) or *working memory* (Baddeley, 1986, 1997). While *working memory* is now favored and captures the brief duration and practical use of retaining the stimulus for comparison with long-term memories and other information, *representational memory* captures the prefrontal cortex function of assembling mental representations through comparisons, the detection of differences and relations, and recognition of the potential significance of some mental representations.

Relational complexity is a proposed framework for understanding prefrontal cortex functions. The common element of these functions is the explicit representation and processing of relational information (Robin & Holyoak, 1995); the prefrontal cortex acquires and uses relational representations to reach a goal. Working memory is central to this concept, as it binds elements into relational structures which guide behavior over time. An instructive feature of this paradigm is that explicit knowledge in the sense used here is developed through slow, effortful, conscious processing utilizing working memory; this is contrasted to implicit, procedural knowledge that uses relatively rapid, effortless, unconscious processing. This relational representation processing occurs at different levels of complexity. Relational complexity refers to the quantity of independently varying dimensions that must be considered jointly to produce an appropriate response, and this conceptual terminology is derived from cognitive development research (Halford, 1993). The relational complexity of tasks is greatest when more novel associations of components are processed, and, as the childhood years are those in which the major relational schemas required in adult life emerge, they also constitute the period of vulnerability to the most detrimental effects of prefrontal cortex damage. Once developed, these relational schemas become part of implicit knowledge that is no longer vulnerable to prefrontal damage.

Two intriguing considerations emerge from these concepts. It is of interest that these capacities develop—or fail to develop—during childhood, when the child is dependent on adult caregivers to nurture cognitive development. This factor, in the context of a second, that the development of specific elements of complex relational representations is effortful, in contrast to the automaticity of the same knowledge once it is learned procedural knowledge, emphasizes that many children would not be expected to expend this effort on their own and would never master complex relational representations. In fact, we know that this is true on a cross-cultural basis, as very large numbers of adolescents do not attain the abstract cognitive capacities which typically emerge in this developmental period, and which depend on the manipulation of complex relational representations. This failure of cognitive development is not mystical, but would be expected to be reflected in subtle brain alterations, such as an underdevelopment of some aspect of prefrontal cortex anatomy (molecular, cellular, or regional) or physiology. This underdevelopment might not always be due to poor nutrition, viral infections, or other acquired etiologies, but also might reflect a lack of the type of instructive environmental stimulation that favors these dawning capacities. These speculations take us in a new direction—having completed a survey of some of the essential components of learning and memory, what do we know about specific functions that might readily be identified as a component of the emerging social interactions of the infant?

☐ Neural Coding of Complex Biological Stimuli: Neural Circuits for Social Cognition and Adaptation

The Developing Recognition of Complex Social Stimuli Assemblies: Face Recognition and Facial Expression

Fundamental to human social functioning is the capacity to recognize faces. "Face recognition" has a singular form, but actually comprises several related components and functions, which themselves reflect the activity of differing underlying neural circuits. It includes the recognition of "face" as a specific category, selective responsivity to the face, perception of the specific features of faces, the recognition of individual faces, the appreciation of categories of faces, the analysis and understanding of facial expressions in order to interpret and predict behavior, emotional responses to faces, behavioral responses to faces, and the imitation of facial expressions. This partial list of components of "face recognition" emphasizes the problem of defining apparently simple functions for clinical observation, allied with the corresponding difficulty of defining the requisite brain systems and their modular or distributed organization. The mapping of these face recognition components onto identifiable brain areas and circuits is an ongoing challenge that is gradually yielding to research (Cohen & Tong, 2001; Downing, Jiang, Shuman, & Kanwisher, 2001; Haxby et al., 2001).

One aspect of these differing face recognition components and neural circuitry that is of special interest is the role of development in their application to building adaptiveness into the infant. Johnson and his colleagues conducted intriguing research in an effort to understand apparently contradictory data, work that has generated an interesting dual phase developmental model of the initial components of face recognition. Responses to faces by neonates occur in the first day of life, suggesting that this could be an innate mechanism, possibly one of those comprising the characteristics essential to human social cognition. However, it is beginning to appear that the earliest preferential orienting to the mother's face is actually orientation to a very few general features which are sufficient to guide the infant because of the predictability of the mother's presence, with the advantage of attachment behaviors linking mother and infant. This initial orienting appears to be under subcortical control, and it assures that, by preferentially tracking faces, the infant has the maximum opportunity to bias subsequent sensory input to the developing cerebral cortex. Cortical architecture is permissive in its initial allocation of cortical areas of refined responsivity, assigning each area to respond to a component of the repeated environmental stimuli to which it is exposed. This enables individual areas to develop the capacity to respond to specific categories of environmental stimuli during this sensitive period, forming representations that act as the initial processing of this class of stimuli. In other words, the cortex is building the preferential, distinct responsivity of specific cortical areas during this early period of synaptogenesis, as discussed above, after which each cortical area remains with a more specific, reduced responsivity to the range of environmental stimuli (Johnson, 1997, chapter 4; Johnson, Dziurawiec, Ellis, & Morton, 1991).

By being exposed to faces over this early sensitive period, especially to the mother's face, the cortical system acquires sufficient information to enable it to continue responding to this category of stimuli and gather further information. Over the second month, the subcortical orienting response diminishes, possibly because cortical inhibitory circuits are becoming sufficiently developed to restrain the activity of the subcortical system, as seems to occur at this time with other subcortical systems. However, the cortical system is maturing, and as it becomes structured through environmentally guided synaptogenesis to respond to facial stimuli, it gradually takes over the responses to faces. As indicated above, the repeated, reliable exposure to faces builds up cortical representations (linked, complex memories) of faces by elaborating increasingly refined synaptic connections in this cortical area. Cortical areas involved are found in the superior temporal gyrus, the middle temporal gyrus, the left orbitofrontal cortex, and Broca's area. The fusiform face area and the superior temporal sulcus are important contributing areas, and other brain regions participate in relation to specific components of face recognition, such as the amygdala (Cohen & Tong, F., 2001; Downing et al., 2001; Haxby et al., 2001; Johnson, 1997).

This is not to say that all of these neural mechanisms have been documented to be a final description of events in a concluding sense, or that other mechanisms do not contribute. For example, there is evidence that the amygdala achieves adult features by 6 to 12 months postnatal age. This is the age at which infants begin to develop the capacity to identify facial expressions, as well as the age at which separation anxiety begins to occur—the latter possibly reflecting the emotion that finally begins to be associated with separation from the mother and the release of regulated physiological and behavioral phenomena in the protest response. Moreover, there are similar developmental events involving biased exposure to native language voices that favor specific speech discrimination capacities. Both of these reflect the tuning of cerebral cortex areas to respond to highly significant and predictably present environmental stimuli, largely contained within the person of the mother. Socially relevant stimuli, such as facial expression and language, gradually, through chronic exposure to relevant stimuli, generate these superordinate systems regulating social interactions and social cognition (Johnson, 1997). We now will consider a brain function that might not so readily be thought of as part of the infant's emerging social capacities, learning through imitation. Nevertheless, it is a pivotal component of social cognition because it comprises a form of learning that releases cascades of abilities for the infant—especially obvious capacities learned through imitation, such as motor abilities. However, more important for our consideration, it has been demonstrated that one element of language learning in early childhood is imitation of facial movements during speaking (see below), and there is reason to believe that imitation is a paramount factor enabling the infant to learn the language of emotions.

The Developing Capacity for Rapid Learning of Complex Social Behaviors: Imitation

Imitation is a category of learning long neglected, possibly due to problems defining it, and certainly because it was outside prevailing classical learning theories (Nadel & Butterworth, 1999; Yando, Seitz, & Zigler, 1978). One definition of imitation is "copying by an observer of a feature of the body movement of a model." This is differentiated from emulation, in which reproduction of the action could be caused by an observed movement of an object, rather than the body movement of the model (Heyes, 2001). Viewed from the brain function perspective, it is obvious that most of the components of imitation are active in other types of learning and behavior. However, one component appears to be unique, which is a mechanism through which visual information about the body movements of another person is translated into matching motor output.

Are there any corresponding brain areas whose activity would seem to match this unique aspect of imitation? In fact, several brain areas have been suggested to have the capacity for imitation. For example, increased activity in areas 44 and 45 of the left inferior frontal gyrus has been observed; area 45 especially appears to be specialized for imitation. Is activation of these areas accompanied by characteristics indicating "imitation" as a unique function? Several features have been identified. First, activity in these areas precedes peak activation in the left primary motor area, so it can be differentiated as a distinct activity (Heyes, 2001; Iacoboni, 1999; Nishitani & Hari, 2000). Second, this brain area is homologous to the F5 area in the monkey, which contains "mirror neurons" activated not only by observation of grasping actions by another individual, but also by his own performance of these grasping actions (Rizzolatti, Fadiga, Fogassi, & Gallese, 1999). Third, activity in this F5 area, responsive to stimulation by hand and mouth movements, is associated with specific motor acts, but is not correlated with other individual movements, such as contracting a discrete muscle group. This essential characteristic reflects the uniqueness of a motor act, which is conferred by the presence of a goal. It suggests that the motor system not only controls movements (muscle contraction, etc.) but also has the capacity of translating a mental state, such as a purpose, into an actuality; thus, it enables the possibility of achieving in reality an outcome responsive to the mental state—for example, "intention"—generated by neuronal circuits from another part of the brain. Example types of neurons described have been "grasping neurons," "holding neurons," "tearing neurons," and "manipulation neurons," (Gallese & Goldman, 1998). These neurons have been described as having the role of acting as a "motor vocabulary" of actions related to prehension (Rizzolatti & Gentilucci, 1988). There was a very strong association, in almost all of the neurons, between what would be the most effective action observed by the monkey (among several observed) and the monkey's motor response, both in terms of the general purpose of the action—such as grasping—and the manner of its performance—such as a precision grip. This appears to be a description of a cortical system with the capacity to match the observation and the execution of motor actions (Gallese & Goldman, 1998).

Research has shown the existence of a system of mirror neurons in humans, apparently functioning similarly to that in monkeys. It also has a location possibly homologous to area F5 in monkeys, in that one area activated in humans is area 45. This includes the anterior portion of Broca's area, which raises the question of why the language area would be involved (Rizzolatti & Arbib, 1998), a topic outside the limits of this discussion but highly relevant. Other brain areas involved in humans are the left superior temporal sulcus (area 21) and the left inferior parietal lobule (area 40). In sum, when we watch someone execute a purposeful action, the brain areas activated in us are the same ones activated during our actual performance of the movement (Fadiga, Fogassi, Pavesi, & Rizzolati, 1995; Grafton, Arbib, Fadiga, & Rizzolatti, 1996; Rizzolatti et al., 1996). Research on imitation raises many additional complex questions, such as its possible role in "theory of mind" functions.

Substantial information is now available about imitation in infancy, much of it generated by the fertile research efforts of Meltzoff and Moore; some of their commentary gives an idea of the role of imitation in the development of the infant. Imitation appears to be a mechanism of learning for which humans have an innate capacity, yet infant imitation is not easy and automatic—as is commonly expected—but is effortful and intentional. Most meaningful for our quest for neural mechanisms is, first, that imitation involves a coupling of perception and action, and determining how it differs from classical types of learning is an objective crucial to understanding early childhood development. Second, the use of imitation suggests some level of understanding of self, other, and the relationship between these two. These two observations are profoundly important to our understanding of the emerging capacity to translate a mental state into action and to apprehend the other person as separate, but "like me" (Meltzoff & Moore, 1999). Infant imitation is similar to several other examples of early perceptual-motor coupling, such as catching moving objects or taking protective actions when encountering looming objects. This phenomenon of linking perception and appropriate motor output without intervening stimulus–response associative learning has been termed *resonance* (Gibson, 1966, 1979; Rizzolatti et al., 1999). Imitation does not involve an inanimate object, and so also has been described as "interpersonal coupling." To accomplish this, infants are required to control their motor output sufficiently to match their own actions to that of a dynamically changing, animated set of activities by the mother (Meltzoff & Moore, 1999).

Meltzoff and Moore also emphasize an observation that underscores that infants are learning through the process of imitation, leading to the conventional end result of memory formation: infants are capable of deferred imitation, one or two weeks later, regulating their actions according to the memory of an event instead of what they are currently observing, which might even be contradictory. Deferred imitation would seem to have notable importance as a mechanism for acquiring culturally relevant adult behaviors, suggesting itself as a means for the transmission of transgenerational behavioral preferences, and for sustaining cultural identity.

Other features of infant imitation have been observed that extend our understanding of this basic brain function in humans. First, facial imitation involves cross-modal matching, which adds a potentially revealing area of investigation to the face recognition research discussed above. Second, infants are faced with the problem not only of recognizing that people exist as distinct things in the world of objects, but also of establishing the identities of individuals in spite of their appearing at different times and in different garb. It has been suggested that one mechanism for distinguishing among individuals is through recognition of the distinctive behaviors of an individual, his "gestural signatures." This aids the infant in his or her attempts first to determine the number of people present, which then leads to subsequent distinctions of individual identity. Finally, it becomes apparent that reciprocal imitation builds and then extends interpersonal interactions and understanding (Meltzoff & Moore, 1999). The topic of imitation has stimulated many other studies, and there is a promise of expanding work in the future; its role in the development of language is one such fertile terrain (Byrne & Russon, 1998).

☐ Language: Learning the Alphabet and Assembling the Dictionary

Perceptual Discrimination of Sound Regularities and Speech Patterns

Nothing is more directly associated with the image of human qualities than language. Language is a brain function that is well known to emerge in early childhood—so it should be a good candidate for supplying information and possibly a generative model for better understanding the overall neural basis for the infant's emerging adaptive capacities. Have affiliated language and developmental neuroscience research spawned such concepts? Rich and extensive research has successfully produced an affirmative answer to this question, but one systematic approach to these questions is especially informative for our purposes. Patricia Kuhl and colleagues carried out a long series of studies which specifies highly important early components of the development of language, as genes and environment exhibit a systematic but complex interplay. Of particular importance to our discussion is that her findings describe the initiation of this process through coding primary language elements and gradually constructing a language map in an ever more complex process. This process is attuned to the perceptual regularities of language input, mapping them, and extruding the irregularities—in this way forming the reservoir of sound units for later word and phrase recognition.

Kuhl's research examined the process of language development in infants, a process uniform in milestones and timing across the languages of the world. Neonates and very young infants can distinguish the differences among all of the phonetic units utilized in the languages of the world, regardless of the language environment to which they are exposed. In fact, this capacity for sound distinctions by the auditory system, enabling the partitioning of the basic elements of speech, has a long evolutionary history and extends to species other than humans (Kuhl, 1991a, 1991b). However, by the end of the first year of life, these perceptual capacities become highly limited, and infants no longer can discriminate contrasts in languages outside the language(s) to which they have been exposed. This is the adult pattern in which the early skills are lost: adults have difficulty distinguishing differences between sounds in a foreign language if these sounds are not discriminants in their own language. This rapid shift in language capacities appears to occur between 6 and 12 months of age. In one of her studies, American 12-month-old infants were much better at differentiating the American English /r/ and /l/ sounds, while Japanese infants, capable of the discrimination at 6 months, had lost the ability by 12 months old (Kuhl, 2000).

Kuhl has demonstrated a parallel transition in speech production, as newborns across the world have the capacity for a universal set of utterances. By the end of the first year of life, however, the infants are becoming limited to distinct speech patterns evident in the phonetic and the prosodic (intonational patterns) characteristics of the language of native speakers around them. Again the question arises, what brings about this shift, causing the infant to lose capacities of speech perception and production over the first year of life. Is this the influence of developmentally programmed genes exerting their effects at the predetermined time? This does not appear to explain the data, because the few cases of socially isolated children with no language input depict a failure to develop normal language. Once again, genetic influences interact with the environment and it is this interplay that needs to be untangled. Kuhl suggests that linguistic experience changes how the brain processes the signal and develops complex mental maps. She describes this by saying that this process "'warps' underlying dimensions" (p. 102) so that perception is changed in a direction that favors distinguishing categories. She judges that this mapping is not like the conventional operant learning of everyday life, and that "neither explicit teaching nor reinforcement contingencies" are required (p. 102). Learning occurs as long as there is exposure to a natural language environment, and it is very durable (Kuhl, 2000).

Tuning and Mapping Neural Circuits for Language: Filtering Signal from Nonsignal by Forming Sound and Speech Category Prototypes

Thus, Kuhl determined from her research that "language experience alters perception" (p. 102), depicting this as occurring through the "perceptual magnet effect." Her research demonstrated the existence of phonetic prototypes, differing according to the native language of the speaker, and functioning like perceptual magnets. Listeners attempting to differentiate a phonetic prototype from surrounding sounds in acoustic space respond as if the prototype attracts the surrounding sounds of the category, pulling them closer to the prototype. It then becomes difficult for the listener to detect differences between the prototype and the nearby sounds of the category. Poor examples of the categories do not function as a prototype and do not have a magnet effect. This "perceptual magnet effect," occurring by 6 months of age, reflects the language to which the baby has been exposed and occurs across all languages. Occurring before word learning, the perceptual system is being tuned and mapped by the ambient language, exaggerating the contrasts of his native language and diminishing those outside it—this means that the process aids in word learning, rather than that it occurs as a result of word learning causing a more meticulous attention to native language sounds. The infant's discrimination of the prototypes actually used in the native language(s) around him help him know what to listen for—the regularities in sounds—which assists in the development of word recognition, the capacity to map sound patterns onto objects and events. This mapping is the foundation of language, as it directs the infant's attention toward the acoustic stimulus features that indicate the sound unit that carries signal value and filters signal from nonsignal, and enables the formation of higher order units (Kuhl, 2000).

Kuhl describes data that demonstrate how infants, slightly after the prototype discrimination capacity is gained, apply this phonetic unit information to the task of recognizing wordlike forms. Just before the appearance of word learning, infants show a preference for word forms that are typical of their native language(s), in which the phoneme combinations and the stress patterns match the pattern of the native language(s) (Jusczyk, Friederici, Wessels, Svenkerud, & Jusczyk, 1993). Similarly, by this time infants are capable of learning something new about sound combinations: when they are put into artificial words, the infant can learn the statistical probabilities of these combinations (Saffran, Aslin, & Newport, 1996). This is important because this knowledge indicates the infant's activity as she uses her increasing knowledge of phonetic mapping to chunk the continuous sound stream into higher order units. Kuhl again makes the point that this process of learning how to discriminate prototypes, map phonemes, and chunk the sound stream is not learning through reinforcement, but that it is automatic and unconscious (Kuhl, 2000). Determining whether this is so, and how the learning takes place, will have an important influence on our understanding of brain development.

Sensitive Periods for Tuning and Mapping Neural Circuits for Language by Forming Sound and Speech Category Prototypes

Once again, however, it is important to recall that the auditory systems of these children retain the capacity to make all of the original acoustic distinctions, yet they no longer attend and respond to the differences; their brain has learned that these distinctions are not relevant discriminations and a new, consistent, prolonged environmental input of these distinctions presumably would be required in order to learn to attend and respond to some of these unattended sound distinctions. These concepts are reflected in emerging information about learning a second language. Research findings indicate that infants exposed to two languages from birth retain the capacity to discriminate sounds and retain the phonetic and prosodic characteristics of spoken language for both languages, especially when two different speakers present the two languages (e.g., mother and father or grandparent or babysitter) (Kuhl, 2000). This can be contrasted to the well-known difficulty that adults encounter when attempting to learn a foreign language. Because the adult has lost the capacity to make the sound distinctions of the foreign language, he is unable to parse the sentence into its component auditory syllables and words, even if these are words that he recently learned in class. His ear does not hear them and his speech mechanisms cannot reproduce the sounds and intonations. Nevertheless, although it will take much longer than a newborn, the adult can learn the language and understand and speak it well; yet, even then, only in rare cases does a native speaker fail to detect an accent. On the other hand, a child who learned two languages as an infant will begin to lose the native accent and much of her vocabulary, even if this was her primary language with her mother for the first years of her life, if at a later age (e.g., upon entering elementary school), she no longer uses the language regularly. An important concrete indication of this difference is that adults who learned two languages in early childhood have overlapping brain regions activated on fMRI during processing of these languages, but adults who acquired a second language during adulthood have two separate regions activated by the two languages (Kim, Relkin, Lee, & Hirsch., 1997). This is evidence that the initial coding for language during infancy does affect brain structure in a permanent manner that registers the distinct brain mechanisms during the readiness of early infancy. Yet, this does not imply a lack of auditory capacity for necessary language sound distinctions or for subsequent learning of a language; the adult can attain the necessary abilities, the tuning of appropriate additional neural circuits in a manner conferring recognition of phonemes and the capacity to build language abilities (Kuhl, 2000).

These deliberations bring up the idea of "critical periods," an intriguing concept in developmental neurobiology which in its original conceptualizations was too sharp-edged. Clinicians and neuroscientists now describe "sensitive periods," emphasizing that exposure of the very young child to stimuli at certain times can lead to more effective learning than at other times, depending on the influence of other factors; there is now substantial data in both animal and human research describing periods in which environmental stimuli have a significantly more pronounced capacity to alter development. For example, Kuhl refers to other components of the systematic research by Knudsen and colleagues on the barn owl described above. This research suggests that the sensitive period is responsive to several influences that reduce or extend it; an example is the observation that experiences taking place in a more natural environment lead to a shorter learning period (Knudsen & Brainerd, 1995; Knudsen & Knudsen, 1990). The underlying mechanisms for sensitive periods are under active investigation, and it appears that early learning might "commit" neural structure, altering the brain through environmental stimuli in such a way that subsequent stimuli are processed differently (Kuhl, 2000).

Learning Language and Other Motor and Social Functions Through Imitation of Perceptual Discrimination and Motor Production

Kuhl describes another perspective from which we can view these developmental processes. This is the importance of hearing the vocalizations of others, as well as one's own sound productions, for the development of vocalizations, both in songbirds—where it is arrestingly evident—and in infants. In both species, the immature are learning the perceptual properties of the signals necessary for communication in their species, and developing the vocal repertoire that allows them to become skilled producers of the signals. These speech motor patterns acquired in infancy are difficult to change later in life, and, as mentioned above, are reflected in the difficulty of eradicating the native language accent when learning a foreign language as an adult. These speech patterns are being formed between 3 and 5 months of age in infants, as shown by definite developmental changes in vowel production during this period.

Of additional interest to our context is the recognition that imitation plays a fundamental role in this process, preferentially reproducing the vowels that they heard in the laboratory sessions. The time of exposure to a vowel in these sessions was only 15 minutes, a profound indication of how rapidly they imitate and learn, and how deeply the ever present ambient language of mother and others must affect their memories of vocal communicative signals and their speech production. Thus, imitation and learning of the continual language of the mother and other principal caregivers is serving to tune the neural circuits for both the memories necessary for auditory signal perception and speech production. This is a pattern of learning and memory evident in a range of very early developmental experiences in which memories of perceptual patterns act as guides for production, including birdsong, prehensile (grasping) movements, facial expressions, tongue protrusion, mouth opening, sign language, and speech. It is difficult to neglect the centrality of imitation in infant learning as this list accumulates. These capacities for perceptual discrimination and for motor production then become the foundation of their capacities, influencing which further perceptual or motor capacities they are capable of acquiring (Cohen & Tong, 2001; Downing et al., 2001; Gallese & Goldman, 1998; Haxby et al., 2001; Johnson, 1997; Kuhl, 2000; Rizzolatti & Gentilucci, 1988).

Imitation of speech production is much more significant than is commonly recognized. Kuhl points out that visual inspection of the speaker's mouth and facial movements during speech is very important to the perception of speech, as we have memories coding for both auditory and visual speech data. When the two modalities are used to send discrepant data, the observers report an intermediate articulation (i.e., /da/ or /tha/, instead of either of the conflicting auditory /b/ or visual /g/ that were presented to them; Green, Kuhl, Meltzoff, & Stevens, 1991; McGurk & MacDonald, 1976). This remarkably replicable observation in which perceptual information from two different channels is discordant, and neural circuits combine the information to produce a unified percept, is an important theoretical principle and a significant reflection on high level perceptual processing that deserves additional study. Moreover, it has been demonstrated that by 5 months of age infants are able to recognize auditory–visual speech matches, a capacity similar to adult lipreading. This attests to the presence of both auditory and visual perceptual information concerning perceptual discrimination and motor production at this early age; other studies suggest that it might be present in newborns (Kuhl & Meltzoff, 1982; Rosenblum, Schmuckler, & Johnson, 1997; Walton & Bower, 1993). Overall, we are pushed to recognize the considerable role of visual information in boosting our capacity for speech perception. The aggregate data testify to the early development of this polymodal representation of speech in humans.

Parents as Educators: Tuning Neural Circuits for Language by Filtering and Repetitive Presentation of Simplified and Exaggerated Sound and Speech Category Prototypes

Having so much information about perceptual and motor learning during the first year of language acquisition in an infant, Kuhl asks if we have any knowledge of how the mother or other caregiver might use special behaviors to optimize the infant's language learning. It might help account for the remarkable success of language learning, when you consider that by age 2 years a toddler is hearing 20,000 to 40,000 words in an ordinary day. In fact, the mother does this in multiple ways, particularly encapsulated in the special "motherese" or "parentese" speaking mode so familiar as a near-universal style and preferred by infants over other complex acoustic signals. Motherese is not random, but has specific characteristics well known to parents, but unconsciously produced: syntactic and semantic simplicity, a slow pace, a high pitch, and exaggerated intonation contours. Kuhl describes an additional quality that her group documented, and which has a very good match with their prior research findings: across three diverse languages (Russian, Swedish, and American English) there is a ubiquitous change in the phonetic units in speech to infants. Parents mold more extreme acoustic models of vowel sounds, "stretching" the acoustic space of what is known as "the vowel triangle" to language investigators. This aids the infant's perceptual discrimination of the acoustic signal, thereby emphasizing decisive spectral parameters that facilitate the infant's own speech production. Here we see that language education for infants is not random, but highly specified information defining the acoustic units, the regularities in sounds that differentiate the signals from nonsignals as the infant moves toward word recognition. Adults are effectively filtering the language input by deepening phonetic distinctions. Research has shown that these techniques are advantageous for aiding language-delayed children, who have improved speech and language capacities following treatment with computer-exaggerated phonetic differences. The benefit for infants is that it draws their attention to the acoustic characteristics essential to language processing. This "hyperarticulation" by adults generates more prototypes, which we have seen are optimal signals for enhancing discrimination and assisting perceptual mapping (Kuhl, 2000).

The Challenge of Defining Neural Modules and Circuits for Language

Localization of the development of neural areas underlying language will be a difficult task, as they appear to be distributed beyond the classical Broca's and Wernicke's areas, and to involve auditory, visual, motor, and other types of information. The lateralization of language functions, predominantly to the left hemisphere, is not evident at birth, but is emerging by 4 months of age—apparently with exposure to linguistically patterned information. It is significant that left hemisphere lateralization appears to be for the communicative function, as it occurs for either speech or sign language, rather than their specific form. Whichever neural circuits are involved, perceptual mapping enabling language creates a map that is based on categories of distinct sound units which develop as ambient language instructs the infant about the sound units significant for her attention, filtering out irrelevant information. These polymodal maps contain auditory, visual, and motor information (Kuhl, 2000). Learning language is a complex task, and we again wonder if motivational reward factors are active at any level. This raises a more basic question: How does the brain supply motivation?

☐ Motivation: Stimulus Significance, Rewards, Memories, and Behavior

Reward Systems

While learning is accepted as essential for adaptation, what is it that leads a child to learn one thing rather than another in situations allowing choice? The brain does not leave this choice to chance, as a complex motivational system guides choices through rewards and a spectrum of accompanying emotions. A direct source of reward can be active during learning, functioning through the activation of specialized centers for reward functions in the brain. Stimulation of such a site elicits a strong feeling of "reward" or pleasure, so that animals will seek repetitive stimulation of the type that originally generated the reward. This can be such an intense reward phenomenon that other activities are neglected. Over a period of more than two decades, the midbrain dopaminergic projection emanating from the ventral tegmental area (VTA) and projecting to the nucleus accumbens (NAC), the prefrontal cortex, and related structures has been identified as a neurochemical substrate of reward, or a reward system in the brain (Wise & Rompre, 1989). However, this view has been altered, with a new perspective favoring the concept that the dopamine system is intrinsically active in the formation of associations between salient contextual stimuli and internal rewarding or aversive stimuli or events. This enables the animal to learn to identify stimuli associated with these events, so that mesolimbic dopaminergic neurons have a significant role in the acquisition of behavior reinforced by natural rewards (Spanagel & Weiss, 1999).

While the search for the underlying "reward systems" continues, it is of no less interest to identify a system that enables an animal to recognize the significant contextual stimuli associated with internal rewarding or aversive events. This implies the presence of motivating reward systems within the brain, but, more significantly, a reward system associated with memory systems capable of pinpointing contextual stimuli predictive of rewards. This establishes a fundamental component of behavior—that children have motivated behaviors, linked to systems that predict reward according to contextual cues recognized through comparisons with memories of similar situations. That the contextual cues will often differ for individual children, according to the contextual stimuli contained within their experiences and related memories, is the key point to be underlined.

However, motivation is a richer and more complex concept than simple reward seeking, because it includes a range of emotions that provide the animal with a rapid, forceful indication of the significance of specific stimuli in a complex environment. This learning activity is at the center of cognitive activity and memory formation during childhood, and it too often preserves a record of regrettable and unpleasant events that carry a signature cue invariably recognized and responded to by the child. Yet, others may have little or no response to the same stimuli. Let us next examine the role of emotions in the brain and mind of a child.

Emotion: The Amygdala and Fear Responses as an Example of Motivational Influences

Amygdala Anatomy and Functions: Manipulating Stimuli, Emotional Motivation, and Memories.   Emotion plays a substantial role in the actions of a child. While identification with significant persons is a means for learning behavior, and memories nourish specific behaviors, each of the child's behaviors eventually occurs for an immediate reason. For a child, an emotion is often the most compelling reason that can be observed. It is, therefore, useful to examine the functions of a brain region mediating some specific emotions as a step toward clarifying how they might affect a child's behavior.

The amygdala is a neuronal complex capable of using experience-dependent emotion to label the significance of stimuli and memories. The amygdala is not the only brain structure capable of generating emotional motivation; other brain regions, such as the orbitofrontal area of the prefrontal cortex, as well as the retrosplenial cortex and the anterior cingulate cortex (Devinsky, Morrell, & Vogt, 1995) also participate in aspects of the emotional guidance of behavior. The amygdala is selected for extended review of its functions and influences on behavior because (1) it has a highly significant regulatory impact on emotion and behavior; and (2) because it is an instructive model due to its participation in stimulus evaluation through multiple levels of stimulus and memory organization: subcortical stimulus responses, cortical memory encoding, and prefrontal elaborated relational memory encoding. Its rich afferent and efferent connections permit its central role in the detection of stimulus significance, its participation in stimulus difference detection through the formation of emotional memories, and its influence on response selection. The amygdala, integrating unimodal and polymodal sensory association information with emotions and memories, is a principal representative of brain regions that integrate the elements of a perceptual–cognitive–effector sequence that contain the experience of emotion; it is the only well-studied such region, and the understanding of other regions with the potential for similar functions is at a more hypothetical stage.

The neuroanatomical meaning of the term *amygdala* has been a source of controversy for many years, as it contains cell groups that appear to be differentiated parts of several nearby regions: the traditional cortex, the claustrum, and the striatum. There is strong evidence to suggest that the amygdala is neither a structural nor a functional unit, so that terms used to describe this clustering of cell groups (e.g., amygdaloid complex, amygdalar complex) appear to be appropriate (Amaral, 1987; Amaral, Price, Pitkänen, & Carmichael, 1992; Swanson & Petrovich, 1998). The amygdala has a primary role in memory and new learning, apparently chiefly associated with the linkage of sensory experiences with emotional states. Afferent (sensory) input from many cortical sensory systems monitoring the external world contributes complex, highly processed sensory information that has converged in unimodal and polymodal association cortices. Efferent output extends to the hypothalamus, brainstem, thalamus, cortex, hippocampal formation, striatum, and cell groups in the basal forebrain (Amaral, 1987).

The amygdala organizes and modulates autonomic, visceral, emotional, and species-specific behavioral responses to environmental stimuli. A relevant example is that activity of specific amygdaloid regions elicits behavioral and autonomic components of species-specific defense responses (Amaral, 1987). Data suggest that the amygdaloid complex has an essential role in remembering the emotional significance of sensory stimuli. Thus, for example, a region monitoring object recognition in central vision within the visual cortex of the temporal lobe projects broadly to an area of the amygdala that is a locus for conferring a specific emotional color (e.g., fear or anger) to a visual sensory experience with a specific object. The cardinal importance of this function is more easily understood by describing the effects of its absence after temporal lobe lesions: an absence of fear when sensory stimuli indicate danger, eating junk or garbage, and choosing anyone who appears as a sexual partner (the Kluver-Bucy syndrome, resulting from bilateral removal of the temporal lobes in monkeys). It no longer links sensory experience with an invariant, preset behavioral output. A particularly illustrative example is that removal of the amygdala in most monkeys leads to a tame, placid monkey, but in submissive monkeys results in unchanged behavior or enhanced aggression. The previously acquired qualitative pattern linking sensory experience and consequent behavior can be altered; it is not a simple quantitative change (Bear, 1991). Here we have an example of how a child's experience, mediated by neural (amygdaloid) mechanisms, confers a specific emotional, motivating meaning on particular stimuli—a meaning that will be highly persistent if the evoking early childhood experiences were sufficiently repetitive, and a meaning that might not be shared by most others when encountered years later.

A common view of the role of the amygdala is that it makes a fundamental contribution to permitting the animal to appreciate the species-specific significance of environmental stimuli. The differing adaptive needs of varied species require that diverse environmental phenomena influence each species. Nevertheless, the generic functions of the amygdala include activities such as facilitating the avoidance of dangerous places or animals, enhancing the selection of foods or safety, or influences on more complex phenomena in humans, even including such activities as the cognitive appreciation of abstract mathematical rules. Once the motivational significance of the sensory experience is established—and experienced by the animal as motivating emotion—how does the amygdala enable the subsequent appropriate behavior of the animal? It does so through several routes, such as by facilitating immediate modifications in bodily state through altered visceral and autonomic mechanisms (via hypothalamic and brainstem structures), affecting functions such as heart rate, blood pressure, micturation, or piloerection. Enhanced selective attention to the environment is also advantageous and is achieved through projections both to neocortical areas. The guidance of possible actions could be realized through projections to the striatum to facilitate the rapid initiation of appropriate behavioral patterns, and to the prefrontal cortex to aid the guidance of choices of behaviors in relation to past experience. Finally, the immediate episode also influences long-term memory, part of the enduring experience of the organism available for guidance of adaptive behaviors in the future (Amaral et al., 1992).

The above descriptions of amygdalar functions fit episodic activities, but the amygdala might exert tonic influences as well, such as affecting the emotional set points, or thresholds, or moods of the person. This fits the observed very high levels of GABA$_A$/benzodiazepine receptors in the amygdala, which might be a primary site of the anxiolytic effects of benzodiazepine drugs. Moreover, brain imaging studies have indicated changes in blood flow in the amygdala in mood and anxiety disorders. These findings suggest that the enduring emotional thresholds distinguishing the amydala of an individual could be important components of his predisposition to behavioral self-control, impulsive aggression, anxiety, or other outcomes (Amaral et al., 1992).

Mediating Neuronal Mechanisms: The Regulation of Behavior by Neuronal Function in the Amygdala

An Animal Model for Fear-Generated Learned Behaviors: Principles of Learning and Neural Circuits. The emotion most frequently examined in animal studies of amygdalar function is fear, which can be measured and manipulated in animal research, and is similar not only to human fear, but to human anxiety. Fear has been demonstrated to be among the frequent stimuli for aggression in ethological studies, and is a common cause of fearful or aggressive behavior in everyday life. The most common approach to the investigation of fear mechanisms is to use aversive classical conditioning, usually called fear conditioning (Davis, 1992). The neuronal circuits defined as being involved in the elicitation of fear have been delineated in substantial detail, particularly in a series of deft studies by LeDoux and his colleagues.

In a discussion of conditioned stimuli, LeDoux considers principles that illuminate why altered brain functioning in response to the environment is so rapid and unceasing and why it is so important to appreciate that the brain is continuously learning about the environment. This again underscores the simple recognition that a child behaves in a perplexing manner because he or she was continuously learning the emotions and behavioral responses in the context of ambient stimuli in infancy and early childhood; when the early stimuli are clarified, the emotions and behavior are understandable. In a discussion of conditioned stimuli (CS), unconditioned stimuli (US), and conditioned responses (CR) he reviews highly significant principles too commonly confused:

> It is important to emphasize that the CRs are not themselves learned. The CRs elicited by CSs are often hard-wired (genetically specified) responses that occur whenever the animal is threatened. . . . Fear conditioning is stimulus learning, not response learning. That is, through fear conditioning, novel environmental events can gain access to neural circuits that control hard-wired responses. The hard-wired responses are naturally activated by stimuli that have acquired meaning through evolutionary learning by the species rather than through individual learning. Fear conditioning opens up this channel of evolutionarily perfected responsivity to new environmental events.
> Conditioned fear learning occurs quickly (in as little as a single trial pairing of the stimuli) and is very difficult to extinguish. Extinction is not permanent and can be overridden. (LeDoux, 1995)

This fits our understanding of a fixed pattern of emotion-generated behavior that can be initiated in response to a variety of stimuli that call forth the emotions and behaviors (e.g., anxiety, oppositional behavior, inattention). The proper emphasis in the study of causes of childhood behaviors is on the varying early childhood stimuli that might spawn these emotions and behaviors.

LeDoux describes basic neural circuits for how a conditioned stimulus (a sound), paired with an unconditioned stimulus (a shock), causes fear. Sensory stimuli pass through the auditory pathway from the ear to the auditory midbrain and the auditory thalamus, from which fibers then project mainly to the auditory cortex. Destroying the auditory cortex does not disturb the fear response because it is mediated by another pathway from the auditory thalamus to the lateral nucleus of the amygdala. In other words, the auditory thalamus projects to two related brain regions. The "lower" area (the amygdala) responds more rapidly and is resistant to extinction, yet is affected by the auditory cortex circuit that participates in more complex appraisal of the stimuli. As the amygdala responds, nerve fibers from the lateral nucleus pass through small nuclei of the amygdala to its central nucleus, which projects to brain areas regulating physiological and behavioral phenomena associated with fear (such as increased heart rate, respiration, and startle reflex, as well as vasodilation, and the animal freezes). There are three principal brain regions sending projections to the lateral amygdala: the hippocampus (providing explicit memory of contextual information about environmental features), the auditory cortex (providing interpretation of more complex stimuli), and the prefrontal cortex (controlling emotional memory expression and inhibiting unneeded emotional responses) (LeDoux, 1996).

LeDoux goes on to make four further points after describing the neural circuits underlying fear conditioning. The first is that either thalamic or cortical projections alone are sufficient to mediate fear conditioning. The second is that the cortical pathway is necessary for discrimination of two different stimuli, and a cortical lesion interferes with this capacity; while the intact thalamic projections to the amygdala continue to mediate a response to the CS, both stimuli evoke a CR, indicating that the thalamic pathway fails to distinguish the two. Third, during the conditioning process, the rats develop fear reactions to the chamber where they received the shocks as well as the CS; this contextual conditioning is mediated by the hippocampus and amygdala. The fourth point is that cortical projections from the medial frontal area appear to mediate extinction of learned fear (LeDoux, 1995). This is an instructive model for brain mechanisms when emotion affects learning. It describes the presence of alternative neuronal pathways, with cortical pathways permitting more refined discrimination of environmental stimuli by retaining more extensive information. Furthermore, learning is not limited to the CS, but includes features of the context of learning as well. Finally, eventual extinction of learned behavior might be mediated by cortical circuits.

The Formation of Emotional Memories. The amygdala is a primary site for learning associations between stimuli and reinforcement, especially when significant for social behavior. This implies an essential role in the child's learned emotional responses, which are emotional states evoked by reinforcing stimuli. The amygdala participates in emotional learning by decoding stimuli to produce emotional states that influence behavior. Both the amygdala and the orbitofrontal cortex distinguish the stimuli that were associated with primary reinforcers in the past, and generate emotional responses to these stimuli. The tuning of thresholds in these neurons (and in structures projecting to them, such as the inferior temporal cortex) appear to regulate the subsequent inputs from the amygdala to associative neuronal networks necessary for the formation of emotional memories, completing the stimulus–reinforcement path underlying learned emotions. This is the link between amygdaloid function and memory, and explication of the elements of this link suggests how emotion influences memory (Rolls, 1992).

Emotions, or enduring mood states, influence the cognitive evaluation of stimuli and memories. Memory storage includes basic stimuli (e.g., visual elements of a fire) and not only their physical context (e.g., a gas range in a kitchen), but their emotional context (e.g., fear). These links develop as associative neuronal networks are elaborated (e.g., in the hippocampus, which receives extensive projections from the lateral and medial amygdala). In this process, stored memories of specific stimuli are formed by augmenting the strengths of active synapses to increasingly activated neurons. Thousands of inputs to a single neuron, and a neuronal network arrangement favoring linkage of essentially arbitrary co-occurrences of inputs to this neuron, create the likelihood that synapses conveying data about the basic stimuli will be accompanied by synapses carrying information about the current emotional state and other contextual features. Retrieval of a memory in these networks is optimal when the "input key" is most similar to the stored original input pattern (e.g., fear aroused upon seeing the normal flames in a gas range in a neighbor's kitchen). This brief description indicates not only how context (including emotion) is stored with the basic stimulus elements of a memory, but also has the capacity to affect memory retrieval. In a sense, given the functional arrangement of associative neuronal networks, the problem of "How can context be stored in memories," is converted to the question "How would it be possible for context not to be stored" given that they provide co-occurring inputs to these synapses? The influence of emotional state on memory formation and retrieval, then, is a specific instance of the effects of context (Rolls, 1992).

The hippocampus is a provisional locus for the influence of emotions on memory storage and retrieval, and another involves projections back from the amygdala and orbitofrontal cortex (centers essential to emotion) to regions of the cerebral cortex involved in the representation of objects (e.g., the inferior temporal cortex). In this manner, forward inputs to these regions from the original regions of less highly processed sensory information, coupled with back projections from the amygdala conveying emotional information, modify the increasingly activated cortical pyramidal cells of the region. This synapse tuning is, in essence, emotional memory storage in the regional associative network involved; an example would be a network generating responses to a competitor's face. Subsequent perception of this stimulus (his face) will activate the cortical pyramidal cells with more strength because it simultaneously is linked with another activating input from back projections carrying emotional information from the amygdala, which repeat the original pattern of activities at the synapses. The matching pattern at the emotion information carrying synapses enhances the capacity of the sensory inputs to activate the cortical pyramidal cells (Rolls, 1992).

In sum, emotions (1) affect the likelihood and strength of memory formation in the hippocampus; (2) are stored as elements of memories in the cortex; and (3) affect memory retrieval and, correspondingly, cognitive processing in general. This provides a mechanism, a pathway of neuronal influences, that could favor a predisposition to the genesis of specific emotions which influence cognitive processes that regulate fearful withdrawal, aggression, or other behavioral choices (Kling & Brothers, 1992).

Strong evidence indicates that the cellular mechanism in the amygdala mediating emotional learning and memory is long-term potentiation (LTP), the enduring form of synaptic plasticity initially described in the hippocampus. NMDA-receptor antagonists block LTP induction in the amygdala, as well as fear conditioning. In addition, fear conditioning leads to increases in amygdaloid synaptic transmission resembling LTP (Maren, 1999). The study of other amygdaloid functions, such as the modulation of explicit memory (McGaugh, Cahill, & Roozendaal, 1996), and its role in attention (Gallagher & Holland, 1994), might extend these findings.

Converging Molecular and Cellular Effects of Stressful Experiences on Neuronal Excitability in the Amygdala and Emotional Memory Formation. The model of LTP- and LTD-induced synaptic plasticity is applicable to amygdaloid neuronal function also, but has different properties of great functional significance. A single high-frequency stimulation to basolateral amygdala neurons produces short-term potentiation (unlike the LTP induced in the hippocampus). However, a second high-frequency stimulation induces LTP, indicating that additional stimulation is necessary to encode amygdaloid long-term memories (Li, Weiss, Chuang, Post, & Rogawski, 1998). Another way of markedly increasing the amplitude of basolateral amygdala neuronal responsivity to stimulation is to utilize noradrenergic potentiation (e.g., using the beta adrenergic agonist isoproterenol). This additional method for enhancing emotional memory formation is in agreement with the data showing that beta blockers reduce emotional memory, but have little effect on other types of memory (McGaugh et al., 1996). It indicates the mechanism for catecholamine-mediated stress responses that include enhanced memory formation during stress.

There is now evidence for history-dependent metaplasticity in amygdaloid neurons. Metaplasticity describes the process of a long-term adaptation by a neuron through which it responds in either of two different directions—potentiation or depression—in response to the identical input, responding according to the prior history of the neuron, including its stimulation characteristics. For example, in the amygdala, following a single high-frequency stimulation adequate to induce short-term potentiation, and the return of synaptic strength to baseline, LTD can be produced by low-frequency stimulation. On the other hand, if the basolateral amygdala had not been stimulated previously, then low-frequency stimulation produces LTP. The earlier history of stimulation of the neuron determines the direction (potentiation or depression) of the long-term adaptation to a specified frequency of stimulation. Therefore, amygdala neurons have elegant adaptive regulatory capacities through molecular mechanisms that relate differential long-term responsivity to the previous stimulation history for the animal. In sum, the long-term adaptive regulatory response of these amygdala neurons is determined by their previous environmental experience (Post et al., 1998).

An extension of this work has a good fit with other frequently observed clinical phenomena. When LTP is elicited by low-frequency repetitive stimulation, or by some high-frequency bursts, it causes heterosynaptic LTP: the induction of enhanced excitability in other synaptic inputs, beyond the synapse originally stimulated. This could be related to highly significant clinically observed phenomena in PTSD, as well as in other disorders. Posttraumatic stress disorder evokes an enduring, heightened excitability not only to stimuli related to the original trauma, but also to other environmental stimuli. This is manifested in augmented arousal and hyperstartle in other neuronal circuits in response to appropriate or inappropriate stimuli in the environment. Heterosynaptic LTP provides an opening to an initial understanding of mechanisms through which information in one neuronal path to a neuron can affect subsequent responses in an unrelated pathway synapsing on the same amygdala neuron (Post et al., 1998).

Neuromodulator influences (e.g., noradrenergic influences) in response to stress are another source of the experience-dependent amygdaloid neuronal responses, either an augmentation or decrement in emotional memory. The noradrenergic system emanating from the locus coeruleus regulates arousal levels, including the bidirectional modulation of hippocampal and amygdala neuronal excitability. Stress produces enduring alterations in the excitability of these neurons through induced NT3 gene expression in the locus coeruleus, conferring yet another means through which lasting hyperarousal might be induced (Smith, Makino, Kim, & Kvetnansky, 1995).

As experience delivers repeated stressful stimuli with a significance breeding the same emotion—fear or anxiety—history-dependent metaplasticity, heterosynaptic LTP, and neuromodulatory noradrenergic systems can act in concert to propagate a state of hyperarousal. Here the vital concept is the convergence of diverse levels of experience-dependent adaptive changes in the function of amygdaloid neurons: molecular (altering gene function), synaptic (altering stimulus-induced excitability), and neuronal circuits (noradrenergic). If the brain has multiple methods for encoding the adaptive significance of an individual's experiences, it is difficult to ignore the significance of continuing early childhood experiences in which a child's anger and fear are repeatedly provoked, requiring that the child develop an adaptive strategy, such as aggression or withdrawal or many other behavioral variants (Post et al., 1998).

☐ Parental Guidance of Adaptation in Infancy and Early Childhood

The Developmental Needs of the Infant and Young Child: Parental Activities Facilitating Adaptation

Several observations about the effects of the immature status of the infant or young child impress themselves upon us. First, the infant is incapable of adapting independently, so all discussions of adaptive mechanisms necessarily include the behaviors of the mother and child, even if the focus here is on the underlying mechanisms in the infant's brain. Second, developmental events in the maturation of the brain during infancy can generate sensitive periods in the development of some capacities, as discussed above. This magnifies the effects of nurturing parental behaviors or unusually depriving or harsh environments during early childhood, so that the effects on the child's later functioning are more prominent. Third, we must be aware of the tendency to search only for the effects of stimuli known to affect mature animals. The immature animal has needs that are different from those of the mature animal; therefore, different environmental stimuli will be salient to the immature animal, and its information processing systems will be oriented toward them. These developmentally attuned needs (e.g., for physical proximity, for emotional validation) play a primary role in maturation if the developing animal is to survive and grow. Fourth, memories guide the appraisal of the significance of a stimulus, and come to be as important in determining behavior in some respects as stimuli, by giving specific contextual and predictive meaning to stimuli. It is important to recall that the information processing systems of the immature animal generate memories related to stimuli salient to its developmental needs. It is these memories, associated with early developmental capacities and experiences, that become the foundation of its experience-guided appraisal of the environment and influence whether or not it will respond adaptively. While the developing animal sheds needs no longer appropriate to its developmental stage, and develops new needs, the older memories exert a continuing influence only gradually modulated by new experiences. It is likely that the influence of earlier memories of unsatisfied needs and emotion dysregulation can be especially significant as a potential source of interference in adaptation.

Attachment Behaviors in the Mother and Infant: The Foundation for Parent-Facilitated Adaptation

How has human adaptation unfolded successfully in spite of the infant's conspicuous dependence? A compensatory solution evolved—maternal and infant attachment behaviors—that has several beneficial outcomes, including indispensable caregiving and protection for the helpless infant, initiation in learning interpersonal interactions, and guidance in cognitive and emotional growth. Attachment behaviors are an appetitive-consummatory sequence of behaviors that are genetically programmed in the immature organism and that complement genetically programmed maternal regulatory behaviors expected to be present in the environment. In the theory of attachment behaviors, initially developed by John Bowlby (1969), *attachment* refers to a motivational system in which the goal is proximity maintenance between mother and infant. Diminished proximity to the attachment object leads to following, searching, clinging, and crying, with the evident goal of restoring proximity. The comfort response follows reunion, and is a cessation of these activities through feedback within this "goal-corrected system." The system confers survival value on infant animals through facilitation of protection from predators and environmental hazards. In this way the protest response to separation is viewed as a highly activated set of attachment behaviors, and the comfort response is the termination of the activation. These behaviors are accompanied by intense emotions, such as love, anxiety, anger, sorrow, and grief (Hofer, 1994).

The essential role of attachment behaviors during infancy commonly guides professional advice to parents (such as avoiding long separations from the mother during infancy), advice that applies to earliest childhood when a parent can feel a special need for guidance—before a child is able to tell us what he or she is thinking or feeling. They cannot verbalize their needs, nor describe whether our actions are harmful or helpful. Instead, we must infer these matters from their behaviors. Yet, how parents nurture infants and toddlers is extremely important, because extraordinary brain growth is occurring during the first three years of life, and developing patterns of neuronal systems will influence the responses of the child for years afterward. Clinical recommendations to parents about the care of infants are not intended to imply that not following the advice ensures poor outcomes, because the brain is subject to multiple influences and is malleable. Instead, these recommendations provide a composite description of how parents can supply fundamental needs of the child and optimize the chances for satisfactory development.

Attachment Behaviors: Maternal Regulation of Infant Physiological and Behavioral Systems

Can we demonstrate the biological significance of parent–infant interactions, especially its relation to brain development and adaptation? In fact, a remarkable, systematic examination of the effects of attachment behaviors on underlying infant physiology and behaviors by Hofer and his colleagues clarified why attachment behaviors are essential to the very young animal. He utilized cross-species similarities, from rats to monkeys, in both the attachment behaviors and the physiological responses of infant animals. To the observer, complex behavior systems appear to be unified in their goals, and suggest adaptive advantages; this applies to "attachment behaviors," which can be observed and monitored. In order to estimate their motivating effects, familiar psychological experiences following separation or loss from a loved one, especially the emotions evoked, are used by clinicians to approximate the experience of the infant during separation or reunion. This replicable configuration of behaviors occurring between infant and mother during separation or reunion is hypothesized to gradually generate an internal working model—meaning a memory or set of related memories—of the primary attachment figure (usually the mother) in the mind of the infant. This mental representation of the mother is associated with emotions that motivate the infant's behavior, therefore qualifying as a set of memories associated with emotional memories (Hofer, 1994).

What did the research with animals by Hofer and others accomplish? They developed a model for the mechanisms governing attachment behaviors, demonstrating an array of regulators of physiological and behavioral systems that are concealed within observable attachment behaviors occurring between rats and their pups during the nursing period. The mother regulates specific behavioral and physiological response systems in the infant through precise mediators (e.g., warmth, olfactory stimuli, or tactile stimuli provided by the mother). If the infant is separated from its mother, all of these regulatory influences vanish, inducing a series of alterations in each system released from its regulator (Hofer, 1994, table 14.1).

Why are these laboratory observations so important? It is because they suggest a new clinical perspective for why the attachment system works. We now conceptualize the system as an array of individual regulatory processes, rather than a centrally inte-

TABLE 14.1. Specific Attachment/Proximity-Related Regulators of Infant Behavior and Physiology

Physiological or Behavioral Process	Regulator	Effect of Regulator
Behavioral-Sensorimotor Regulators		
Behavioral reactivity (searching behavior)	Intermittent tactile or mother-specific olfactory stimulation	Presence: decreased reactivity Absence: increased reactivity
Rhythmic nutritive sucking	Gastric distention by milk	Presence: decreased rhythmic sucking Absence: increased rhythmic sucking
Arrhythmic nonnutritive sucking	Orosensory stimulation by nursing interaction	Presence: decreased nonnutritive arrhythmic sucking Absence: increased nonnutritive arrhythmic sucking
Growth hormone (GH) level	Interaction with non-lactating foster mother Vigorous tactile stimulation High ambient temperature A factor in milk	Presence: increased GH level Absence: decreased GH level
Basal corticosterone levels and Corticosterone response to novelty or saline injection	Passive contact with mother (tactile/olfactory) and Milk delivery	Presence: decreased levels Absence: increased levels
Thermal-Metabolic Regulators		
Activity level	Warmth	Presence: hyperactivity, mediated by increased cathecolamines Absence: hypoactivity, mediated by reduced cathecolamines
Nutrient-Interoceptive Regulators		
Heart rate	Milk, via gastric interoceptors	Presence: normal heart rate Absence: low heart rate (up to 40% below normal)
Metabolic response to cold	Nutrient, via gastric or intestinal interoceptors	Presence: thermogenesis Absence: central inhibition of thermogenesis

(Continued)

TABLE 14.1. Continued

Physiological or Behavioral Process	Regulator	Effect of Regulator
Sleep-wake states	Timing of intermittent nutrient and tactile stimulation	Presence: normal sleep-wake cycles Absence: fragmentation of sleep-wake cycles, including arousals and less REM sleep

(Adapted from Hofer, 1994)

grated pattern guiding attachment. Although viewing the attachment process as centrally coordinated continues to have highly practical value for counseling parents and organizing our clinical work, due to its simplicity (e.g., do not leave your infant for more than brief periods if this is possible), when we are investigating the developmental needs of immature animals we need more physiological specificity. Most important is that an understanding of the array of individual regulatory processes confirms the biological foundation of the clinical focus on attachment behaviors.

The components of attachment behaviors, and the "hidden regulators" of behavioral and physiological processes controlling them, are discussed further elsewhere, as are the behaviors of the infant animal when "attachment" is achieved (i.e., they successfully maintain proximity to the mother; Hofer, 1970, 1984, 1994; Hofer & Shair, 1980; Young, 1999). The critical point is that by maintaining proximity to the mother, the rat pup is available for specific behaviors and ministrations of the mother that have discrete behavioral and physiological effects on the rat pup, varying according to the specific regulator made available by the mother (e.g., warmth, milk in the rat pup's stomach, or vigorous tactile stimulation). Table 14.1 surveys the regulators, the regulated behavioral and physiological processes in the rat pup, and the effects of the regulators that have been investigated by Hofer and others. "Hidden regulators" contained in the mother's behaviors (stimuli) control the biological components of the behavioral and emotional states associated with attachment and separation in infancy, such as behavioral, autonomic, endocrine, and sleep–wake cycle phenomena. These biological components are the sensory and motor-building blocks of early mental representations. Evolving over time, these mental representations become internal working models that organize the growing child's inner experience and expectations in relation to significant nurturing figures (Hofer, 1994).

This information, however, led Hofer to recognize something unanticipated: The mechanism underlying separation behaviors can be conceptualized as a group of processes undergoing release from regulation. The mother–infant interactions incorporate multiple regulators of infant behavior and physiology that are active when they are close to one another. Separation causes the simultaneous loss of this cluster of regulators supplied by the mother, and the physiological transduction mechanisms are no longer activated. The response to separation in the immature animal is that the group of processes is suddenly released from regulation, altering their direction, frequency, intensity, and timing. Levels of function increase or decrease following separation, according to whether the regulator had inhibited or enhanced the activity level of a system. The later sequence of separation responses involves recovery after an initial intense reaction through replacement by new regulatory relationships and interactions, increasingly effective self-regulatory systems, and long-term effects, despite recovery. For the parent or clinician, the early phase of these adjustments, after the initial protests of crying and fitful movements, is distinguished as a more subdued state which evokes a sense of infant "depression" in the eyes of the adult observer (Hofer, 1994).

Are these features of attachment behaviors what we commonly identify as "stranger anxiety"? It turns out that the phenomena are not necessarily identical, although the two concepts are commonly merged and are at least behaviorally related. Studying the two by examining attachment specificity and discrimination, Hofer and colleagues identified proximity-maintenance behaviors: Rat pups encountering any object that provides the appropriate olfactory, tactile, and thermal characteristics will approach, huddle against it, and cease vocalizing. On the other hand, olfactory discrimination of attachment objects at a distance has been documented: Rats younger than one week old discriminate their own dam in preference to another lactating female, their own littermate in preference to a pup from another litter, their biological father from an unrelated male rat, and degrees of relatedness among unfamiliar rats (Hepper, 1986). Both responses utilize chemical signal detection of scent cues, some scents reflecting genetic similarities and other scents associated with prior experience. This indicates that infant rats are capable of high discrimination of attachment objects and comfort can be given by a much larger group of individuals. How these discrimination and prior attachment experience systems are related remains unclear; it is possible that infant rats have highly specific attachment objects and comfort responses *or* that there is parallel maturation of a separate behavioral system (e.g., in humans at approximately seven months of age) related to fear of strangers ("stranger avoidance") that makes attachment (comfort) objects appear to be highly discriminated. The degree of integration of the attachment (proximity maintenance/comfort) system with individual discrimination (stranger avoidance) is variable during development (Hofer, 1994).

To sum up some of the main points of Hofer's research, we observe behaviors associated with proximity maintenance or separation from the mother as comfort and protest responses in the infant which reflect, respectively, either multiple processes undergoing regulation or release from regulation. The comfort response ensues from regulation of the infant's level of affective arousal. The regulation occurs through specific sensorimotor interactions with the mother during contact and close proximity, through which predictable patterns of stimuli (tactile, textural, thermal, olfactory, vestibular, auditory, and visual) act in a graded manner to modulate arousal within a range from quiet alert to sleep, associated with emotions of comfort and security. When separation occurs, the sensory interactions cease, arousal and accompanying affect are no longer regulated to remain at low levels, and the protest response occurs. Table 14.2 describes a component of the protest response and gives an example of specific regulators (Hofer, 1994).

The research by Hofer documented a correlation between the amount of time pups maintained contact with various test stimuli (i.e., the amount of contact elicited by the stimuli) and the degree of reduction in vocalization. We see that the conceptual framework differs from the usual: Rather than thinking of arousal and distress as inevitably stimulated by events, we think of arousal and distress as being contained or modulated (regulated) by predictable patterns of events. This is not unusual in physiology, however, as it fits a common physiological pattern in which the long-term effect of inter-

TABLE 14.2. Example of a Component of the Protest Response and Ineffective and Effective Regulators

Component of the protest response:
    Regulated behavior: Separation-distress vocalization response
    Effects of regulators: Regulators act in a graded manner according to
      • the number of familiar sensory modalities and
      • their arrangement in model surrogates resembling the pup's
        littermates to varying degrees

Specific regulators:
    Ineffective: Warm rubber model, not soft, and lacking familiar
        olfactory cues
    Somewhat effective: Piece of fur laid flat on the floor
    Very effective: Flashlight battery warmed to 36 degrees C, wrapped
        in fur, and scented with home cage shavings
    Most effective: An anesthetized littermate

(Adapted from Hofer, 1994)

mittent stimulation is often to *reduce* the level of functions. Release from regulation (escape phenomena) leaves excitatory mechanisms unopposed (Hofer, 1994).

Attachment Experiences and the Development of Mental Representations That Guide and Motivate Later Adaptive Choices

While we have reviewed attachment processes in detail in order to emphasize how essential they are for the dependent infant's survival and development, their vital significance does not end in infancy. The power of their influence on continuing development is attained through the role of attachment experiences in the formation of memories, building mental representations of their environment, and particularly to features and emotions related to social interactions and social cognition. Mental representations of the environment are derived from sensorimotor experiences embedded in long-term memory, meaning those experiences selected from working memory as significant in some manner. The sensorimotor experiences most susceptible to being designated as significant are those related to interpersonal interactions with the person (or persons) who provide nurturance (in the most general sense) and have maximum survival value. The mother–infant interaction, encompassing its intrinsic regulatory processes, together with the emotions associated with both the regulated state and release or escape state, becomes the matrix for the most enduring mental representations (memories). Hofer points out that this cluster of memories gradually is transformed into internal working models of the infant's relationship with the mother and other important aspects of the environment. Emotions associated with the attachment experiences, now associated with the surviving memories, are intrinsic to the internal working model. These emotional memories act as motivational influences when current experiences are contrasted to internal working models for guidance about choice of attitudes and actions (Hofer, 1994).

The elaboration of associative memories gradually enables the child to function at a symbolic level, and internal working models are organized mental structures that attain additional symbolic value. Mental representations, including symbols, become higher order regulators of the physiological systems related to emotion and motivation, gradually replacing the sensorimotor, nutrient, and thermal regulators of infancy. In this sense, seeing a flag, or watching a dog and her puppy, or seeing one's lover, can elicit a subset of emotions drawn from attachment experiences with one's mother and explain why older children and adults threatened by separation experience the "same" emotions that actual separation elicits in infants (Hofer, 1984, 1994).

Frequent humor about mothers can make us forget the obvious: A relationship between mother and child enduring over 20 years provides an opportunity for powerful maternal influences on the child. Activation of the regulators responsive to their interactions can elicit preferential responses to certain classes of environmental stimuli, preadapting the child to conditions that the child has not yet encountered—an example of vertical transmission of the effects of experience (mother to child to grandchild) to subsequent generations, conveying a selective advantage to mother–child pairs with strong attachment systems (Hofer, 1994). The neural systems underlying emotions are regulated by the mother–infant interaction even prior to the infant's differentiation of emotion expression, so it is not surprising that emotions are so strongly affected by social interactions. Moreover, some emotions in both early and later life are regulated by relationships, and what we describe as the self-regulation of emotion is linked to a concept of self that is rooted in internal symbolic relationships emerging from early interactional experiences (Hofer, 1994).

Clinical Applications of Research on Attachment Behaviors: Comfort and Affect Attunement

It is not surprising that significant clinical applications emerge from this understanding of attachment behaviors and their regulatory influences, particularly the importance of facilitating mother–child attachment behaviors in early childhood. This is a simple prescription for nurturing the development of mother–child interactions that are mutually satisfying. Attachment behaviors provide comfort by promoting contact and physical proximity, which activate the transduction mechanisms of sensorimotor-physiological regulators that contain or modulate overarousal and distress. *Comfort* is no longer a vague, warm, sentimental term, but an indication of the presence of affect attunement, the optimal state for the development of well-adapted children.

These interactions between mother and child are dynamic and changing, not static. Infant capacities are observable and are active determinants of his or her adaptation. The idea that a baby's needs and behaviors can be read and understood by the mother, and used by her to predict future needs and behavior (Osofsky, 1976) is fundamental to responsive maternal care for an infant. It reflects the recognition that the infant is continually responding to the demands of the environment, and that his or her capacity to recover and organize himself following significant changes (e.g., delivery, new environments, new caregivers) becomes an indicator of the infant's learning and coping capacities (Brazelton, 1979). Such factors can be examined in a preliminary manner even in the first weeks of life, when using a standardized instrument, such as the Neonatal Behavioral Assessment Scale (Brazelton, 1984; Brazelton, Nugent, & Lester, 1987).

Commonsense application of findings from animal studies is reasonable, but is there evidence that human infants respond to separation in a manner similar to that of other immature animals? Several research groups have conducted relevant clinical investigations, such as examining the responses of infants undergoing separation in different circumstances. Infants and mothers might utilize some regulators already described, but we also might find new regulators related to the differing sensorimotor capabilities and higher cortical processes of humans. It is important to examine these factors carefully, for they are embedded in the mother–child interactions that are the focus of professional recommendations.

Brazelton monitored mother–infant interactions by plotting rhythmic cycles of the mother's activity and the infant's attention, and determined that mothers respond variably to the needs of infants: (1) adjusting their rhythms to the infant's and following his or her gazing-away cues with increases and decreases in stimulation; (2) not responding to the infant's rhythm but instead continuing their own stimulation and reinforcing the time the infant spends looking away; or (3) attempting to impose their own rhythm to regulate the child's rhythm (Brazelton, Koslowski, & Main, 1974).

Brazelton and his colleagues subsequently developed systems for coding behaviors and the affective quality of interactions (Tronick, Als, & Brazelton, 1977), quantifying mother–infant interactions by scaling behavioral states according to an attentional-affective dimension: disengagement to engagement or negative to neutral to positive states, for each member of the mother–infant pair. The data are reviewed to determine how much time the mother and child share the same behavioral state. *Harmonious interactions* describe when mothers and infants experience and share the same behavior states, and cycle together across these behavior states, apparently sharing rhythms of interaction. Continuous coding of videotapes, using computer programs, has been used by Field and colleagues to examine whether a behavior cycles with another behavior in rhythm (is in *synchrony*). Behavioral and physiological rhythms can be described according to cycles, periods, frequencies, and amplitudes. *Synchrony* is the degree of concordance or coherence between the behavioral–physiological cycles of the two individuals. Cross-spectral analysis, using two time series generated from the behaviors of mother and infant, is used to assess whether there are shared rhythms between the two partners (Field, 1994). Stern observed that nearly half of a sample of mothers' behaviors consist of mirroring and echoing the infants' visual and vocal behavior in either the same or a different modality. He described this as *affect attunement*. Stern coded attunement according to whether the mother's behavior matched the infant's behavior according to shape, intensity, contour, or temporal features (duration, beat, or rhythm). He suggested that this reflected a matching of inner states of the infant and mother (Stern, 1977, 1985). This burgeoning knowledge about maternal–infant interactions did not remain isolated from applications: Klaus and Kennell described the necessity for mothers to have contact with their newborn infants, generating studies of bonding and practical solutions to common problems, such as doula support (Klaus & Kennell, 1982).

Clinical investigators (e.g., Brazelton, Stern, Kennell, Sander, & Field) have generated sufficient data about infant–mother interactions to establish the comparability of clinical phenomena to the animal model. For example, Field and her colleagues investigated how infants establish behavioral and physiological organization, and, therefore, develop emotion regulation, within the context of mother–infant interactions. The mother's role is to read the infant's signals, which permits her to provide optimal stimulation (involving modality, form, intensity, variability, contingency) and to regulate arousal levels in the infant. Moreover, the mother models behaviors to be imitated by the infant and models the contingent responsivity of the behavior (the mother simplifies and imitates the infant's behavior) which leads to reinforcement of the infant's behaviors. The infant's role is to remain physiologically and behaviorally organized, alert, attentive, and receptive to stimulation, and to read the mother's signals during social interactions. Additionally, the infant must seek out and approach optimal stimulation (this depends on the infant's stimulus threshold, as well as his sleep–wake state and ability to regulate himself without the parent's modulation; all of these depend on the infant's maturity and previous experience) and withdraw and avert from nonoptimal stimulation. Finally, the infant needs to respond contingently to the mother's behaviors, largely through imitation, which reinforces the mother's behaviors (Field, 1978, 1994).

When these roles of the mother and infant are carried out effectively during early life, the mother–child interactions appear harmonious and synchronous. The behavioral and physiological coordination existing between mother and infant has been designated as *attunement*. Many alternative terms have been used by clinical investigators, such as *entrainment* (emphasizing the important clinical concept of the mother setting rhythms of the child; see Sander, 1969), *bonding, synchrony, affect matching, behavior meshing*, or *concordance*.

It is as if over the course of evolution gradually there has been a shift to include long distance sensory cues as regulators more prominently, so that the visible and audible expression of needs by the infant gains in significance, and "reading" the other in the mother–infant pair becomes increasingly effective for mutual regulation. Clinical investigators, therefore, focus observations on these regulators' transition between (1) the basic physical–metabolic maternal regulators described in rats by Hofer, and comparable regulators described in infants by Brazelton, Field, Stern, and others, and (2) the symbolic regulators of later childhood and adulthood.

Clinical Research on Emotion Dysregulation in the Infant: The Mother as Regulator of Escapee Phenomena

When the mother is physically or emotionally unavailable for a significant period of time, the infant is deprived of the mother's role as a regulator and there is emotion dysregulation. During synchrony, the mother modulates the optimal stimulation and arousal level of the infant, but, when the mother is unavailable, the mother's and infant's physiological and behavioral rhythms become asynchronous and the infant becomes behaviorally and physiologically disorganized: release from regulation leaves the excitatory mechanisms unopposed. Substitute caregivers often appear to be less familiar with the infant's signals, thresholds, personal preferences for stimulation, and other characteristics. They are, therefore, less able to provide optimal stimulation and act as an external regulator of arousal for the infant. The ensuing behavioral and physiological disorganization in the infant affects heart rate, body temperature, affect, activity level, crying, clinging, aggressive behaviors, sleep, and play behavior during the separation, and sometimes into the postreunion period (Field, 1985, 1994). Thus, physiological and behavioral processes responding to all three of the major categories of maternal regulators in rats described by Hofer (behavioral–sensorimotor, thermal–metabolic, and nutrient–interoceptive) are affected by the infant's separation experience. It is important to clarify here that we are describing the inherent advantages of maternal care and attunement with the infant developed through evolution, and not stating that other caregivers cannot provide appropriate, attuned care. In fact, we all have seen instances in which a substitute caregiver achieves greater attunement and harmony with the infant than the biological mother. Instead, we are suggesting that the process of evolution has resulted in biological mechanisms in the mother and child that favor specific behaviors most likely to facilitate the infant's adaptation.

This dysregulation during separations from the mother becomes particularly evident around 9 months of age. By 12 months of age, the infant has begun to master some self-regulatory behaviors that modulate stress and arousal, such as gaze aversion or thumb-sucking. Infants also develop strategies for emotion regulation adapted to the behavioral patterns of specific partners or circumstances. It is probable that very familiar partners, such as the father or a live-in nanny or grandparent, in the context of the familiar surroundings of the child's own home, make it more likely that a substantial degree of attunement with a person other than the mother will be achieved. These individuals and circumstances make it most likely that the infant's own preferred rhythms will be followed (Field, 1994).

Emotion dysregulation follows from physical unavailability or emotional unavailability. Physical unavailability, for example, might occur because of a mother's business trips, the illness of a mother's relative, or a mother's hospitalization for the birth of another baby. Other factors converge with physical unavailability to affect its influence on the infant; for example, the cumulative effect of the mother's hospitalization for a baby is more negative than that for a conference trip, probably because the mother is less emotionally available due to the arrival of another baby (Field, 1994). Similar research paradigms have been used by several research groups to capture the infant's response to an emotionally unavailable mother, such as occurs in maternal depression or when a mother is preoccupied with a new baby (Tronick, Als, Adamson, Wise, & Brazelton, 1978; Stoller & Field, 1982). Emotional unavailability can be mimicked in the laboratory through the momentary absence of the mother, or through the still face paradigm (Tronick et al., 1978), the effect of which is more negative than momentary separation from the mother, probably because the mother's presence excited the anticipation of expected interactions, but the mother's still face disrupted the interaction. Clinically, a common source of emotional unavailability is maternal depression, which causes very negative effects in the infant because the infant's behavioral and physiological disorganization is more prolonged. The mother supplies disruptive, noncontingent stimulation, and there is ineffective arousal regulation.

The fact that reduced synchrony is achieved in samples of preterm infants (Lester, Hoffman, & Brazelton, 1985) indicates that infant behavior altered by constitutional factors also can interfere with the quality of mother–infant interactions. There is also research evidence that the temperament of the infant (e.g., uninhibited vs. inhibited) can influence the meshing between mother and infant, as has been observed by many clinicians. In general, the degree of mother–infant match or mismatch in rhythm and temperament is a fundamental influence on emotion regulation and dysregulation.

In sum, the mother–infant interactions of humans described as attachment behaviors are quite well defined and stable. They enable the activity of regulators of behavioral and physiological processes in the infant, and in the absence of mother–infant interactions infants lack these regulators and are subject to emotion dysregulation. This emotion dysregulation can be among the sources significantly influencing mood and behavior in the developing child, not only immediately, but more significantly in the future. Thus, the concept of emotion dysregulation fits well with the conventional understanding of general sources of the disorganization of behavior during development: Behavior becomes disorganized when basic needs are not satisfied (and behavioral and physiological systems lose their regulators); when the child is overstimulated, exceeding a threshhold for predictable responses by regulators or their regulated systems; and when the child is stimulated to behave in ways that are maladaptive in his or her environment or developmental stage.

While these applications of knowledge about attachment behaviors are highly important, the salient issue discussed here is the interface of the infant's behaviors and the underlying neural mechanisms. Further observations and data from clinical research validating the equivalence of the animal research findings to those in humans, and the relevance for parent counseling and clinical care, is reviewed elsewhere (Young, 1999).

☐ The Other Partner in Attachment Behaviors: Genetic, Neural, and Hormonal Influences Guiding Maternal Facilitation of Infant Adaptation

The extensive participation by the mother in the adaptation of her "helpless" infant implies strong genetic, learning, and motivational influences within the mother if she is to carry out these complex, sustained, and sometimes arduous tasks. Only brief examples of the regulation of these influences can be given here, with the purpose of highlighting the complex influences: genetic, molecular, neural circuits, neuroendocrine, social, and cultural. This systematic interplay at so many levels within and between the mother and child once again illuminates how central attachment behaviors are to infant adaptation, learning in childhood, and cultural transmission.

Maternal behavior in mice is regulated by two imprinted genes, *Mest* and *Peg3*. *Mest* is of paternal origin and acts to regulate maternal behavior and growth of the pups. *Peg3* is also a paternally expressed gene, and mutant mothers show deficits in pup retrieval, nest building, and warming pups by crouching over them. Pups of these *Peg3* mutant mothers have growth retardation and often die. Examining the possible mediating factors for these observations, it was found that *Peg3* expression occurs in brain regions essential to maternal behavior, such as hypothalamic nuclei, medial amygdala, bed nucleus of the stria terminalis, hippocampus, and the olfactory bulb. Mutant mothers have a lactation defect, which appears to result from an inadequate oxytocin surge and subsequent impaired milk ejection. Why does this occur? There are a reduced number of oxytocin-positive neurons and altered neuronal connectivity in the mutant mothers (Li, Keverne et al., 1999). Infusion of oxytocin is known to induce maternal behaviors (Caldwell, Greer, Johnson, Prange, & Pedersen, 1987).

The neural circuits influencing maternal behaviors are complex, as they include regulation of response systems to multisensory stimulation in the female following exposure to pups. Even virgin females can be induced to show maternal behaviors by sensory exposure to pups. Induction of maternal behavior in postpartum females occurs through both the hormonal priming occurring during pregnancy and contact with pups following birth (Calamandrei & Keverne, 1994; Li, Keverne et al., 1999).

This example makes the simple point that, just as there are multiple levels of regulatory influences guiding the infant's responses to the mother and general environment, so there are corresponding multiple levels of intense regulatory influences guiding the mother's behaviors, especially in the early period of attachment behaviors. This coordinated interaction is not left to chance, yet it remains highly responsive to various environmental features.

These environmental influences are highly complex in human mothers. As humans are "cooperative breeders," the environment extends beyond the mother and the infant's capacities must reflect this. Similarly it is essential for parents and cultures to consider this need for cooperative help for young children in their family arrangements and policy planning, so as to maximize the infant's adaptive capacities. These capacities are developed over the very long period of dependency and continuing requirement for provisions, and they entail sustained effort and care from adults. Survival and adaptation require adult commitment, love and the matrix of emotional capacities that enable it, and the capacity to see the world from the other's perspective that is developed during early childhood (Hrdy, 2001). These are demanding requirements.

Moreover, when viewed from a cultural perspective there is even greater complexity. Social cognition, so intensely fostered during human infancy, is clearly necessary in specific forms in species other than primates (Wilson, 1975). For example, the oldest female elephant living in a typical matrilineal family unit is known as the *matriarch*. The matriarch develops, over many years, enhanced social discriminatory abilities that have an impact on the reproductive success of the entire female group. The presence of the matriarch provides a level of social knowledge within the group that affords superior ability for discriminating the calls of close associates from the calls of distant associates, influencing the appropriate use of defensive tactics (McComb, Moss, Durant, Baker, & Sayialel, 2001).

☐ The Influence of Stressful Experiences on Development and Adaptation in Early Childhood

Emotional Arousal and the Formation of Memories

One route of validation for descriptions of neural mechanisms underlying early childhood behavior, and the vital role of the interactive behavioral systems of mother and child, is to examine whether a failure of these complex systems in early childhood has an anticipated impact on later behavioral outcomes. Because memories are central to the brain function and attachment behaviors described, it is appropriate to begin this discussion of disrupted infant needs with a consideration of memory. An implied question pertains to the link between early childhood experiences of emotion dysregulation and later "maladaptive" behavior: Why will the child remember early experiences that are painful? Why will they not be forgotten, along with so many other childhood experiences? While it is reasonable to hypothesize the adaptive importance of remembering salient events that interfere with the child's comfort and adaptation, validation requires specification of mediating mechanisms. This question occupies a central position among those arising from clinical observations indicating the deleterious effects of varied and chronic stress on the developing child. It also drives an important sector of neuroscience research, and regulatory factors are beginning to be identified.

One example of underlying mechanisms is evidence that enhanced memory is associated with emotional arousal. This results from activation of beta-adrenergic stress hormone systems during and after an emotional experience. A placebo or propranolol (a beta-adrenergic receptor antagonist) was given before subjects read an emotionally arousing short story, or a closely matched but more emotionally neutral story, and long-term memory for the story was tested in the groups one week later. Propranolol significantly impaired memory of the emotionally arousing story but did not affect memory of the emotionally neutral story. The enhanced memory associated with emotional experiences involves activation of the beta-adrenergic system (Cahill, Prins, Weber, & McGaugh, 1994). Chronic emotion dysregulation in a young child, including unopposed excitatory mechanisms, implies the more frequent occurrence of emotional arousal during frustration, which would facilitate memory formation. Memories of frequent frustration, coupled with the child's lower threshold for emotion dysregulation, would readily ignite aggressive or other "maladaptive" responses in later disappointing relationships and frustrating circumstances.

Early Experience and the Modulation of Genetic Vulnerability to Stress

There is now significant evidence that experiences in infancy and early childhood have a significant influence on the adult response to stress. For example, research with rat pups showed that their early postnatal handling changed mother–pup interactions, leading to increased grooming and licking of the rat pups. The outcome in adult rats was similar to adult outcomes when the mothers naturally provided more grooming and licking: the pattern of behavioral (e.g., fearfulness) and neurochemical changes indicated a diminished response to stress (Calddji et al., 1998).

In another set of experiments two types of modified early experience were assessed for their impact on the genetic vulnerability to stress-induced gastric ulcers in adult rats. Neonatal handling for 21 days reduced the size of stress-induced ulcers equally in both the vulnerable and the less vulnerable strains. In contrast, an enriched environment for 90 days reduced the stress-induced ulcer size in the adults only in the less vulnerable strain. Moreover, there was evidence of diminished stress effects on behavior following each of the early experience modifications, but the effects were more prominent in the less vulnerable strain (Pare & Kluczynski, 1997). In this research, as might be theorized, early experiences reducing the stress response were less effective in the animal that was genetically more vulnerable.

Reducing the Impact of Stress and Inadequate Resources During Development: Modulation by Maternal Behaviors and Cultural Guidelines

Adults often assume a neglectful attitude toward the existence of stress in the lives of children, commenting that "life isn't perfect" and that their own childhood was more difficult. However, as a society, we must recognize the suffering and expense entailed if we fail to develop improved knowledge about the role of chronic stressful experiences in the development of children. Parallel to the dramatic advances in molecular and clinical genetics, and their application to better understanding of psychiatric disorders, there have been numerous research reports indicating the major role of environmental stresses in the genesis of serious psychiatric disorders during adulthood. These have been conceptualized within a model encompassing all types of risk and protective factors, and summed in the concept of vulnerability.

For example, it has been shown that there may be subtle ways in which individuals interact with others in their environment that makes them more vulnerable to a psychotic illness. It was found that if an individual has a higher level of familial risk for psychosis, this is associated with greater emotional reactivity to daily life stresses. The nature of the stresses utilized in this research was that they were "events and small disturbances in the natural flow of daily life," but the investigators comment that they "assessed frequently occurring exposures in daily life, the cumulative effects of which may be considerable" (Myin-Germeys, van Os, Schwartz, Stone, & Delespaul, 2001, p. 1142). This is a more realistic assessment of the effects of cumulative small stresses during the day than is usually given, and more closely approximates the experience of urban dwellers with busy lives. Certainly, it would appear that this is a more genuine attempt to consider stresses from the point of view of the patient, a perspective too often neglected (Strauss, 1994).

While such findings are readily interpreted as genetic in origin, it additionally could reflect social inheritance of familial styles of interpersonal interactions and child-rearing techniques. Our recognition of the pronounced receptivity of the cerebral cortex to experience during infancy suggests this as a contributing element in the causal chain, a point at which maternal behavior might lead to enduring changes in the brain and behavior of the infant as she develops into a child and adult. A child who was unable to achieve adequate state regulation as an infant, and whose escape mechanisms went unopposed too often would be expected to react differently later in life. Similarly, if her mother was unable to give consistent, repeated, graded environmental stimuli and "teaching" responsive to the infant's state and capacities, she would be expected to respond quite differently later in life to minor stressful stimuli. This is because stressful stimuli have a different meaning to someone who has been burdened with too many unregulated stimuli, and because the individual might have a different threshold of reactivity due to how the thresholds were set during an infancy characterized by repeated episodes of escape phenomena and emotion dysregulation.

These clinical data reflect observations at a temporal and perceptual level better fitting brain function, both in its stimulus detection and stimulus significance modes. This temporal and perceptual level has long been examined and understood by psychoanalysts and psychodynamically oriented clinicians, who observed, commented on, and based therapy upon these minute but highly revealing and significant interactional components. It is similarly small and discrete interactions that occurred during synaptogenesis and arealization of the brain, structuring the dictionaries of the infant that later will be adaptive or maladaptive.

Behavioral and Physiological Alterations Following Early Childhood Stress

If the presence of an attentive mother appears to be so important for the infant's comfort and for avoiding escape from the regulation of his or her physiology and behavior, is there evidence that there are significantly detrimental effects later in life if the attentive mother is lacking? In recent decades a substantial amount of research with animals (including primates) and humans has defined quite serious and replicable effects of early life stress on brain function and adult outcome. Severe childhood stress leads to an increased risk of developing recurrent major depression and posttraumatic stress disorder. When children who are abused reach adulthood they have small hippocampal volumes, indicating actual changes in brain morphology following stress during early childhood. When adults with recurrent major depression and posttraumatic stress disorder are examined, they too have small hippocampal volumes. What is the cause of these hippocampal changes? It has been suggested that the reduced hippocampal volume is caused by stress-related disorders, a concept that is implied by research describing stress-related changes in the hippocampal morphology of rodents.

Relevant to our examination of maternal–infant attachment behaviors, the investigation of stress effects on the brain in primates has centered on maternal deprivation as the prototypical early childhood stress. The maternal deprivation produced not only behavioral problems in Rhesus macaque monkeys analogous to those in humans—behavior similar to depression, disrupted sleep patterns, and inordinate alcohol consumption—but also altered physiology and brain function, including changes in the regulation of autonomic activity, magnified responses to stress in the hypothalamic-pituitary–adrenal axis (HPA), and increased sensitivity in the brain to dopamine and norepinephrine. The nature of such stressful experiences for primate or human infants is complex, and among the many studies reported there are varying results; moreover, it is essential to dissociate genetic effects (Lyons, Yang, Sawyer-Glover, Moseley, & Schatzberg, 2001). While the sources of alterations are unclear, we can unquestionably say that severe stresses in infancy, especially prolonged or repeated separation of the infant from his mother, lead to unequivocal changes in brain morphology, physiology, and behavior. Moreover, there is now substantial evidence that there are significant effects of many childhood, especially early childhood, stressful experiences.

☐ Culture and Cultural Identity: Guiding Influences on Maternal Sculpting of the Infant's Experiences and Memories

It would be convenient if we need only direct our recommendations for baby care to a pregnant woman, train her through repetition, and await the beneficial result. This is not possible, of course, due to her appropriate reliance on her own conscious and unconscious adaptive strategies. In addition, there are a range of other influences, many of which can usefully be encapsulated in the concept of *culture*. The conceptual and research distance between brain function and "culture" has narrowed considerably, and now permits preliminary comments about the nature of their interactions. A more detailed account is available elsewhere (Young, 2002a, 2002b).

The concept of *culture* has been notoriously difficult to define. Nevertheless, the perspectives on culture are expanding rapidly. The standard social science model of culture is giving way to a far more inclusive consideration of the subject that draws from many more disciplines and establishes its biological and psychological roots (Tooby & Cosmides, 1992). Writers commonly refer to the definitions of others, in this way avoiding the pitfall of being captured by the complexity of the concept. For example, "Culture has been variously defined as a social construction, a 'text,' social behaviours, artifacts or the mental entities (ideas/beliefs/values) in people's heads" (Aunger, 2000b, p. 7). Another author, Plotkin (2000), comments on the diversity of opinions when defining "culture," but emphasizes the importance of the definition. He describes Tylor's attempt as a "shotgun" definition: "knowledge, belief, art, morals, law, custom, and other capabilities and habits acquired by man as a member of a society including every artefact of cultural behaviour," yet any piece subtracted from this mix would spawn arguments from some defender. Similarly, he recalls Goodenough's definition ("Whatever it is one has to know or believe to operate in a manner acceptable to that society's members"), remarking that it at least has the virtue of having some focus—shared knowledge and beliefs (Plotkin, 2000, p. 74). It is import to our topic that these definitions emphasize that culture is fundamentally contained within the domain of knowledge, ideas, or beliefs. These terms, in turn, reflect mental constructs that are, fundamentally, complex, integrated, and interacting memories. *Memory* is a concept that brings us back to a fundamental focus for understanding how best to help a developing child. Possibly more important, it reminds us how to conceptualize our approach to prospective parents, who will soon be joining their infant in building memories.

The new breadth of approach to the concept of *culture* has been both spurred and aided by the emergence of the concept of *memes*. Commenting that genes need not be the only replicators, Richard Dawkins, in his 1976 publication *The Selfish Gene*, gave birth to the idea of memes:

> We need a name for the new replicator, a noun that conveys the idea of a unit of cultural transmission, or a unit of imitation. . . . Examples of memes are tunes, ideas, catch-phrases, clothes fashions, ways of making pots or of building arches. Just as genes propagate themselves in the gene pool by leaping from body to body via sperms or eggs, so memes propagate themselves in the meme pool by leaping from brain to brain via a process which, in the broad sense, can be called imitation. (Dawkins, 1976, p. 192)

Like *culture*, however, the definition of *meme* is controversial; moreover, the idea of memes hatched unrelenting debate among scientists about whether or not a meme exists or is a concept with sufficient conceptual rigor to be useful (Blackmore, 1999; Aunger, 2000a). However this debate concludes, we realize that, with this definition, we have not only the concept of an entity very much related to memories, but also find "imitation" to be a central component. Two of the elements that this chapter emphasizes as fundamental to understanding the developing infant, memories and imitation learning, are carried within the concept of *memes*. We can use it as a preliminary, viable concept for the transmission of culture, and a useful approximation of a conceptual language that will aid us in our understanding of how culture affects the infant.

It is clear by now that an infant does not learn about his or her environment by chance encounter. The infant's view is the view selected by the parents, particularly the child's mother. Part of this is genetically and biologically determined, for example, just as the prolactin surge influences genetically programmed and hard-wired breast-feeding behaviors. Part is determined by cultural influences, because the mother decides what to say to the infant, how to say it, and how frequently; who might hold the infant, for how long, and how often; whether the baby goes outside the house or meets others outside the family; how the infant's crying will be responded to; how often he or she will be fed; how his or her sleep cycle will be responded to; and endless other large or small decisions. How the mother feels about her ministrations to the baby is determined to a large extent by how well it fits the expectations of her family, friends, and culture—and sometimes appropriate maternal actions cause unhappiness because the mother's culture prescribes less beneficial alternatives.

At the same time, these parental–infant interactions are molding the beginnings of a cultural identity within a child, a growing expectation of what is to be done and how and why in so many important or insignificant situations. This cultural identity will differ in unpredictable ways from his or her parents' identity, and will then be transmitted to the next generation; the components of this transmitted culture will in part be novel memes, in part identical memes, and in part similar, but not identical memes. With each generation, the tools of adaptive success may be improved.

☐ Successful Adaptation: Competence, Self-Esteem, and Identity in Adulthood

This has been an extended account of infants, their developing brains, and their welfare. How can we characterize the goal toward which this trajectory of planful care is directed? Can we describe the functional characteristics of a young adult whom we would judge to be the product of solicitous, beneficial, and successful caregiving? Are global characterizations of personality features that we use to describe "well-adapted" adults useful, or are they pretentious, vague abstractions? Considered from the developmental perspective, they achieve a useful integration of observations concerning both developmental influences and an individual's currently functioning brain. Viewing clusters of childhood memories that retain guiding parental influences—including emotional memories—from different perspectives, we can identify features that define highly significant elevated, integrated components of the personality. These are composite characterizations of overlapping sectors of the adaptive capacity of the brain and mind.

Parental–child interactions initiate and amplify a cascade of beneficial or unfortunate effects on the neuronal circuits, molding adaptive capacities carried in the child's memories. These include:

- The mother's combined capacities to instill a feeling of effectiveness, to teach or delegate teaching for the child, and to help him or her respond to stress, lending what we call *competence* to the child.
- The child's experience of adequate self-regulation, of reasonable gratification, of a tolerable mood, and of effective capacities to adapt to stress, that we call *self-esteem*.
- The child's authoritative knowledge of who he or she is, where the child comes from and belongs, and who he or she belongs to; we call this *identity*.

These characteristics sum up many of the goals that parents have as they anticipate the outcome of their child's development. Competence, self-esteem, and identity—each is carried in the memories and emotional memories, implicit and explicit, of the late adolescent venturing into the world. When solidly present, these characteristics suggest neuronal circuits tuned to an adaptive harmony with his or her culture, family, and friends, yet sufficiently flexibly adaptive to coping and surviving even the most devastating catastrophes in an altered ecology.

To achieve this, a child needs the good fortune of one or more adults who accompany him or her along the way and who have the capacity to understand deeply this child's unique experiences and respect them.

"It is evening. We are seated on the steps of your palace. There is a slight breeze," Marco Polo answered. "Whatever country my words may evoke around you, you will see it from such a vantage point, even if instead of the palace there is a village on pilings and the breeze carries the stench of a muddy estuary." (Calvino, 1974, p. 27)

☐ References

Abbott, L. G., Varela, J. A., Sen, K., & Nelson, S. B. (1997). Synaptic depression and cortical gain control. *Science, 275*, 220–224.

Amaral, D. G. (1987). Memory: Anatomical organization of candidate brain regions. In F. Plum (Ed.), *Handbook of physiology: Neurophysiology–higher functions of the brain* (pp. 211–294). Bethesda, MD: American Physiological Society.

Amaral, D. G., Price, J. L., Pitkänen, A., & Carmichael, S. T. (1992). Anatomical organization of the primate amygdaloid complex. In J. P. Aggleton (Ed.), *The amygdala: Neurobiological aspects of emotion, memory, and mental dysfunction* (pp. 1–66). New York: Wiley-Liss.

Anderson, D. J., & Jan, Y. N. (1997). The determination of the neuronal phenotype. In W. M. Cowan, T. M. Jessell, & S. L. Zipursky (Eds.), *Molecular and cellular approaches to neural development* (pp. 26–63). New York: Oxford University Press.

Antonova, I., Arancio, O., Trillat, A.-C., Wang, H.-G., Zablow, L., Udo, H., Kandel, E. R., & Hawkins, R. D. (2001). Rapid increase in clusters of presynaptic proteins at onset of long-lasting potentiation. *Science, 294*, 1547–1550.

Ashby, F. G., & Ell, S. W. (2001). The neurobiology of human category learning. *Trends in Cognitive Sciences, 5*, 204–210.

Aunger, R. (Ed.). (2000a). *Darwinizing culture: The status of memetics as a science.* Oxford: Oxford University Press.

Aunger, R. (2000b). Introduction. In R. Aunger (Ed.), *Darwinizing culture: The status of memetics as a science* (pp. 1–23). Oxford: Oxford University Press.

Baddeley, A. (1986). *Working memory.* New York: Oxford University Press.

Baddeley, A. (1997). *Human memory: Theory and practice* (Rev. ed.). Hove, UK: Psychology Press.

Barinaga, M. (1998). Owl study sheds light on how young brains learn. *Science, 279*, 1451–1452.

Bear, D. (1991). Neurological perspectives on aggressive behavior. *Journal of Neuropsychiatry, 3*, S3–S8.

Bhalla, U. S., & Iyengar, R. (1999). Emergent properties of networks of biological signaling pathways. *Science, 283*, 381–387.

Blackmore, S. (1999). *The meme machine.* Oxford: Oxford University Press.

Bliss, T. V. P., & Lomo, T. (1973). Long-lasting potentiation of synaptic transmission in the dentate area of the anaesthetized rabbit following stimulation of the perforant path. *Journal of Physiology, 232*, 331–336.

Bourgeois, J. P., Goldman-Rakic, P. S., & Rakic, P. (2000). Formation, elimination, and stabilization of synapses in the primate cerebral cortex. In M. S. Gazzaniga (Ed.), *The new cognitive neurosciences* (2nd ed., pp. 45–53). Cambridge, MA: MIT Press.

Bowlby, J. (1969). *Attachment and loss: Vol. 1. Attachment.* New York: Basic Books.

Brazelton, T. B. (1979). Behavioral competence of the newborn infant. *Seminars in Perinatology, 3*, 35–44.

Brazelton, T. B. (1984). *Neonatal behavioral assessment scale* (2nd ed.). London: Blackwell.

Brazelton, T. B., Koslowski, B., & Main, M. (1974). Origins of reciprocity: The early mother–infant interaction. In M. Lewis and L. Rosenblum (Eds.), *The effects of the infant on its caregiver* (pp. 49–76). New York: Wiley.

Brazelton, T. B., Nugent, J. K., & Lester, B. M. (1987). Neonatal behavioral assessment scale. In J. D. Osofsky (Ed.), *Handbook of infant development* (2nd ed., pp. 780–817). New York:

Wiley.

Butler, L. T., & Berry, D. C. (2001). Implicit memory: Intention and awareness revisited. *Trends in Cognitive Sciences, 5,* 192–197.

Byrne, R. W., & Russon, A. E. (1998). Learning by imitation: A hierarchical approach. *Behavioral Brain Science, 21,* 667–721.

Cahill, L., Prins, B., Weber, M., & McGaugh, J. L. (1994). Beta-adrenergic activation and memory for emotional events. *Nature, 371,* 702–704.

Calamandrei, G., & Keverne, E. B. (1994). Differential expression of fos protein in the brain of female mice dependent on pup sensory cues and maternal experience. *Behavioral Neuroscience, 108,* 113–120.

Calddji, C., Tannenbaum, B., Sharma, S., Francis, D., Plotsky, P., & Meaney, M. (1998). Maternal care during infancy regulates the development of neural systems mediating the expression of fearfulness in the rat. *Proceedings of the National Academy of Sciences, U.S.A., 95,* 5335–5340.

Caldwell, J. D., Greer, E. R., Johnson, M. F., Prange, A. J., & Pedersen, C. A. (1987). Oxytocin and vasopressin immunoreactivity in hypothalmic and extrahypothalmic sites in late pregnant and postpartum rats. *Neuroendocrinology, 46,* 39–47.

Calvino, Italo (1974). *Invisible cities.* New York: Harcourt, Brace. (Original work published 1972)

Cohen, J. D., & Tong, F. (2001). The face of controversy. *Science, 293,* 2405–2407.

Davis, M. (1992). The role of the amygdala in conditioned fear. In J. P. Aggleton (Ed.), *The amygdala: Neurobiological aspects of emotion, memory, and mental dysfunction* (pp. 225–306). New York: Wiley-Liss.

Dawkins, R. (1976). *The selfish gene.* Oxford: Oxford University Press.

Devinsky, O., Morrell, M. J., & Vogt, B. A. (1995). Contributions of anterior cingulate cortex to behaviour. *Brain, 118,* 279–306.

Downing, P. E., Jiang, Y., Shuman, M., & Kanwisher, N. (2001). A cortical area selective for visual processing of the human body. *Science, 293,* 2470–2473

Fadiga, L., Fogassi, L., Paresi, G., & Rizzolatti, G. (1995). Motor facilitation during action observation: A magnetic stimulation study. *Journal of Neurophysiology, 73,* 2608–2611

Field, T. (1978). The three Rs of infant–adult interaction: Rhythms, repertoires, and responsivity. *Journal of Pediatric Psychology, 3,* 131–136.

Field, T. (1985). Attachment as psychobiological attunement: Being on the same wavelength. In M. Reite and T. Field (Eds.), *Psychobiology of attachment and separation* (pp. 415–454). New York: Academic.

Field, T. (1994). The effects of mother's physical and emotional unavailability on emotion regulation. The development of emotion regulation: Biological and behavioral considerations. *Monographs of the Society for Research in Child Development, 59*(2–3, Serial No. 240).

Freedman, D. J., Riesenhuber, M., Poggio, T., & Miller, E. K. (2001). Categorical representation of visual stimuli in the primate prefrontal cortex. *Science, 291,* 312–316.

Friedrich, R. W., & Laurent, G. (2001). Dynamic optimization of odor representations by slow temporal patterning of mitral cell activity. *Science, 291,* 889–894.

Fuster, J. M. (1989). *The prefrontal cortex: Anatomy, physiology, and neuropsychology of the frontal lobe.* New York: Raven Press.

Gallagher, J., & Holland, P. C. (1994). The amygdala complex. *Proceedings of the National Academy of Sciences, U.S.A., 91*(11),771–776.

Gallese, V., & Goldman, A. (1998). Mirror neurons and the simulation theory of mind-reading. *Trends in Cognitive Sciences, 2,* 493–501.

Geertz, Clifford (1973). *The interpretation of cultures.* New York: Basic Books.

Gibson, J. J. (1966). *The senses considered as perceptual systems.* Boston: Houghton Mifflin.

Gibson, J. J. (1979). *The ecological approach to visual perception.* Boston: Houghton Mifflin.

Goldman-Rakic, P. (1987). Circuitry of primate prefrontal cortex and regulation of behavior by representational memory. In F. Plum (Ed.), *Handbook of physiology: The nervous system—Higher functions of the brain* (pp. 373–417). Bethesda, MD: American Physiological Society.

Goldman-Rakic, P., Bourgeois, J.-P., & Rakic, P. (1997). Synaptic substrate of cognitive development: Life-span analysis of synaptogenesis in the prefrontal cortex of the nonhuman primate. In N. A. Krasnegor, G. R. Lyon, & P. S. Goldman-Rakic (Eds.), *Development of the prefrontal cortex: Evolution, neurobiology, and behavior* (pp. 27–47). Baltimore: Paul H. Brookes.

Grafton, S. T., Arbib, M. A., Fadiga, L., & Rizzolatti, G. (1996). Localization of grasp representations in humans by PET: II. Observation compared with imagination. *Experimental Brain Research, 112*, 103–111

Green, K. P., Kuhl, P. K., Meltzoff, A. N., & Stevens, E. B. (1991). Integrating speech information across talkers, gender, and sensory modality: Female faces and male voices in the McGurk effect. *Perceptual Psychophysiology, 50*, 524–536.

Halder, G., Callaerts, P., & Gehring, W. J. (1995). Induction of ectopic eyes by targeted expression of the eyeless gene in *Drosophila. Science, 267*, 1788–1792.

Halford, G. S. (1993). *Children's understanding: The development of mental models*. Hillsdale, NJ: Erlbaum.

Haxby, J., Gobbini, M. I., Furey, M. L., Ishai, A., Schouten, J. L., & Pietrini, P. (2001). Distributed and overlapping representations of faces and objects in ventral temporal cortex. *Science, 293*, 2425–2430.

Hepper, P. G. (1986). Kin recognition: Function and mechanisms. *Biological Review, 61*, 63–93.

Heyes, C. (2001). Causes and consequences of imitation. *Trends in Cognitive Sciences, 5*, 253–261.

Hofer, M. A. (1970). Physiological responses of infant rats to separation from their mothers. *Science, 168*, 871–873.

Hofer, M. A. (1984). Relationships as regulators: A psychobiologic perspective on bereavement. *Psychosomatic Medicine, 46*, 183–197.

Hofer, M. A. (1994). Hidden regulators in attachment, separation, and loss. *Monographs of the Society for Research in Child Development, 59*(2–3, Serial No. 240).

Hofer, M. A., & Shair, H. N. (1980). Sensory processes in the control of isolation-induced ultrasonic vocalizations by 2-week-old rats. *Journal of Comparative Physiology and Psychology, 94*, 271–299.

Holden, C. (2001). Single gene dictates ant society. *Science, 294*, 1434.

Hrdy, S. B. (2001). Mothers and others. *Natural History, 110*, 50–62

Huttenlocher, P. R., & Dabholkar, A. S. (1997). Regional differences in synaptogenesis in human cerebral cortex. *Journal of Comparative Neurology, 387*, 167–178.

Iacoboni, M. (1999). Cortical mechanisms of human imitation. *Science, 286*, 2526–2528

Johnson, M. H. (1997). *Developmental cognitive neuroscience*. Oxford: Blackwell.

Johnson, M. H. (1999). Cortical plasticity in normal and abnormal cognitive development: Evidence and working hypotheses. *Development and Psychopathology, 11*, 419–437

Johnson, M. H., Dziurawiec, S., Ellis, H. D., & Morton, J. (1991). Newborns' preferential tracking of face-like stimuli and its subsequent decline. *Cognition, 40*, 1–19.

Johnston, D. (1997). A missing link? LTP and learning. *Science, 278*, 401–402

Jusczyk, P. W., Friederici, A. D., Wessels, J. M. I., Svenkerud, V. Y., & Jusczyk, A. M. (1993). Infants' sensitivity to the sound patterns of native language words. *Journal of Memory and Language, 32*, 402–420

Kim, K. H. S., Relkin, N. R., Lee, K. M., & Hirsch, J. (1997). Distinct cortical areas associated with native and second languages. *Nature, 388*, 172–174.

Klaus, M. H., & Kennell, J. H. (1982). *Parent–infant bonding* (2nd ed.). St. Louis, MO: C. V. Mosby.

Kling, A. S., & Brothers, L. A. (1992). The amygdala and social behavior. In J. P. Aggleton (Ed.), *The amygdala: Neurobiological aspects of emotion, memory, and mental dysfunction* (pp. 353–377). New York: Wiley-Liss.

Knudsen, E. I. (1998). Capacity for plasticity in the adult owl auditory system expanded by juvenile experience. *Science, 279*, 1531–1533.

Knudsen, E. I., & Brainerd, M. S. (1995). Creating a unified representation of visual and auditory space in the brain. *Annual Review of Neuroscience, 18*, 19–43.

Knudsen, E. I., & Knudsen, P. F. (1990). Sensitive and critical periods for visual calibration of sound localization by barn owls. *Journal of Neuroscience, 10,* 222–232.

Krieger, & Ross. (2001). Identification of a major gene regulating complex social behavior. *Science, 294,* 1411.

Kuhl, P. (1991a). Human adults and human infants show a "perceptual magnet effect" for the prototypes of speech categories, monkeys do not. *Perceptual Psychophysiology, 50,* 93–107.

Kuhl, (1991b). Perception, cognition, and the ontogenetic and phylogenetic emergence of human speech. In S. E. Brauth, W. S. Hall, & R. J. Dooling (Eds.), *Plasticity of development* (pp. 73–196). Cambridge, MA: MIT Press.

Kuhl, P. (1994). Learning and representation in speech and language. *Current Opinion in Neurobiology, 4,* 812–822.

Kuhl, P. K. (2000). Language, mind, and brain: Experience alters perception. In M. S. Gazzaniga (Ed.), *The new cognitive neurosciences* (2nd ed., pp. 99–115). Cambridge, MA: MIT Press.

Kuhl, P. K., & Meltzoff, A. N. (1982). The bimodal perception of speech in infancy. *Science, 218,* 1138–1141.

LeDoux, J. E. (1995). In search of an emotional system in the brain: Leaping from fear to emotion and consciousness. In M. S. Gazzaniga (Ed.), *The cognitive neurosciences* (pp. 1049–1134). Cambridge: MIT Press.

LeDoux, J. (1996). *The emotional brain.* New York: Simon & Schuster.

Lester, B., Hoffman, J., & Brazelton, T. B. (1985). The rhythmic structure of mother-infant interaction in term and pre-term infants. *Child Development, 56,* 15–27.

Li, H., Weiss, S. R., Chuang, D. M., Post, R. M., & Rogawski, M. A. (1998). Bidirectional synaptic plasticity in the rat basolateral amygdala: Characterization of an activity-dependent switch sensitive to the presynaptic metabotropic glutamate receptor antagonist 2S-alpha-ethylglutamic acid. *Journal of Neuroscience, 18,* 1662–1670.

Li, L.-L., Keverne, E. B., Aparicio, S. A., Ishino, G., Barton, S. C., & Surani, M. A. (1999). Regulation of maternal behavior and offspring growth by paternally expressed *Peg3. Science, 284,* 330–333.

Lisman, J. E., & Fallon, J. R. (1999). What maintains memories? *Science, 283,* 339–340.

Liu, L., Wolf, R., Ernst, R., & Heisenberg, M. (1999). *Nature, 400,* 753.

Lynch, G. (2000). Memory consolidation and long-term potentiation. In M. S. Gazzaniga (Ed.), *The new cognitive neurosciences* (2nd ed., pp. 139–157). Cambridge, MA: MIT Press.

Lyons, D. M., Yang, C., Sawyer-Glover, A. M., Moseley, M. E., & Schatzberg, A. F. (2001). Early life stress and inherited variation in monkey hippocampal volumes. *Archives of General Psychiatry, 58,* 1145–1151.

Magee, J. C., & Johnston, D. (1997). A synaptically controlled, associative signal for Hebbian plasticity in hippocampal neurons. *Science, 275,* 209–213.

Malenka, R. C. (1995). LTP and LTD: Dynamic and interactive processes of synaptic plasticity. *The Neuroscientist, 1,* 35–42.

Maren, S. (1999). Long-term potentiation in the amygdala: A mechanism for emotional learning and memory. *Trends in Neuroscience, 22,* 561–567.

Markram, H., Lübke, J., Frotscher, M., & Sakmann, B. (1997). Regulation of synaptic efficacy by coincidence of postsynaptic Aps and EPSPs. *Science, 275,* 213–215.

Martin, K. C., Bartsch, D, Bailey, C. H., & Kandel, E. R. (2000). Molecular mechanisms underlying learning-related long-lasting synaptic plasticity. In M. S. Gazzaniga (Ed.), *The new cognitive neurosciences* (2nd ed., pp. 121–137). Cambridge, MA: MIT Press

McComb, K., Moss, C., Durant, S. M., Baker, L., & Sayialel, S. (2001). Matriarchs as repositories of social knowledge in African elephants. *Science, 292,* 491–494.

McGaugh, J. L., Cahill, L., & Roozendaal, B. (1996). Involvement of the amygdala in memory storage: Interaction with other brain systems. *Proceedings of the National Academy of Sciences, U.S.A., 93,* 13508–13514.

McGurk, H., & MacDonald, J. (1976). Hearing lips and seeing voices. *Nature, 264,* 746–748.

Meltzoff, A. N., & Moore, M. K. (1999). Persons and representation: Why infant imitation is important for theories of human development. In J. Nadel & G. Butterworth (Eds.), *Imitation in infancy* (pp. 9–35). Cambridge: Cambridge University Press.

Murphy, G. G., & Glanzman, D. L. (1997). Mediation of classical conditioning in *Aplysia californica* by long-term potentiation of sensorimotor synapses. *Science, 278,* 467–471.

Myin-Germeys, I., van Os, J., Schwartz, J. E., Stone, A. A., & Delespaul, P. A. (2001). Emotional reactivity to daily life stress in psychosis. *Archives of General Psychiatry, 58,* 1137–1144.

Nadel, J., & Butterworth, G. (1999). Introduction: Immediate imitation rehabilitated at last. In J. Nadel & G. Butterworth (Eds.), *Imitation in infancy.* Cambridge: Cambridge University Press.

Nishitani, N., & Hari, R. (2000). Temporal dynamics of cortical representation for action. *Proceedings of the National Academy of Sciences, U.S.A., 97,* 913–918.

Nowakowski, R. S., & Hayes, N. L. (1999). CNS development: An overview. *Development and Psychopathology, 11,* 395–417.

Oliet, S. H., Malenka, R. C., & Nicoll, R. A. (1996). Bidirectional control of quantal size by synaptic activity in the hippocampus. *Science, 271,* 1294–1297.

Osofsky, J. D. (1976). Neonatal characteristics and mother-infant interaction in two observational situations. *Child Development, 47,* 1138–1147.

Pallas, S. L. (2001). Intrinsic and extrinsic factors that shape neocortical specification. *Trends in Neurosciences, 24,* 417–423.

Pare, W., & Kluczynski, J. (1997). Developmental factors modify stress ulcer incidence in a stress-susceptible rat strain. *The Journal of Physiology, 91,* 105–111.

Plotkin, H. (2000). Culture and psychological mechanisms. In R. Aunger (Ed.), *Darwinizing culture: The status of memetics as a science* (pp. 69–83). Oxford: Oxford University Press.

Post, R. M., Weiss, S. R. B., Li, H., Smith, M. A., Zhang, L. X., Xing, G., Osuch, E. A., & McCann, U. D. (1998). Neural plasticity and emotional memory. *Development and Psychopathology, 10,* 829–855

Puelles, L., & Rubenstein, J. L. (1993). Expression patterns of homeobox and other putative regulatory genes in the embryonic mouse forebrain suggest a neuromeric organization. *Trends in Neuroscience, 16,* 472–479.

Rakic, P. (2000). Setting the stage for cognition: Genesis of the primate cerebral cortex. In M. S. Gazzaniga (Ed.), *The new cognitive neurosciences* (2nd ed., pp. 7–21). Cambridge, MA: MIT Press.

Reich, D. S., Mechler, F., and Victor, J. D. (2001). Independent and redundant information in nearby cortical neurons. *Science, 294,* 2566–2568.

Rescorla, R. A. (1988a). Pavlovian conditioning: It's not what you think it is. *American Psychologist, 43,* 151–160.

Rescorla, R. A. (1988b). Behavioral studies of Pavlovian conditioning. In W. M. Cowan (Ed.), *Annual Review of Neuroscience, Vol. 11,* 329–352.

Richmond, B. (2001). Information coding. *Science, 294,* 2493–2494.

Rizzolatti, G., & Arbib, M. A. (1998). Language within our grasp. *Trends in Neurosciences, 21,* 188–194

Rizzolatti, G., & Gentilucci, M. (1988). Motor and visual-motor functions of the premotor cortex. In P. Rakic & W. Singer (Eds.), *Neurobiology of neocortex* (pp. 269–284). New York: Wiley.

Rizzolatti, G., Fadiga, L., Matelli, M., Bettinardi, V., Bulesu, F., Perani, D., & Fazio, F. (1996). Localization of grasp representations in humans by PET: I. Observation versus execution. *Experimental Brain Research, 111,* 246–252

Rizzolatti, G., Fadiga, L., Fogassi, L, & Gallese, V. (1999). Resonance behaviors and mirror neurons. *Archives of Italian Biology, 137,* 85–100.

Robin, N., & Holyoak, K. J. (1995). Relational complexity and the functions of prefrontal cortex. In M. S. Gazzaniga (Ed.), *The cognitive neurosciences* (pp. 987–997). Cambridge, MA: MIT Press

Rolls, E. T. (1992). Neurophysiology and functions of the primate amygdala. In J. P. Aggleton (Ed.), *The amygdala: Neurobiological aspects of emotion, memory, and mental dysfunction* (pp. 143–165). New York: Wiley-Liss.

Rosenblum, L. D., Schmuckler, M. A., & Johnson, J. A. (1997). The McGurk effect in infants. *Perceptual Psychophysiology, 59,* 347–357.

Saffran, J. R., Aslin, R. N., & Newport, E. L. (1996). Statistical learning by 8-month old infants. *Science, 274,* 1926–1928.

Sander, L. W. (1969). The longitudinal course of early mother–infant interaction: Cross-case comparisons in a sample of mother–child pairs. In B. Foss (Ed.), *Determinants of infant behavior.* London: Methuen.

Sanes, D. H., Reh, T. A., & Harris, W. A. (2000). *Development of the nervous system.* San Diego: Academic Press.

Sejnowski, T. J. (1997). The year of the dendrite. *Science, 275,* 178–179.

Shimizu, E., Tang, Y.-P., Rampon, C., & Tsien, J. Z. (2000). NMDA receptor-dependent synaptic reinforcement as a crucial process for memory consolidation. *Science, 290,* 1170–1174.

Smith, M. A., Makino, S., Kim, S. Y., & Kvetnansky, R. (1995). Stress and glucocorticoids affect the expression of brain-derived neurotropic factor and neurotrophin-3 mRNAs in the hippocampus. *Journal of Neuroscience, 15,* 1768–1777.

Spanagel, R., & Weiss, F. (1999). The dopamine hypothesis of reward: Past and current status. *Trends in Neurosciences, 22,* 521–527.

Squire, L. R. (1992). Memory and the hippocampus: A synthesis from findings with rats, monkeys, and humans. *Psychology Review, 99,* 195–231.

Squire, L. R., & Knowlton, B. J. (2000). The medial temporal lobe, the hippocampus, and the memory systems of the brain. In M. S. Gazzaniga (Ed.), *The new cognitive neurosciences* (2nd ed., pp. 765–779). Cambridge, MA: MIT Press.

Stern, D. N. (1977). *The first relationship.* Cambridge, MA: Harvard University Press.

Stern, D. N. (1985). *The interpersonal world of the infant: A view from psychoanalysis and developmental psychology.* New York: Basic Books.

Stoller, S., & Field, T. (1982). Alteration of mother and infant behavior and heartrate during a still-face perturbation of face-to-face interaction. In T. Field & A. Fogel (Eds.), *Emotion and early interactions.* Hillsdale, NJ: Erlbaum.

Strausfeld, N. J., Hansen, L., Li, Y., Gomez, R. S., & Ito, K. (1998). *Learning and Memory, 5,* 11.

Strauss, J. S. (1994). The person with schizophrenia as a person. II. Approaches to the subjective and complex. *British Journal of Psychiatry, 23*(Suppl.), 103–107.

Stuss, D. T., & Benson, D. F. (1986). *The frontal lobes.* New York: Raven Press.

Swanson, L. W., & Petrovich, G. D. (1998). What is the amygdala? *Trends in Neuroscience, 21,* 323–331.

Tang, S., & Guo, A. (2001). Choice behavior of *Drosophila* facing contradictory visual cues. *Science, 294,* 1543–1547.

Thorpe, S. J., & Fabre-Thorpe, M. (2001). Seeking categories in the brain. *Science, 291,* 260–263.

Tong, Y. C., Busby, P. A., & Clark, G. M. (1988). Perceptual studies on cochlear implant patients with early onset of profound hearing impairment prior to normal development of auditory, speech, and language skills. *Journal of the Acoustical Society of America, 84,* 951–962.

Tooby, J., & Cosmides, L. (1992). The psychological foundations of culture. In J. H. Barkow, L. Cosmides, & J. Tooby (Eds.), *The adapted mind: Evolutionary psychology and the generation of culture* (pp. 19–136). Oxford: Oxford University Press.

Tronick, E. Z., Als, H., & Brazelton, T. B. (1977). Mutuality in mother–infant interaction. *Journal of Communication, 27,* 74–79.

Tronick, E. Z., Als, H., Adamson, L., Wise, S., & Brazelton, T. B. (1978). The infant's response to entrapment between contradictory messages in face-to-face interaction. *Journal of Child Psychiatry, 17,* 1–13.

Tulving, E. (2000). Introduction: Memory. In M. S. Gazzaniga (Ed.), *The new cognitive neurosciences* (2nd ed., pp. 727–732). Cambridge, MA: MIT Press.

Walton, G. E., & Bower, T. G. R. (1993). Newborns form "prototypes" in less than 1 minute. *Psychological Science, 4,* 203–205.

Wenning, A. (1999). Sensing effectors make sense. *Trends in Neurosciences, 22,* 550–555.

Wilson, E. O. (1975). *Sociobiology: The new synthesis.* Cambridge, MA: The Belknap Press of Harvard University Press.

Wise, R. A., & Rompre, P. P. (1989). Brain dopamine and reward. *Annual Review of Psychology, 40,* 191–225.

Wolpert, D. M., Ghahramani, Z., & Flanagan, J. R. (2001). Perspectives and problems in motor learning. *Trends in Cognitive Sciences, 5,* 487–494.

Yando, R., Seitz, V., & Zigler, E. (1978). *Imitation: A developmental perspective.* Hillsdale, NJ: Erlbaum.

Young, J. G., Brasic, J. R., Ostrer, H., Kaplan, D., Will, M., John, E. R., Prichep, L., & Buchsbaum, M. (1996). The developing brain and mind: Advances in research techniques. In M. Lewis (Ed.), *Child and adolescent psychiatry: A comprehensive textbook* (2nd ed., pp. 1209–1234). Baltimore: Williams & Wilkins.

Young, J. G., Kaplan, D., Pascualvaca, D., & Brasic, J. R. (1995). Psychiatric examination of infants, children, and adolescents. In H. I. Kaplan & B. J. Sadock (Eds.), *Comprehensive textbook of psychiatry* (Vol. 6, 6th ed.). Baltimore: Williams & Wilkins.

Young, J. G. (1999). Stress and violence in childhood and youth: The brain, genes, environment and experience during development. In J. Gomes-Pedro (Ed.), *Stress e Violência na Criança e no Jovem/Stress and Violence in Childhood and Youth* (pp. 577–623). Lisbon: Clínica Universitária de Pediatria, Departamento de Educação Médica.

Young, J. G. (in press, a). The concept of culture. In J. G. Young, P. Ferrari, S. Malhotra, S. Tyano, & E. Caffo (Eds.), *Brain, culture, and development.* New Delhi: Macmillan India.

Young, J. G. (in press, b). Neural mechanisms mediating etiological influences: The developing brain, evolution, and culture. In J. G. Young, P. Ferrari, S. Malhotra, S. Tyano, & E. Caffo (Eds.). *Brain, culture, and development.* New Delhi: Macmillan India.

Zhang, F., Endo, S., Cleary, L. J., Eskin, A., & Byrne, J. H. (1997). Role of transforming growth factor-ß in long-term synaptic facilitation in *Aplysia. Science, 275,* 1318–1320.

Zola-Morgan, S., & Squire, L. R. (1993). Neuroanatomy of memory. *Annual Review of Neuroscience, 16,* 547–563.

J. Gerald Young

The Cradle of Adaptation: Models Describing the Experience-Responsive Development of Neural Structure and Adaptive Capacities in Infancy and Early Childhood

"Papà," Giannina asked again, "why is it that ancient tombs are not as sad as new ones?"

Giorgio Bassani
The Garden of the Finzi-Continis (p. 5)

The question of a 9-year-old girl in a novel echoes in the mind of a clinician who has experienced a variation of the phenomenon she refers to. Reading a pitiful story about the abuse of a 5-year-old child in the newspaper in the morning, along with descriptions of the subsequent intense concern of adults trying to unravel how this could have happened, I later consider the story from a new perspective while seeing a patient. This patient might be a child or teenager of any age, but what is of special interest in relation to the newspaper story is that, while my patient was abused, physically or psychologically, when a very young child, the adults in his life show surprisingly little concern about this as they complain about his current behavior. The present behavior—whether aggressive behavior, or visible depression, or palpable anxiety—reflects adaptive responses learned when he was abused, behaviors solidified in the child's mind and brain in such a way that it has become automatic, habitual, unconscious behavior. The child remains a victim, just as a Holocaust survivor was still a victim 15 years later, and should be expected to behave in a manner that reflects his past. Yet, we must admit the truth: we are less concerned with an old victim, who misbehaves or appears chronically despondent, than a new victim, shattered and confused. In short, we have difficulty appreciating the indisputable significance of effects occurring after a long time interval, no matter how poignant the events. There are many reasons for this, such as the growing recognition that there are so many of these children. Yet, a substantive part of our neglect is ignorance about these genuine causal influences from early childhood. Perhaps, if we were to understand better how the infant's brain and mind are formed, and why early childhood memories endure, we would be more responsive to the older victim's needs.

☐ A Model for the Formation of Primary Memory Prototypes in Infancy and Early Childhood: Forming and Tuning Neural Circuits Through Predictive Signal Mapping

Candidate Stimuli, Processing Units, and Predictive Signal Mapping

In order to understand the links between early childhood experiences and later behavior, we must review the purposes and functions of the brain, beginning in infancy. If the infant is to survive and develop within the loving embrace of her family, she must gradually learn to decipher the meanings of the shower of stimuli flooding her daily. In essence, this means that she must learn which stimuli are predictive in some manner that is useful for guiding her adaptive responses. This is a daunting task, so complex that adults forget how little an infant knows at birth. At the risk of providing too much detail and unfamiliar terminology, we shall construct models for how the brain of the infant makes sense of its surroundings and gains the capacity to apply this knowledge for its own needs.

When we observe the behavior of infants, and attempt to understand the purposes and adaptive functions of what a baby is doing, there is a common source of misconception. It is usual for us to respond to stimuli as composite or aggregate stimuli (e.g., a chair, a clock, a skier)—forgetting that we spent months to years learning to do so a very long time ago, at the beginning of our lives. Long since forgotten is that these perceptual capacities were built up gradually, from initially responding to myriad individual stimuli (and whatever limited group of more complex stimuli for which we have a genetically programmed response capacity); this was a tedious, and now uninteresting, effort of the past. There are many other examples of our ready misconceptions about what the infant is doing. For example, research on the development of face recognition capacities in the infant has uncovered multiple component processes underlying the development of the capacity for face recognition, warning us to be cautious about assigning adult-conceptualized content or purposes too readily to infant responses to faces just after birth. Simpler neural and cognitive mechanisms for responding to stimuli can be utilized during development, at least temporarily (Johnson, 1997; Johnson, Dziurawiec, Ellis, & Morton, 1991). This reflects the problem of our own learning. To return to our initial example, we view things as composites of characteristics that we no longer identify separately unless there is a reason (e.g., someone asks what the color of a sweater is). Infants are building identities through recognition of recurring composites, whether of animate or inanimate objects. Their strategies can seem obvious in retrospect, yet surprising when it is first realized how the infant was approaching a perceptual "problem."

Nevertheless, like it or not, when attempting to help our patients, whether infant or adult, we must reawaken our awareness of minute stimuli—in the infant nursery, in the consulting room, and in our theoretical formulations. Stimuli arrive at our sensory receptors as "individual" candidate stimuli and percepts are formed; predictive stimuli are selected from among them if determined to be significant signals, and these percepts are subjected to ever-higher, more complex processing—passing through neural circuits as newly formed processing units that carry more complex information. As memory templates are formed and sculpted into primary memory prototypes, new stimuli are compared with these increasingly complex memory templates—and the brain begins to have the capacity to respond to aggregate stimuli that have predictive value, increasing the rapidity of response and sophistication of adaptation. The higher order "processing units" presumably pass through the same processes for predictive signal mapping that simple percepts do, and they themselves become familiar: a category, like "sonatas," or a symbol, like the word *piano*.

These thoughts raise the problem of how we retrospectively define "context"; what we call *context* is really shorthand for all of the candidate stimuli in the environment other than a few we have selected. When we say that a child responded to something, such as a bullying 5-year-old classmate months ago, we commonly add the comment that he now also seems to respond to something else, such as the school itself, or a specific classroom, parts of the original scene that we view as the "context" of what occurred. We wonder why the boy is very reluctant to go to school. Without thinking about it, we have already selected, in retrospect, what we determine to be the significant stimulus, which is the boy who hit him. The full picture might be more complex, possibly including the humiliating laughter of others, or the facial expression of a teacher ready to scold him. While the bullying classmate might no longer threaten him, he is less sure about the thoughts of the previously taunting classmates or the current intentions of the now-frightening teacher. At the time of the original incident, his brain did not respond to our postevent selection of stimuli, but instead was responding to a broad canvas of candidate stimuli, among which a group of stimuli, not just one, were selected as possible predictors of something significant that would occur. Later on, adults tend to ignore these other relevant stimuli and comment that his nervousness around the other students and his teacher is unreasonable. But his brain is functioning too well to ignore these stimuli; it must learn about its environment if it is to survive and adapt. Adults can aid in this learning process, but not if they ignore stimuli which are too powerfully relevant to be neglected.

Paying attention to context is not a novel idea—this is what therapists have been doing for many years: attending to the details of an individual's experience and his associations to an experience, whether infant or teenager or adult, and attempting to determine *the relevant stimuli in his memories or recent life experiences*. Moreover, context reflects what a large group of investigators, led by Bronfenbrenner, have for many years identified as the "ecology" of the developing child (1979). With these thoughts in mind, let us review the pathway of these individual predictive signal stimuli, from whatever environmental source, as they enter into sensory systems and activate sequential neural structures. We do so with the objective of understanding the structural regularities of these neural functions, and how they might inform our understanding of how the baby learns about the physical reality of the world, about emotions, and about the social world and so many other phenomena, all within his mother's arms.

Predictive Signal Mapping

Reviewing the specific hypothetical steps involved in the processing of a "processing unit" in the brain is ponderous and interrupts our chain of thought, but it is necessary if we are to illuminate infant care and enjoy a fresh view of a baby's development. It also contains inherent uncertainty due to the nature of this complex series of events: The molecular and cellular events are the physical reality underlying all else, and comprise sequential signaling at synapses chained through neural structures recruited in response to the environmental stimulus. The translation of these events into functional concepts like *memory templates* or *significance determination*, let alone higher level concepts like *attachment behaviors* or *emotional language*, is hazardous. Nevertheless, in order to make sense of these events, and the adaptive activities of the infant, which is the locus of our ultimate interest, we are encouraged to assemble viable hypothetical models, and a corresponding functional terminology, for the processes that the neural circuits utilize to predict environmental events in an adaptive manner. In other words, it is important to indicate that there now is sufficient data so that we can hazard a serious attempt at a model for predictive signal mapping using processing units. This hypothesized model describes an efficient method for processing different units in a similar manner (as examples, see the application of this model to perceptual stimuli, categories, and symbols in Tables 15.1, 15.2, and 15.3). Some of the essential components of this model can be rendered briefly as follows:

TABLE 15.1. Predictive Signal Mapping: Hypothetical Model for the Formation and Tuning of Primary Memory Prototypes for Perceptual Stimuli

---

Processing Unit: Perceptual Signal

Perceptual Stimulus Discrimination and Significance Detection, Generating Primary Memory Prototypes

Perceptual Stimulus *Detection*: Detection of Candidate Perceptual Stimuli

Signal (Perceptual Stimulus) *Discrimination*: Discrimination of Predictive Perceptual Stimuli from Candidate Perceptual Stimuli

    Species-Specific Perceptual Discrimination Capacities (e.g., to auditory characteristics of human voice or to faces) (initially, genetically programmed neural capacity)

    Determination of Perceptual Stimulus *Significance* (initially, genetically programmed neural capacity)

        Reward or Pain

        Emotion

    Signal *Memory Template Matching* According to Perceptual Stimulus Significance (Working Memory)

    Signal *Memory Template Formation* (Long-Term Memory)

Signal (Perceptual Stimulus) Primary Memory Prototype Formation

    Signal *Primary Memory Prototype Matching and Tuning* (Long-Term Memory)

    Signal *Secondary Memory Prototype Matching and Tuning* (later memory tuning alterations)

Filtering of Perceptual Stimulus Signal Primary Memory Prototypes from Perceptual Stimulus Candidate Primary Memory Prototypes (Automation/Implicit Memory)

TABLE 15.2. Predictive Signal Mapping: Hypothetical Model for the Formation and Tuning of Primary Memory Prototypes for Categories

Processing Unit: Category

  (Category: Reliable to Perfect Occurrence of Grouping Feature(s) with Stimulus Prototypes)

Category Discrimination and Significance Detection, Generating Primary Memory Prototypes

Category *Detection*: Detection of Candidate Category Features (Stimuli)

Signal (Category Feature) *Discrimination*: Discrimination of Predictive Category Features (Stimuli) from Candidate Category Features (Stimuli)

    Species-Specific Perceptual Discrimination Capacities (initially, genetically programmed neural capacity)

    Determination of Category Feature *Significance* (initially, genetically programmed neural capacity)

      Reward or Pain

      Emotion

    Category Signal *Memory Template Matching* According to Category Significance (Working Memory)

    Category Signal *Memory Template Formation* (Long-Term Memory)

Signal (Category Features) Primary Memory Prototype Formation

  Signal *Primary Memory Prototype Matching and Tuning* (Long-Term Memory)

  Signal *Secondary Memory Prototype Matching and Tuning* (later memory tuning alterations)

Filtering of Category Features Signal Primary Memory Prototypes from Category Features Candidate Primary Memory Prototypes (Automation/Implicit Memory)

Predictive Signal Mapping:
  Hypothetical Model of Sequential, Component Events during the Formation and Tuning of Primary Memory Prototypes:
    Detection
    Discrimination
    Significance Determination
    Memory Template Matching
    Memory Template Formation
    Primary Prototype Memory Matching and Tuning
    Secondary Prototype Memory Matching and Tuning
    Filtering and Automation

Perceptual Discrimination: Separating Predictive Stimuli (Signals) from Candidate Stimuli Using Stimulus Significance Detection.   The predictive stimulus (i.e., the signal) can be a single stimulus element or aggregate stimuli (stimulus assemblies, such as a face, etc.). It must be detected and discriminated from all similar candidate stimuli in order to become a perceptual processing unit. Perceptual unit formation and discrimination reflect the nature of the signal method—whether using the

---

TABLE 15.3. Predictive Signal Mapping: Hypothetical Model for the Formation and Tuning of Primary Memory Prototypes for Symbols

---

Processing Unit: Symbol

(Symbol: Reliable to Perfect Coincident Occurrence of an Arbitrary Stimulus with a Stimulus Prototype or a Category Prototype)

Symbol Discrimination and Significance Detection, Generating Primary Memory Prototypes

Symbol *Detection*: Detection of Candidate Symbol Features (Stimuli)

Signal (Symbol Features) *Discrimination*: Discrimination of Predictive Symbol Features (Stimuli) from Candidate Symbol Features (Stimuli)

> Species-Specific Perceptual Discrimination Capacities (initially, genetically programmed neural capacity)
>
> Determination of Symbol Feature *Significance* (initially, genetically programmed neural capacity)
>
> Reward or Pain
>
> Emotion, especially in relation to social interactions
>
> Symbol Signal *Memory Template Matching* According to Symbol Significance (Working Memory)
>
> Symbol Signal *Memory Template Formation* (Long-Term Memory)

Signal (Symbol Features) Primary Memory Prototype Formation

> Signal *Primary Memory Prototype Matching and Tuning* (Long-Term Memory)
>
> Signal *Secondary Primary Memory Prototype Matching and Tuning* (later memory tuning alterations)

Filtering of Symbol Features Signal Primary Memory Prototypes from Symbol Features Candidate Primary Memory Prototypes (Automation/Implicit Memory)

---

firing rate of the neuron or another signal system—and the tuning involves the gradual setting of the signal threshold and an adequate stimulus range for response while responding to the statistical probabilities of the percept formation. The stimulus is discriminated on the basis of stimulus significance, meaning that the stimulus is found to predict the presence of consequences (i.e., reward or danger) in the environment, activating reward systems and emotion-generating neural structures of the brain. Subsequent repeated stimulus detection can lead to "experience-altered perception" if it is possible to "tune" the response of the neurons in the sensory or perceptual area (some neurons are "untuned"). Repetitive discrimination of a stimulus as significant leads to memory formation and consolidation (LeDoux, 1996; Lynch, 2000; Martin, Bartsch, Bailey, & Kandel, 2000).

Early Learning in Infants: Memory Template Formation, Comparisons of Stimuli with Templates, and the Formation of Primary Memory Prototypes. As matching of percepts with prior percepts in working memory occurs, a long-term memory for the percept might be formed if the stimulus—now a percept—is significant.

This can become the locus, if there is a repetitive appearance of similar stimuli, for more comparison and matching with memory templates, and the gradual transformation into a primary memory prototype in the infant. As the latter is the first consolidated, sculpted template, it functions as a prototype that has a guiding effect on the response to subsequent similar stimuli as signal mapping continues. A primary memory prototype is not immutable, but carries an advantage for durability as the initial memory that predicts environmental meanings. It sets a tone of expectation that subsequent stimuli will be the same, reflected in analogous terms sometimes used in reference to (less durable) percepts such as *expectancy wave,* or "search image." These terms refer to the neural template generated in expectation of an odor after training, which is altered if the stimulus proves to be different than expected or predicted from experience, as observed in electrophysiological studies of the olfactory system (Freeman, 1979, 1981, 1983). While the primary memory template tends to endure, if subsequent environmental responses are consistently altered, the new experiences might change the prototype during the period of brain development in early childhood; this might be a source of the loss of early childhood memories as neuronal systems are altered. Moreover, continuing developmental neural processes, such as synaptic pruning, offer new opportunities to consolidate only those stable memory prototypes receiving sustained reinforcement. Primary memory prototypes in long-term memory, typically in the cortex, thus, begin to dominate the response to related stimuli; if there was subcortical perceptual capacity, it remains, but is increasingly overridden by cortical responses. A memory template does not consist of a perfect replication of all features of the stimulus. Thus, a "best" representation, the memory template, is gradually molded; part of the process necessarily includes removing what does *not* fit the general form of the stimuli—thus, retaining what matches and omitting what does not.

> And yet each piece of information about a place recalled to the emperor's mind that first gesture or object with which Marco had designated the place. The new fact received a meaning from that emblem and also added to the emblem a new meaning. Perhaps, Kublai thought, the empire is nothing but a zodiac of the mind's phantasms. (Calvino, 1972/1974, p. 22)

This is a system constructed for rapid response to environmental stimuli by using comparisons of current stimuli with memory templates of previous experiences. We should step back from the formal language of memory templates and processing units, which is transitional between neural mechanisms and clinical applications of this knowledge, and recall the phenomena which emphasize how directly experience guides the specification of function within neocortical areas during infancy, and are the foundation of our model. While there are multiple developmental events affecting brain structure that might affect clinically observable functions in a profound manner (such as synaptic pruning or the elimination of neurons, which suggest the temporary presence of another sensitive period), we have focused on the impact of synaptogenesis. As we discussed in the previous chapter, it is possible to transform one primary sensory cortical area presumed to be the locus for one function (auditory cortex neurons utilized for hearing) to another function (becoming visual cortex neurons for sight), by redirecting visual inputs to the auditory thalamus, which then projects to the auditory cortex. This indicates how experience-induced activity patterns determine the function of the neural circuits of these cortical areas during synaptogenesis. This open receptivity to experience confers a period of remarkable plasticity in the functional specification of the cortex, a responsivity to the infant's unique experiences during this early period that guides the formation of synaptic connections in cortical areas that underlie memory formation and influence later stimulus appraisal. In other words, the modular organization of the sensory cortex mirrors the type of sensory-thalamic projections reaching the cortex, and their activity patterns, during this sensitive period. These projections continue to participate in the later changes, as well as the stability, of these neural circuits. Moreover, it is a sufficiently extended process to permit the infant to have ample "confirming" interactions with the actual environment in which he will live, maximizing adaptive potential (Bourgeois, Goldman-Rakic, & Rakic, 2000; Goldman-Rakic, Bourgeois, & Rakic, 1997; Johnson, 1997; Rakic, 2000; Sanes, Reh, & Harris, 2000).

Matching and tuning continue, and with increased experience with the environment, progressively higher order perceptual processing units are formed (e.g., through feature combination or cross-modal linking to another sensory modality). Ultimately, formal cognition begins as memories for increasingly abstract phenomena are formed, such as for categorization and symbol formation. These complex memories are formed in response to the regular presentation of stimuli that discriminate more complex relationships of the cooccurrence of stimuli, generating grouping or pairing on this basis. For example, when a symbol is encountered, the reward or motivation is extended from the primary source, the perceptual signal(s) (e.g., a red, rounded fruit), to include a secondary source, the symbol for the perceptual signal(s) (the written word, *apple*). Complexity also is added through perceptual symbol combinations, with relational cognitive elements, including rules and a temporal component. In this manner, sentences and paragraphs can be formed in conventional written or spoken language, or a social interaction can be completed (such as congratulating a friend on her success). Finally, as the regularities of the processing of very repetitive "familiar" stimuli are evident to the neural circuits, it is inefficient to allocate this complex response system in its entirety each time the familiar stimuli occur, so a system for filtering primary memory prototype-matching stimuli and responding to them automatically is enacted, enabling automation of the process of separating predictive signals from stimulus candidates and responding to them outside of awareness (e.g., utilizing basal ganglia, cerebellum, and other structures).

The Concept of Processing Units.   Running through this discussion is the term *processing unit*, a hypothetical construct used to aid us as we trace the progress and transformation of what originates as a sensory stimulus, and is sequentially recoded within specific neural pathways—so it is important to ensure that the term is understood. A primary sensory cortex feature map (e.g., for visual cortex) indicates individual cellular responses, each to a specific feature. As continued perceptual processing occurs, the processing unit appearing in other cortical areas, further downstream in the brain pathways, becomes a composite signal composed of multiple features, eventually including crossmodal feature information. Processing units, therefore, build first in perceptual complexity, and then in other types of complexity, especially in order to assemble categorical, symbolic, and relational information. In this sense, higher level processing units are aggregate stimuli or stimulus assemblies. Table 15.4 gives some examples of different levels of processing units.

Moreover, processing units can have another level of complexity, which is related to the coupling of both the discrimination and response functions within the same cell.

TABLE 15.4. Examples of Processing Units

---

1. Initial Sensory–Perceptual Stimulus
2. Category (e.g., fireplaces)
3. Symbol (e.g., a letter or word)
4. Face
5. A Smile
6. Signs of Anxiety or Anger in Another Person
7. Preparations for Feeding

This is the concept of perceptual–motor coupling described earlier in the discussion of imitation. Just as a single sensing effector neuron can respond to an altered physiological status (e.g., external osmolality or blood sugar levels) by both processing the new information and adjusting its response to the single cue that it regulates (Wenning, 1999), a neuron utilized for imitation responds to specific aggregate stimuli (e.g., a moving arm) by transforming the perception into activation of the primary motor cortex and immediate motor activity without intervening neurons. For example, specific neurons have been identified for specific hand movements, such as grasping, so that a perceptual–motor "vocabulary" can be fashioned, suggesting yet another type of language that the brain assembles (Rizzolatti & Arbib, 1998; Rizzolatti & Gentilucci, 1988; Rizzolatti, Fadiga, Matelli, Bettinardi, Paulesu, Perani, & Fazio, 1996). In these instances, a perceptual processing unit is converted within the cell recognizing the stimulus to a processing unit that carries the command for the motor cortex to initiate a movement without the usual intervening neurons (e.g., the basal ganglia).

In sum, all of these developmental designs foster the opportunity for the infant brain to adapt to the *actual environment in which he is born*—not only an average expectable environment as determined by evolution—and to retain some plasticity of response to the environment, yet a plasticity that is constructed on a foundation of stable responsivity. This is not to say that new variations on this class of templates—primary memory prototypes—cannot be formed, but anyone learning a foreign language, or making a change of profession, or moving to a new culture, as an adult, knows how difficult this process can be as we struggle against the expectations from our past that no longer pertain to the current situation. Once again, it would be a mistake to interpret these processes as conferring immutability on the primary memory prototypes. The circuits of the brain are continuously active, and the experiences of the day spawn neural activity even as we sleep. For example, the cortico–thalamic–cortical circuits interacting with one another play a major role in synapse formation and tuning from infancy onward, even during sleep: Steriade comments that "the rhythmic spike-bursts of thalamic and neocortical neurons that are present during non-REM sleep oscillations could assist in specifying and reorganizing the brain circuitry, and could contribute to the strengthening of synaptic contacts that carry behaviorally relevant information" (Steriade, 1999, p. 338). Following the formation of the full range of primary memory prototypes, the basic synaptic architecture is stable, and this stability is necessary for the very young child to have a predictable view of the world—a stable anatomical structure of neural circuits and synaptic connections which is formed in infancy and is functionally adaptive for the child. As environmental stimuli, favorable and unfavorable, emerge and the child responds in relation to his needs, the stable synaptic connections are tuned, gradually sculpted to reflect stable changes in the environmental stimuli confronting him. With good fortune—largely meaning thoughtful caregiving by parents—the neural circuits and adaptive capacities are continually sculpted in a manner conferring skillful adaptability.

Categorization

A word about higher levels of processing—formal cognition—is necessary to indicate some strategies for unraveling the perplexing conceptual and research problems that any individual component of higher intellectual activity presents to the investigator. The increasing complexity of these processes suggests that they differ in some ways from the processing models described here, but we should not jump too quickly to any conclusions. We can use the relatively straightforward cognitive activity of "categorization" to examine possibilities for elucidating puzzling brain activities in these cognitive functions. Categorization is a complex concept whose processes and underlying neuronal circuits continue to be investigated. However, enough is known to suggest outlines of possible organization. For example, different types of categorization can occur. One type uses exemplars—the most similar objects recalled in memory—for comparison with the test object, while another compares the test object to a prototype (an abstracted model, as if an average of each relevant feature). On the other hand, the comparison might be to whether the test object fits the application of a set of rules (Smith & Jonides, 2000).

Experiments examining the underlying cognitive neuroscience of categorization suggest that these three types of categorization may have validity, but the results are complicated, particularly due to differing localization on neuroimaging according to the content of the representations. Nevertheless, there is evidence that the procedures of categorization, not just the content of the test objects, guide the observed neural activation. For example, categorization by rule activation involves attention and working memory in the prefrontal cortex, while categorization by exemplars employs retrieval from long-term, explicit memory (with activation in posterior brain areas) and categorization by prototype involves implicit memory, with the brain areas involved less well defined (Smith & Jonides, 2000).

How might these findings be applied to aid our understanding of the developing adaptive capacities of the infant? This perspective on categorization suggests alternative views; for example, of the processes involved in language acquisition, either spoken or emotional language. One type of categorization might require an initial application of rules to define the category of words or facial expressions, while another might involve explicit, long-term memory of the objects in the category as perceptual wholes—exemplars—the end process of extensive processing, and available for comparison with test objects for analytical purposes as needed. A third type of categorization, the use of prototypes, might exist for rapid, automatic, procedural processing and responses. After a period of time it is no longer beneficial to an infant to examine the components of a smile and analyze them; a quick, unconscious response is necessary in order to pursue other information or goals. Of course, all of these considerations take on their special importance because infants initially are naive to the environment, so this is a period of extensive and rapid formation of new categories, and the inherent determination of boundary definitions. As mentioned previously, categorization links perception and cognition—thinking uses knowledge (memories) about the feature-defined classes of things that are perceived in order to plan, classes which might be straightforward or ambiguous. Categories of emotions have more nebulous boundaries than classical perceptual categories, so we could expect a more complex transition in neural activity when defining boundaries.

☐ Learning the Language of Emotions: Predictive Signal Mapping Guiding the Development of Emotional Language

Emotion, Language, and Social Cognition

If the conventional spoken language system is built using the tools described up to this point, selecting and enhancing relevant perceptual information from the environment, and generating auditory, visual, and motor capacities for language, then can we anticipate that this developmental pattern can serve as a model for other emerging capacities? There is reason to believe that similar developmental events in the brain frame the development of emotions, emotional language, and the social cognition and interactions that are dependent on emotional language, and it is of particular importance if this model were to fit. These are essential adaptive capacities that have a distinct human core and permit the development of elaborate responses to stress, an understanding of the personal view of others, the genesis of culture, and other similarly complex topics. We first need to examine emotions, and their production by neural systems, in relation to their adaptive utility. As the complexity of all of these interacting brain functions expands, we also need to establish how an organizing, protective, and facilitating system might be developed for the infant, who is establishing these extensive and varied mental representations of the world around her.

When examining brain function in a developmental context, we observe sequential phases of brain development in which specific, increasingly complex, functional capacities are dominant; these capacities, in turn, determine which environmental features the brain is preferentially attuned to. For example, as described above, Johnson and colleagues describe a brief postnatal period during which the neonate's attention is responsive to the general outlines and features of the human head and face, sufficient to ensure attention to facial features. When the next phase emerges, this preferential orientation to the face, in effect, selects the sensory stimuli that will determine the processing units to be mapped to an area of the cerebral cortex, causing this locus to acquire memories of increasing detail about facial features (Johnson, 1997; Johnson et al., 1991). These emerging developmental capacities enhance the infant's abilities to predict the meaning of environmental stimuli in relation to danger or gratification by using the new tools (i.e., such as facial expression). In the previous chapter we discussed the vital communicative capacities that are emerging, and that dramatically boost the infant's adaptative skills: (1) the expressive activities of the human face (and later of gesture and body posture, as well), (2) the denotative and connotative (expressive) activities of the human voice, both initially mirroring primarily the mother's voice. Most important is that (3) these capacities are learned in coordination with the experience of the infant's own emotions, helping the infant to recognize and eventually "label" emotions within herself, and increasingly to predict intention, emotion, action, and outcome—her own or that of others. This conceptualization of emerging social cognition retains our perspective that the brain has an essential predictive function for adaptation, and begins to specify the infrastructure for social cognition.

The Attachment Situation: A Standard Reference System for Language Learning

Attention to contextual details is characteristic of animal brain function, but there is a highly significant shift in infants. The persistent orientation, through attachment behaviors, toward the human face and human voice, ensures that contextual details are much more standardized. Because of the reliable occurrence of this orientation from the first postnatal moments, this standard reference system—secured by the mother's own attachment behaviors—makes it highly probable that certain stimuli will reliably be present and that resulting predictive signal information will be transmitted to and embedded structurally in an associated cortical area, ensuring its efficient and persistent function. Such a standard reference system for learning to make better predictions about the future can subsequently be utilized for the development of standard information coding systems, also using other novel capacities, such as imitation and developing language capacities.

Essential to all of this is that emotions take on a new meaning. If emotions were previously stimulus significance detectors, they now have an expanded function. The repeated association of the infant's own emotion with specific maternal facial expressions permits the development of a shared language: the mother's facial contours and vocal inflections become codes predicting what is useful for the infant to attend to, whether he is responding correctly, and, increasingly, what the outcome of these behaviors will be—gratification or danger, and an evolving gradation between the two that will encompass increasing sophistication of outcome prediction. It is obvious from these comments that this is a description of the emergence of a formal language as the codes become increasingly standardized, a language that will be utilized by mothers, families, and cultures. A meaningful issue is that the shared language between infant and mother is actually broader than we typically consider it to be in everyday life. The denotative aspect of spoken language is so pragmatically and efficiently powerful in its cognitive uses that it is easy to overlook or dismiss the other components of the language codes more directly associated with emotions. This consists of facial expression, gestures, body posture, and vocal intonations as indicators of intention and prediction. This is a firm and necessary language for social cognition and general adaptation, but it is burdened with inherent problems that hide its power: it is vulnerable to the individual codes and knowledge of the mother and to the uses of deception—even if this is emotional self-deception by the mother. Here the problem is that variations of the shared emotional language are used by innumerable small groups of people (mirroring the dispersion of major languages and their dialects among the peoples of the world), and are only gradually observed, modified, and slowly subject to a consensus agreement that leads to a willingness to conform to agreed-upon emotional meanings. Even then, the private adaptive styles of families and individuals sustain variations of meanings within emotional languages.

Learning Emotional Languages

These developing languages have an additional importance: they allow the child to view language as having primacy over other contextual details, which can be so abundant and so variably associated with outcome that they are more difficult to use for prediction. Moreover, once this primacy is accepted, it becomes a vehicle for cultural learning (i.e., for cultural and social transmission), for the social inheritance of information and the rapid accrual of a useful knowledge of meanings and predictors. Language development is the development of higher level processing units—for example, primary memory prototypes of spoken words or facial expressions—that bear a notable similarity to the concept of *memes* discussed earlier as socially transmitted, replicating units of culture. The relation of these replicative units (i.e., the mother's actions, and associated emotions, representing her perspectives on experience, are conveyed to the infant) to the idea of "memes" will benefit from further study (Young, in press a, in press b).

We recall that language building does not require that the brain change how it processes the signal, but that it adds a new capacity that supersedes the old without altering or destroying the original capacity. The neuronal capacities for responding to the full range of phonemes remains, but the initial open receptivity of the cerebral cortex for "effortless," rapid learning, conferred by synaptogenesis, has been lost. Learning a new language now requires the gradual building up of synaptic changes no longer eased by an unusually plastic synaptogenesis phase; language learning for an adult takes place by utilizing the slower synaptic changes associated with adult learning. The learning will be imperfect or incomplete—as accents will remain, whether of intonation in a conventional language or of personality style in one's emotional language—because the speech production system has been constructed in relation to the first language and there will be a need for years of "comparative work," as the person compares output with exemplars in the environment.

The cardinal point is that the reduced pace of learning a new spoken language as an adult also describes the slower pace of learning emotional language as an adult. It will be learned only when fueled by substantial motivation and effort, as the adult overcomes the biased "expectations" of the childhood synaptic connections and memory prototypes. Just as inborn sound discrimination capacities can be "lost" for a long period, so inborn emotion discrimination capacities can be "lost." A final point is that our relative neglect of constructing emotional categories and descriptors leaves us with a relative poverty of emotional language, and when we attempt to use a broader emotional vocabulary we risk the appearance of using odd-sounding words. This reflects the lack of familiarity that most people have with the terminology of emotions. An instructive parallel example is the vocabulary of wine tasting. The limited vocabulary sets that most people have for gustatory or olfactory sensations means that someone deciding to use their taste and smell sensations seriously must develop additional language. This is done, typically by utilizing adjectives from other types of olfactory sensations, causing the wine taster to sound "affected" (using such adjectives as *graphite, saddle leather, dried herbs,* etc.). Yet, this is the same playful origin of new vocabulary for a new field that we witnessed in the development of the language of computer programmers and developers: *boot up, mouse, cut and paste,* etc. You develop vocabulary as you learn about a topic and the need arises. As the topic of emotions generally bears the burden of assumed nebulousness, the acceptance of new vocabulary is a more difficult undertaking.

It is worthwhile to consider these matters from another perspective: Imitation is a profound influence on and facilitator of language development. This rapidly performing perceptual–motor translation instrument is extremely well adapted to nurture these essential human capacities of conventional spoken language and emotional language (Byrne & Russon, 1998; Meltzoff & Moore, 1999). For cognitive, ordinary, descriptive language, imitation is very useful because the child first learns phonemes, the smallest sound units that make up the words used in any language. The teacher is primarily the mother, although the father and others play strong roles in this language teaching. The mother teaches through simple repetition of the sounds of the one or more languages that she speaks, and the listening infant gradually tunes the cortical neurons to recognize the set of sounds characterizing the language (Kuhl, 2000). Moreover, the mother is also teaching the grammar and syntax of the language through its repetition. The success of this language teaching method is very much associated with the linked maternal–infant attachment behaviors, and the consequent consistent, repetitive information presentation and profound maternal control over the presentation of rewards to the infant.

Less obvious, but no less important, is the emotional language taught to the infant during attachment behaviors. Her mother presents repeated, consistent alphabet and vocabulary information from two principal types of emotional language, facial expression and vocal inflection. Each time an actual word is stated, it is accompanied by vocal intonation and facial expression, but it is also attended by emotions within both the mother and the infant. The consistent repetition of these stimuli makes use of the infant's imitation: As the infant listens, he also begins to imitate, and even when the mother is speaking repetitively the infant can begin to imitate quietly or out loud, developing the function of the imitation neuronal circuits. This perceptual–motor linking makes rapid learning possible, and the linked facial expression and vocal intonation melded with an emotion concurrently teach the meaning—the alphabet and dictionary—of emotions.

Other thoughts on this topic might include another question: We have gathered together many details about mother–child attachment behaviors, as well as about the teaching of conventional spoken language to infants and its possible basis in the specific events of early cortical development. This prompts us to ask, how likely is it that another, completely separate, system would exist for the development of emotional language and understanding, and for social cognition and social interactions? Obviously it is possible, but given the "fit" with the standardized structures for learning conventional spoken language, it seems less likely. Moreover, a component that Kuhl appears to view as missing—Kuhl makes the point that this process of learning how to discriminate prototypes, map phonemes, and chunk the sound stream is not learning through reinforcement, but that it is automatic and unconscious—is not so definitively absent. Her comments, while correctly highlighting the unique nature of learning in infancy, seem to neglect the very pleasurable responses of the mother during the highly structured teaching within the attachment situation—lending an exceptionally rewarding element to the infant's learning. Once again, the attachment system appears to structure these predictable rewards in such a powerfully predictable manner that it favors the idea that both spoken and emotional languages use similar systems for infant learning.

A final reflection is that these languages are not necessarily fully separate. The proximity of conventional spoken and written languages to emotional language is reflected in one of the major spoken language elements, pragmatic language (as contrasted to syntactic and semantic language elements). Pragmatic language is that aspect of formal spoken language that reflects emotional and social communication elements, and, therefore, has strong elements of both conventional spoken language and socioemotional language. However separate from conventional spoken language, the significance of emotional language is prodigious. Learning emotional language has wide-ranging ramifications for the developing infant, for this language is a basis for interpersonal interactions, social cognition, and cultural inheritance.

Ambiguities Due to the Use of Multiple Emotional Language Dictionaries

Of course, the restriction is that the alphabet and dictionaries used by the mother and infant are agreed upon by smaller groups of people. While it might be true that there are core emotional meanings that are agreed upon, because they are either genetically endowed or so "obvious" that they are the same across all cultures, in general the mother is teaching a specific emotional language whose dictionary might or might not conform sufficiently to those of others to make her emotional language adaptive and useful for the infant as he enters the wider world.

Thus, one unspoken activity in life is learning as many of these emotional languages as possible from individuals and groups with whom one interacts, and through this learning develop a broad knowledge of interpersonal interactions. This activity brings the pleasure of new knowledge, and also the wish to develop this emotional language system to a level sufficient to make its predictive capacity as powerful as the "more cognitive" denotative spoken language system. The fact that emotional language has less clarity than other languages (because it is standardized among smaller groups who commonly disagree with each other—often due to deception and self-deception) makes us less willing to accept this emotional language as a true language, in spite of its simultaneous emergence in the infant. No one changes the alphabet of a language, even though dictionaries change. Similarly, the alphabet of emotional language is agreed upon across cultures and does not change. But the words and dictionaries of an emotional language are controversial and used somewhat differently by small groups, and they change according to the needs of the emotional language users—again mirroring features of spoken language.

We are simultaneously describing the genesis of the use of symbolization, because the use of contextual details takes on new functions and complexity. The association of a contextual emotional detail with an outcome no longer means only that the next time that this detail is among the ambient stimuli the child can use it to select behavior with relative confidence in the beneficial outcome. Contextual details can be variably associated with outcomes, and the infant or toddler uses her mother's signaling to assist in determining the meaning of contextual features at specific times. For example, the mother's smile typically is associated with an activity (e.g., eating or looking or reaching or grasping or uttering a noise). In contrast, the mother's look of fear or anger or dismay or frustration may be associated with other stimuli, such as the electrical plug. The next time that food—or an object to be looked at, or reached for, or grasped—or an electrical plug appears, the mother might not be there, but her facial expression remains as a memory and a symbol associated in the baby's mind with a predictive meaning that guides actions, including further experimentation about the consistency of a symbol's meaning. Thus, we recognize the primal importance of "negativism" in the child's development as a way of gradually accruing, from repeated exposure, the validation or invalidation that lends a stable meaning for the symbol.

The two paths of language development now diverge: Emotional languages are vastly more difficult to learn because of their multiple dictionaries, and we spend a lifetime, especially intense in college dormitories at two in the morning, engaging in elaborate attempts to validate and extend our hopefully shared meanings of consensual emotional experiences and linking of alphabet (facial expression, vocal intonation, etc.) to a dictionary of accurate meanings. On the other hand, cognitive activities that assign meaning to concrete objects have the advantage of their relatively unchanging nature. In this instance we participate in the propagation of ever larger dictionaries of standard spoken languages that occurs with fewer impediments. If mother says "milk" many times before milk appears, and the child eventually says "milk" to find that it appears soon, and repeats this with essentially the same result most of the time, then a highly reproducible chain of events has occurred between them that leads to a valued reward, which, in turn, ensures repetition. Once again, though, this phase in the evolution of a system is one in which the original stimulus is not actually repeated—there is no milk in sight. The mother and infant have, though, inserted a new contextual, but symbolic feature: the sound of the word *milk* is now a highly predictive phenomenon in the child's life and among the initial elements of his or her emerging dictionary.

But, when we take up the emotional language dictionary, matters are not so clear—we enter into a domain of controversy that has been protracted but interesting. A few summary comments about one component of emotional language, the facial expression of emotions, will help us to understand its current status. There is strong evidence that a universal set of facial expressions exists. Paul Ekman comments that "While robust, the evidence is limited to just a handful of emotions: anger, disgust, sadness, enjoyment, and fear/surprise. I agree with Darwin in believing that fear and surprise do have separate distinct expressions, but the evidence for it comes only from literate cultures" (Ekman, 1988, p. 390). A bit later Ekman makes the following remarks:

> Darwin's central point is well established: a number of emotions have a universal expression. This would have pleased Darwin, for he acknowledged that not *every* emotion has an expression, let alone a universal one. But to find evidence of universals for six to eight emotions is consistent with an evolutionary view.
> To have shown that there are universals in facial expressions of emotion does not mean that expressions are universal in every regard. Our evidence, and that of others, shows only that when people are experiencing certain strong emotions, and are not making any attempt to mask their expressions (display rules), the expression will be the same regardless of age, race, culture, sex, or education. That is a powerful finding.
> There are a number of ways in which cultures do differ in their emotional expressions. I have already mentioned one—the display rules which specify who can show which emotion to whom and when. Cultures differ also in some of the specific events which are likely to call forth an emotion. (p. 390)

Ekman makes a final comment about "one more way in which cultures differ in emotional expression," stating that "I expect that languages differ in the words they have for emotions, not only in terms of the numbers of words for each emotion, but the extent to which a word gives subtle nuances or combines emotions or tells us what caused the emotion" (p. 392). Moreover, we must wonder whether it might be possible for us to lack words for some emotions, similar to the situation of the wine tasters who needed to invent new terms to extend their dictionary to a useful size. The discovery of the right description of an elusive emotion is a pleasant experience, and welcomed by others. In part, this is the essence of art—that undescribed emotions, or complex emotions, are elicited and in this way are made to exist, even though they might not be easily definable. They are recognizable to the audience as they reexperience a set of emotions in relatively pure form, therefore having experiences in a safe, identifiable, and pleasurable manner. However, it is also true that not everyone would be happy with the discovery and naming of an emotion. Conflicts within oneself, particularly when they involve self-deception and deception of others about our emotions, are very common occurrences and make emotions difficult to define and to "read."

Another perspective on this discussion concerns the conspicuous potential for conflicting information in emotional language. The importance of *visual* information determined to be present in the perception and production of speech (Kuhl & Meltzoff, 1982), alerts us to the recognition that more is being perceived by children and adults than we might have guessed—we focus, of course, on the auditory channel for spoken language—and that the amount of information about emotions being perceived and processed by the brain at any one time is vast, and not a myth. The potential for contradiction among these channels and these pieces of information is correspondingly massive and presents a momentous challenge not only to the developing child but to any parent or culture that becomes aware of it. The production of an illusion when conflicting perceptual data from auditory and visual channels are presented to an observer, described in the previous chapter, is a highly important observation, because it suggests a significant contribution to our understanding of the exceedingly common contradictions in emotional signals presented to children and adults, and one of the possible origins of illusory phenomena reported by them.

Having considered the problematic ambiguities in emotional language, we now return to our original purpose, which is to explain our emphasis on the existence of a profound emotional language that is underappreciated in daily life, although certainly not underused. To validate the function and status of emotional expression as a language, we will examine its components and structure in relation to conventional spoken language.

Parallel Structures of Conventional Spoken Language and Emotional Language

We have an increasingly large set of tools to apply to our attempts to look again at emotional development and attempt a new understanding; these include our understanding of the neural mechanisms underlying the infant's development of primary memory prototypes and increasing adaptive skills in the first year of life, an instructive model for language development, and a description of the neural mechanisms utilized for the genesis of emotions. Emotional responses, such as pain or fear, guided adaptation through eons of evolution before the appearance of human language and reasoning. We can add that emotional influences on behavior have not diminished to an insignificant role, and higher cognitive processing and language are superimposed on and interactive with emotional influences. We need to understand better how emotional responses have evolved in their adaptive roles. To do so, we search for structuring principles for the development and organization of emotional responses. Kuhl's description of the developmental processes for spoken language are particularly useful, because they can be recast in terms of primary memory prototype sculpting occurring during synaptogenesis and other events of brain development (described by Rakic, Goldman-Rakic, Bourgeois, and others), and generative parallels emerge. A model for the development of neural and adaptive functions fits well for processing units ranging from percepts in the primary visual cortex to symbol formation in long-term memory in varied cortical regions, and applies to both emotions and spoken language. In fact, we find that analogous processes are observed in the genesis of conventional spoken and written language when compared to the development of emotional language. In this sense, the development of conventional spoken language becomes a generative model for the development of emotional language.

Emotional responses are generally judged not to have the clarity of a language, so it is worthwhile to examine the conspicuous points of similarity. We are encouraged to do so by the explication of the neural basis for emotion generation by LeDoux and others, some of which was discussed in the previous chapter (LeDoux, 1996). This work breaks down the apparent ambiguity of emotion into a chain of specific neural processes, steps that conform to the manipulation of other processing units and to learning spoken language. In order to clarify how emotional language is systematically organized, and corresponds at each level with a conventional spoken or written language, the language elements for each are specified in Table 15.5. The cardinal point to be recognized here is how language elements build on the prior language element— they add another level of complexity while utilizing the language elements of previous levels. This corresponds to the systematic manner in which processing units are built up, bit by bit, through the activities of neural circuits responding to ambient stimuli. While emotional language might lack the comparatively crystalline clarity of conventional written language, it has its own clear and distinct set of meanings that might or might not be learned well by an individual, and it is characterized by a highly compelling significance conferred on emotions through the long molding of evolution. Just as a child may or may not learn a second spoken language, she may or may not learn emotional language well. Yet, it is imperative to recognize the highly significant role of emotional language in a child's life. A recent study examining adult decision-making when confronting a morally ambiguous dilemma found that a specific type of decision made by the individuals—when the dilemma generated intense internal conflict and the decision was difficult to explain in spite of attempts to make it appear rational— was based upon emotional influences, as determined by neuroimaging (Greene, Sommerville, Nystrom, Darley, & Cohen, 2001).

Does emotional language have specificity, even if it is more ambiguous than spoken language? In fact, the emotional language elements indicated in Table 15.5 are quite explicit, although we tend to underestimate the precision of visual recognition of both spoken and emotional languages. For example, the smallest language element in conventional written language is a letter of the alphabet. For emotional language a corresponding language element would be an emotional expression element (EEE), which is a discriminated element assigned to a particular emotional meaning and identified as separate (e.g., a gestural expression element, such as the shoulder movement in a shrug, excluding whatever hand and arm movements might complete the act of shrugging). A group of these smallest elements (EEE), through the consistent guidance and modeling of the mother, are gradually discriminated as consensually assigned emotional expres-

TABLE 15.5. Language Elements: Parallel Structures of Spoken and Written Languages and Emotional Language

Language Element	Spoken Language	Written Language	Emotional Language
Smallest Language Element	Sound of a Letter	Written Letter	Emotional expression element (An EEE, e.g., a facial expression component, such as a down-turned mouth)
The Complete Set of Consensually Assigned Language Elements	Sounds of the Alphabet	Alphabet	Collection of all consensually assigned emotional expression elements (e.g., all consensually recognized facial expression components)
Single or Combined Language Elements with a Consensual Symbolic Meaning	Sound(s) of a Word	Written Word	Consensual sign of emotional meaning (e.g., depressed facies)
Class of the Group of Language Elements	Sound of the Part of Speech	Part of Speech (e.g., noun)	Class of the consensual sign of emotional meaning (e.g., facial expression, posture)
Language Element Combinations with Rules, a Temporal Component, and a Consensual Symbolic Meaning	Sounds of a Sentence	Written Sentence	Social interaction sequence (e.g., an exchange of social greetings, including facial expressions, gestures, vocal intonations, etc.)
Consensually Organized Collection of Symbolic Meanings	Sounds of Words in a Written Dictionary and Their Meanings	Written Dictionary with the Meanings of Words	Collection of consensual signs of emotional meanings (e.g., the meanings of specific facial expressions or vocal intonations)

sion elements that correspond to the letters of the alphabet; they are the basic building blocks for emotional language, which are used to form a language element corresponding to a word in spoken language. In spoken or written language, the *word* (or the sound of *word*) is the meaning of a combination of letters, while for emotional language it is a conventional sign of emotional meaning (such as outstretched arms as a sign of welcome and affection), which is made up of identifiable emotional expression elements. Another example is the smile, a combination of facial expression elements which are analogous to letters of the alphabet.

The dictionary for the consensual signs of emotional meaning appears to be much smaller than the conventional word dictionary, although it is possible that it would be larger if the signs were more consistent across groups, there was less deception, and more attention was given to recognizing subtle signs of emotional meaning. As with conventional spoken or written languages, the alphabets of emotional languages can differ. An illustration is in the gestural group of emotional language elements; some ethnic groups, such as those within the broad Mediterranean culture, utilize gestures with the hands much more than other cultures, such as Anglo-Saxon groups, and with specific, consensual meanings for their hand gestures that have a specificity of meaning that can be surprising to Americans, for example.

The dictionary is a consensually organized collection of symbolic meanings (e.g., for emotional language, a collection of the meanings of various facial expressions, vocal intonations, etc.); therefore, it is made up of a large group of words or, for emotional language, the meanings assigned to signs of emotional expression that are consensually agreed upon. In spite of this consensual agreement, it is clear that there can be competing dictionaries, such as British English versus American English. This becomes exceedingly important for emotional language, because competing dictionaries are not only formed by different cultures, but families within a culture commonly assign differing meanings. In spite of the primary role that emotional language plays in our lives, it remains implied rather than defined and accepted as a guiding force in our decisions and behavior. Suspected as "irrational," we attempt to deny that emotion affects our important decisions. Moreover, the lack of formal agreements concerning meanings in the competing dictionaries of emotional language is further complicated by disagreement that is actually due to deception or self-deception. Parents regularly deny an "unacceptable" emotion (e.g., sadness or depression) in spoken language, when their emotional language unquestionably indicates the true emotion. Adults learn to expect and adjust to these competing dictionaries—or alternative rules systems, which can be quite purposefully employed, as described by Stendhal:

> "A court," said the Contessa to the Marchesa, "is quite a ridiculous thing, but it is amusing. It's a game that interests you, but in which you have to conform to the rules. Whoever thought of protesting against the absurdity of the rules of whist? And yet, once you are accustomed to the rules, it is delightful to beat your opponent by winning all the tricks." (Stendhal, 1839/1958, p. 114)

Such deception does not always have results in actual life that are as amusing as in novels, of course, and children attend carefully to the problem of understanding the rules. Children grow up expecting this discordant information between spoken and emotional language, and learn to make predictions about intention and behavior using both sources. The problem persists, however, because the children have learned that they are not to consciously define, or use spoken language to articulate, their use of emotional language when judging the intent of others. The competing dictionaries for emotional language are readily passed from one generation to the next. Families continue to define emotional language in ways that differ somewhat, and psychotherapists become experts and judges who help individuals recognize and be attentive to emotional language within themselves and others. In this context, we recall that emotional language learning begins during infancy, and it is during infancy that we can most efficiently improve the quality of this education in a preventive manner.

Some special qualities of learning emotional language deserve comment. First, the rapidity of learning of emotional responses can be notable, including two trial learning for some amygdalar responses, as described in the previous chapter (Post et al., 1998). It is less clear how quickly an infant learns conventional language elements, although there is evidence that infants rapidly learn spoken language elements (reproducing vowel sounds after 15 minutes of laboratory exposure) at five months of age (Kuhl, 2000). A second illuminating perspective is that conventional spoken language is a novel activity, and there is no requirement to override subcortical precursors. The development of emotional language, in contrast, involves emerging cortical inhibition of subcortical emotional influences, and a tenuous balance remains. As LeDoux comments, extinction of an adaptively "inappropriate" fear response mediated in the amygdala, for example, is never complete (LeDoux, 1995). The tension between subcortical and cortical control of emotional expression is considerable and the struggle entailed for the growing child continues as a challenge throughout development—aggravated by the inconsistent meanings of apparently shared emotional vocabulary that undermines his regulation of emotionally charged, impulsive responses. In essence, the child learns primary memory prototypes for emotional language as an infant, but is required to supplement this with subsequent education using different dictionaries— which might be compared to the difficulty of learning a conventional foreign language as an adult. The initial efforts in this learning process are reflected in the developing affect "attunement" with her mother (Brazelton, Koslowski, & Main, 1974; Field, 1985); this terminology suggests what is actually occurring—a continuous neural tuning in her developing cortex, reflecting the mother's effort to achieve emotional understanding, empathy, and emotional equilibrium with her infant—and the baby gradually absorbs her mother's emotional language while cradled by her.

☐ An Expanded Model for Attachment Functions: The Regulation of Infant Experiential Learning and Primary Memory Prototype Formation During Synaptogenesis and Other Developmental Processes

Regulating Infant State, Motivation, and Attention to Predictive Stimuli

In addition to the regulatory effects on infant physiology and behavior provided by attachment behaviors (Hofer, 1970, 1984, 1994), the predictable presence of her mother is immensely beneficial to a child's development in other ways. If her mother enjoys making sounds and the baby imitates them, both are happy. If her mother now changes the game, and favors establishing meanings by the designation of joint attributions to things, then memory of language meanings—and subsequently cognition—begins to develop. What will become selective attention in the child is already mother-selected attention for the infant, and there will be a long transition until the child is "fully" selecting what he will attend to. Mother's continuing presence makes it possible for her to select the stimuli and environments for the infant to attend to, and repeat the stimuli and environments in a manner that will give to the infant what she values emotionally and intellectually—in other words, teach the infant and transmit culturally valued information and experiences. This selection of stimuli for the infant does not end after one or two years; her mother will continue to guide the growing child in learning what to pay attention to at different ages, although gradually relinquishing maternal control over the years. Moreover, the infant is simultaneously learning about a relationship, and how relationships work, regardless of whether this specific relationship is a good model for generalization.

An initial concern, however, is that the concepts discussed here are easily distorted. They do not imply that no caregiver other than the mother can be helpful or a significant caregiver. Instead, they describe an attachment system, forged by evolution, that takes advantage of biologically based drives in a mother and infant to nurture the flourishing of the infant's developing adaptive capacities. Others, such as the father, an older brother or sister, a grandparent, or a nanny, can occupy highly important and contributing subsidiary roles, or even the primary role. The critical elements for any of these caregivers to occupy such roles are consistent availability and adequate satisfaction of the baby's fundamental needs. Our focus is on the neural systems underlying these behaviors, and our discussion centers on the mother as the biologically prepared and most common person to occupy the role of primary caregiver.

Cortical synaptogenesis, while enabling open functional specification of cortical areas during its brief span of prominence, is a fountain of opportunities for guiding basic experiential learning during infancy. Protected in the cradle of attachment behaviors, the infant responds to the mother's teaching by learning through repetition, with a special emphasis on maternal selection and reliable presentation of significant stimuli, maternal judgment of the infant's state and readiness to learn, the infant's learning the meanings of facial expression and vocal intonation, and learning through imitation. Attachment behaviors can be viewed as a scaffold for guiding the transduction of maternally selected experiences into neuronal mechanisms that form primary memory prototypes; this is the basis for learning conventional spoken language, emotional language, and fundamental elements of social cognition. Attachment behaviors transmit maternal and cultural influences on the child's developing adaptive responses. As these processes are elaborated, symbols bit by bit become important predictors that increasingly substitute for concrete objects or activities.

The Attachment Situation as a Standard Reference System for Learning

Within our remarks about the genesis of emotional language between mother and infant were vital observations about the conditions that permit and facilitate these developments. We recall our emphasis on the infant's preferential orientation to the mother's face, in this manner selecting the sensory stimuli to be transformed into the processing units eventually mapped to an area of the cerebral cortex—which becomes the site of memories of facial features. Unlike in other animals, the infant's attention to contextual details is more limited and focused, because attachment behaviors induce a persistent orientation toward the human face and human voice over a long period, ensuring that the stimuli attended to are more standardized. The mother's own attachment behaviors ensure the reliable occurrence of this orientation, creating a standard reference system that preselects certain groups of stimuli that will predictably be present; this, in turn, determines the resulting signal information to be transmitted to the associated cortical area. This control of the stimuli to which he or she is exposed ensures a consistent, repetitive presentation of the elements to be learned, creating the best opportunity for rapid learning—as well as ensuring that the basic elements are learned at the outset. The standard reference system, in turn, takes on an expanded function for learning, as it comes to play a pivotal role in the development of preeminent maternal-infant educational activities, such as the development of conventional spoken language and emotional language, the introduction of the use of symbols, and the easing of all these activities through the ready application of imitation as a means of learning.

If physiological functioning is stable and the infant is able to enjoy a state of quiet alertness, then he is optimally prepared to learn about the salient aspects of his environment that will optimally guide his adaptation. If his physiological and behavioral functioning is erratic and unpredictable, then his learning will be "tuned" by these experiences, as well; however, of particular importance are the disruptive effects of these dysregulated states on his receptivity to learning during this crucial early period of cortical synaptogenesis.

As the infant finds himself on the launching pad of life, he is also, in a sense, held within a protective control module which is largely controlled externally by another, who uses it to sustain his life and guide his explorations. For example, the control module helps to control the balance among stimulus appraisal, working memory activity, and possible distractions while directing the infant's attention to salient features of the environment. In addition, no student who is hungry, or has had inadequate sleep, can be attentive to the learning materials presented to him or her; this is also true if the student is an infant. The infant's mother is able to make reasonable judgments about the infant's state—whether he or she is awake, drowsy, in pain, hungry, or seeking stimulation. She determines and fulfills the child's needs, readying him for his novel explorations by ensuring that he has an optimal capacity to be attentive. Within his control module, he observes displays selected for him by his mother as most beneficial for his mission at that particular time. His mother, therefore, simultaneously regulates the infant's life support system and his exploratory trajectory.

Moreover, we must not ignore the artful maternal abilities to quietly and patiently encourage the infant as he gropes for understanding of the vast array of stimuli confronting him. Through a combination of this patient, repetitive positive feedback, and occasionally more intensely motivating rewards (e.g., special laughter and hugs, picking the infant up and dancing with him or her), the baby's energy for learning is kept at a maximum level. As this learning progresses, we recognize that the mother is actually aiding the infant to forge new primary memory prototypes, and these templates are, in turn, used as a basis for comparison with later, novel stimuli in new cycles of learning. These new cycles include the combination of the basic elements already learned into more complex stimuli and associated meanings. Parents, if they can be patient, allow the child to learn these more complex concepts through trial and error, so that the infant's knowledge is more inclusive. The infant learns to experience activity as a means to influence the environment in order to produce the desired outcome: The baby's observation of his or her mother's responses (e.g., her smile, her gestures, etc.) is an aid; they act as mediators predicting the outcome to determine which behaviors lead to a desired result. Similarly, to the degree that a parent is conscious of her teaching role, she might model more consciously the practical use of information as she gives it to an infant (e.g., after naming a spoon that she is using, she might show how it is used). This also recalls how the mother is a stable source of teaching by providing the modeling so central to the infant's learning by imitation, which is used as a wonderfully effective shortcut for learning behaviors that have a maximum capacity to induce specific maternal responses, and, later, specific responses of others in the environment. All of these maternal activities foster the infant's development in increasingly complex ways, as the infant profits from consensual validation of these maternal activities from her family and culture about what the infant should learn; in this manner, the mother and infant receive the beneficial wisdom of a broad cumulative experience concerning optimal methods for teaching very young children. Nevertheless, it is also true that this same selection and validation process can lead to biased teaching to very young children who receive the views and prejudices—for better or worse—of a small group of people.

We might pause in our discussion and list those features of the learning situation that are well known to facilitate it. If we do so, we find that the attachment situation fulfills these needs extraordinarily well (see Table 15.6). And as we consider how well adapted to learning the attachment system is, it is worthwhile reviewing and comparing (see Table 15.7) what are commonly described as the optimal conditions for the

---

TABLE 15.6. An Expanded Model for Attachment Functions: Mechanisms for Regulating Experimental Learning and Primary Memory Prototype Formation During Synaptogenesis and Other Developmental Processes

---

1. Provide reliable, consistent, repetitive exposure to a stable source of learning
2. Provide reliable satiation of the infant's basic needs, facilitating adequate attention
3. Restrict and preselect the range of stimuli for learning
4. Provide a reliable presentation of basic elements to be learned
5. Provide patient, positive feedback in response to accurate learning
6. Provide reliable source of additional motivating rewards for learning
7. Facilitate production and molding of primary templates through repetition
8. Nurture further learning through comparison with primary templates
9. Provide consistent combination of basic elements as they are elaborated into more complex but reliable stimuli and their associated meanings
10. Provide the opportunity for learning through actions on a reliable world, using a trial-and-error paradigm with available rewards
11. Provide a continuity of modeling of the practical use of the information being presented, and how it produces rewards
12. Provide reliable, repetitive exposure that stabilizes the source of learning by imitation
13. Nurture transition to the use of mental representations and symbols to guide adaptation
14. Provide reliable, repetitive exposure to sources of conventional (spoken) language
15. Provide reliable, repetitive exposure to sources of emotional language
16. Provide reliable, repetitive exposure to sources of social interactions, social cognition
17. Provide reliable, repetitive exposure to sources of self-regulation, competence, self-esteem, and identity
18. Provide reliable, repetitive exposure to familial and cultural selections of adaptive knowledge

---

TABLE 15.7. Optimal Educational Conditions for Learning a Language

---

1. Attendance at class with a reliable, consistent teacher
2. Reliable satiation of the child's basic needs, permitting him or her to achieve adequate attention
3. Thoughtful, focused selection of an appropriate range of materials for learning
4. Presentation of a consistent alphabet and words to be learned
5. Continuing patient and positive feedback concerning accuracy of the language use, associated with rewards
6. Reliable availability of highly desirable rewards to encourage accurate learning efforts
7. Facilitate production and molding of memory templates for the words of the new language through repetition
8. Promote additional learning through comparison of new words with earlier memory templates
9. Consistent combination of alphabetic elements to produce reliable language components and associated meanings
10. The opportunity to study and learn through action—experiential learning—using a trial-and-error paradigm
11. Continuing demonstration of the practical utility of the language and its capacity to generate rewards (i.e., it is neither a dead language nor one not used among familiar people)
12. Repeat the language exposure through teacher modeling, language tapes, and language CDs in order to enhance learning by imitation
13. Provide reliable, repetitive exposure to models using the language in social interactions
14. Provide reliable, repetitive exposure to familial and cultural uses of the language

---

language learning process; these conditions match the attachment conditions quite well, indicating how beneficial a situation it is for learning emotional language.

It is an interesting contrast to wonder how much of the difficulty of learning a language as an adult is due to the inferior techniques for teaching adults when compared to infant education. The infant's education is full-time, meticulously attuned to her needs (e.g., the vocal qualities and timing of the teacher), and tied to purposeful rewards (e.g., the adult's big, congratulatory smile and encouraging laughter versus the response of amused laughter *at* the adult learner's poor attempt at pronunciation). Similarly, the educational desk for the infant optimizes the infant's attention and her teacher is the most favored person in the infant's world.

A final thought is that this framework suggesting a relative restriction of the infant's perceptual world, favoring a focus on his mother and those stimuli selected (or permitted) by her, will increasingly be better understood by uncovering contributing developmental neural changes. A possible example is the phenomenon of "sticky fixation," in which infants between 1 and 3 to 4 months of age (peaking at 2 months) have difficulty disengaging fixation on a central stimulus in order to orient to a peripheral target (Hood, Atkinson, & Braddick, 1998). Is it possible that this aspect of neural development favors the infant's early learning about his mother's face and voice? Improved understanding of attentional development during the first year of life will contribute to knowledge about the expanded functions of attachment behaviors.

Enhancing Maternal Well-Being and the Mother's Capacities for Regulating Infant State and Learning

We should not neglect the needs of the teacher in any educational situation. If she is to be effective, her own sense of reasonable stable comfort is essential. A list comparable to Table 15.6 might be prepared for the baby's mother if we seek to optimize the baby's learning. One significant element on the list might be mentioned—the need for a supportive partner to share the joys, confusion, work, frustration, contemplation, problem solving, decision making, and many other activities of the mother. Increasing numbers of mothers must cope as single parents, a demanding and unforgiving commitment, as the developmental needs of the child appear regardless of the mother's capacities on any single day. In order to regulate the physiology and behavior of the infant, the mother must be physically present, which might be impossible if she must work, or if she herself is exhausted or depressed. Similarly, if she is to function as teacher for her child, she needs a sense of satisfaction with herself and her life to be able to energetically attend to the needs and responses of the infant and reward him sufficiently to sustain his motivation for learning. If the mother is depressed, for example, then the baby will be imitating a different set of behaviors than if the mother is chronically angry or if she is enthusiastic and buoyant. These comments are not intended to be critical of single mothers, or pessimistic about the developmental progress of their children. Instead, these observations intend (1) to use the difficult challenges confronting single parents as a common example of how neglect of the mother's needs profoundly affects the infant, and (2) to urge the support of maternal needs as an essential element of child care by recalling that the mother's emotional and behavioral status has an inevitable, biologically determined, transforming influence on the infant.

The Development of Loving Attachments and Social Understanding

The experiences of well-being, gratification, and predictable tension resolution are associated with the mother's face, reflecting the exquisitely refined response of the amygdala and other neuronal systems to the predictably repeated details of the context of the baby's life. His dependence limits the horizons of his life and increases his need for his mother's presence, in this way necessarily increasing the portion of time in which the context of his experience will include his mother and various other stimuli related to her. This is highly important when considering how it nourishes a preference for humans and the tendency to turn to others in order to reach goals; this is most evident in the constellation of motivating emotions experienced when falling in love. However, it is less obvious in another of its effects, which is to foster the tendency to communicate with other humans and to agree to trust in shared meanings for a variety of symbols used for languages or other purposes. This orientation to people, first evident in the inborn tendencies to recognize faces or to imitate others, is essential to group cooperation and communication, so fundamental to the adaptive success of humans. For this reason the recommendations for infant care given to parents by professionals (e.g., that emphasize the importance of the infant's proximity to her parents, or the value of persistent thoughtful maternal interactions with her infant) might seem to be unscientific to some observers, or precious or silly or "too obsessive" to others, yet, can have a pivotal impact on the development of children. One only has to consider the emotions and expectations of a 3-year-old who has grown up in a household character-ized by neglect of these considerations, spawning unpredictability, frequent parental absences, and abrupt, verbally aggressive behaviors. It is disheartening to think of such a context influencing the cognitive and emotional memories of this 3-year-old, but it is not uncommon. Another way to say this more generally is that inconsistent, contradic-tory information, or a lack of information because data are rarely repeated in an orga-nized manner (due to disorganization, poverty, fighting among adults, unavailability, etc.), leads to an inability to merge the various social maps that are being created in the child's developing cortex.

This prolonged period of complete, and later relative, infant dependence, structured and relieved by maternal–infant attachment behaviors, is the foundation of our human adaptive success, focusing us from our first days on interest in and love for others, intense emotional responses to them, and a desire to center our attention on them through communication, shared thoughts, and cooperation. This dependent situation nourishes a more plastic adaptive capacity, as the brain and adaptive abilities are formed while the child's actual environment influences elements of neuronal circuit develop-ment, especially the developing synaptic connections. In short, maternal–infant at-tachment behaviors help the child adapt optimally to his specific environment, as he has the advantage of the best judgments of his mother and other relatives, and of his culture, about how he should be cared for, understand others and his environment, and learn to adapt. While we might be frustrated with the problem that individual families can provide exposure to adaptive behaviors that become maladaptive in later life and other circumstances, we should not forget the marvel of how this maternal guidance of developing adaptive capacities is so plastic and responsive, permitting flex-ibility and the utilization of modeling by family and others, as well as the transmission of the wisdom of decades or centuries of cultural judgments about how best to nurture the infant's development.

These reflections on the framework of maternal–infant interactions echo decades of clinical psychoanalytic observations and commentary describing related concepts, such as "the holding environment," the centrality of "trust"—which might be conceptualized as the experience of adequate maternal regulation and infrequent escape from regula-tion—and "the separation–individuation" process as events that now can be viewed in the context of the infant's increasing capacity for self-regulation, while interrupted by increasingly less frequent episodes of dysregulation as he relies less and less on his mother for physiological and behavioral regulation. Thus, we add one more group to the long list of psychoanalytic observations that were predictive of the data later pro-duced in neuroscience research. Many psychoanalysts were remarkably astute observ-ers, although not as successful as scientific investigators—largely working prior to the development of scientific methods applicable to clinical settings and prior to the avail-ability of genetic or cognitive neuroscience research data.

In summary, Hofer described the "hidden" regulation of physiological and behav-ioral behaviors as the foundation of attachment behaviors (Hofer, 1970, 1984, 1994). We argue that attachment behaviors also comprise a felicitous, suitable, and effective educational situation, including the advantage that they subsume a profound reward system in which the mother regulates not only the physiology of the child, but also the related comfort and escape responses, including their associated discomfort and pain. This consistent reward system does not occur in other animals for such a prolonged period postnatally. For the child it ensures that the infant is extremely attentive to this unique, and in ideal circumstances, predictable and frequently present, part of the environment. Such attention is one of the essentials of the language learning process, including emotional language learning, as is the profoundly rewarding power that the mother possesses and distributes according to the baby's responses while he or she is learning.

We underscore the importance of these phenomena in relation to providing an optimal matrix for developing other types of social cognition essential to human development, such as face recognition, social imitation, social interactions, and empathy. The infant is literally in his or her mother's arms, receptive to and dependent on her actions—making her embrace the germinating ground for sensory and emotional experiences that develop into these other forms of social activities and social cognition. While the infant will someday achieve the goals of separation, individuation, and independence, the emerging adult will continue to carry within him- or herself this framework for adaptation, embedded within a network of emotional memories centered on his or her mother.

> But while other men displayed their courage to win glory for themselves, Marcius's motive was always to please his mother. The delight that she experienced when she saw him crowned, and the tears of joy that she wept as she embraced him—these things were for him the supreme joy and felicity that life could offer. (Plutarch, 1965, p. 18)

☐ References

Bassani, Giorgio (1977). *The garden of the Finzi-Continis* (W. Weaver, Trans.). New York: Harcourt Brace. (Original work published 1962)

Bourgeois, J.-P., Goldman-Rakic, P. S., & Rakic, P. (2000). Formation, elimination, and stabilization of synapses in the primate cerebral cortex. In M. S. Gazzaniga (Ed.), *The new cognitive neurosciences* (2nd ed., pp. 45–53). Cambridge, MA: MIT Press.

Brazelton, T. B., Koslowski, B., & Main, M. (1974). Origins of reciprocity: The early mother–infant interaction. In M. Lewis & L. Rosenblum (Eds.), *The effects of the infant on its caregiver* (pp. 49–76). New York: Wiley.

Bronfenbrenner, U. (1979). *The ecology of human development: Experiments by nature and design.* Cambridge, MA: Harvard University Press.

Byrne, R. W., & Russon, A. E. (1998). Learning by imitation: A hierarchical approach. *Behavioral Brain Science, 21,* 667–721

Calvino, I. (1974). *Invisible cities.* New York: Harcourt, Brace. (Original work published 1972)

Ekman, P. (1998). Afterword: Universality of emotional expression? A personal history of the dispute. In Charles Darwin, *The expression of the emotions in man and animals* (3rd ed., pp. 363–393). Oxford: Oxford University Press.

Field, T. (1985). Attachment as psychobiological attunement: Being on the same wavelength. In M. Reite & T. Field (Eds.), *Psychobiology of Attachment and Separation* (pp. 415–454). New York: Academic.

Freeman, W. J. (1979). EEG analysis gives model of neuronal template-matching mechanisms for sensory search with olfactory bulb. *Biological Cybernetics, 35*(4), 221–234.

Freeman, W. J. (1981). A physiological hypothesis of perception. *Perspectives in Biology & Medicine, 24*(4), 561–592.

Freeman, W. J. (1983). The physiological basis of mental images. *Biological Psychiatry, 18*(10), 1107–1125.

Goldman-Rakic, P., Bourgeois, J.-P., & Rakic, P. (1997). Synaptic substrate of cognitive development: Life-span analysis of synaptogenesis in the prefrontal cortex of the nonhuman primate. In N. A. Krasnegor, G. R. Lyon, & P. S. Goldman-Rakic (Eds.), *Development of the prefrontal cortex: Evolution, neurobiology, and behavior* (pp. 27–47). Baltimore: Paul H. Brookes Publishing Co.

Greene, J. D., Sommerville, R. B., Nystrom, L. E., Darley, J. M., & Cohen, J. D. (2001). An fMRI investigation of emotional engagement in moral judgment. *Science, 293*, 2105–2108

Hofer, M. A. (1970). Physiological responses of infant rats to separation from their mothers. *Science, 168*, 871–873.

Hofer, M. A. (1984). Relationships as regulators: A psychobiologic perspective on bereavement. *Psychosomatic Medicine, 46*, 183–197.

Hofer, M. A. (1994). Hidden regulators in attachment, separation, and loss. *Monographs of the Society for Research in Child Development, 59* (Nos. 2–3, Serial No. 24).

Hood, B. M., Atkinson, J., & Braddick, O. J. (1998). Selection-for-action and the development of orienting and visual attention. In J. E. Richards (Ed.), *Cognitive neuroscience of attention: A developmental perspective* (pp. 219–249). Mahwah, NJ: Erlbaum.

Johnson, M. H. (1997). *Developmental cognitive neuroscience.* Oxford: Blackwell.

Johnson, M. H., Dziurawiec, S., Ellis, H. D., & Morton, J. (1991). Newborns' preferential tracking of face-like stimuli and its subsequent decline. *Cognition, 40*, 1–19.

Kuhl, P. K. (2000). Language, mind, and brain: Experience alters perception. In M. S. Gazzaniga (Ed.), *The new cognitive neurosciences* (2nd ed., pp. 99–115). Cambridge, MA: MIT Press.

Kuhl, P. K., & Meltzoff, A. N. (1982). The bimodal perception of speech in infancy. *Science, 218*, 1138–1141.

LeDoux, J. E. (1995). In search of an emotional system in the brain: Leaping from fear to emotion and consciousness. In M. S. Gazzaniga (Ed.), *The cognitive neurosciences* (pp. 1049–1062). Cambridge: MIT Press.

LeDoux, J. (1996). *The emotional brain.* New York: Simon & Schuster.

Lynch, G. (2000). Memory consolidation and long-term potentiation. In M. S. Gazzaniga (Ed.), *The new cognitive neurosciences* (2nd ed., pp. 139–157). Cambridge, MA: MIT Press.

Martin, K. C., Bartsch, D., Bailey, C. H., & Kandel, E. R. (2000). Molecular mechanisms underlying learning-related long-lasting synaptic plasticity. In M. S. Gazzaniga (Ed.), *The new cognitive neurosciences* (2nd ed., pp. 121–137). Cambridge, MA: MIT Press

Meltzoff, A. N., & Moore, M. K. (1999), Persons and representation: why infant imitation is important for theories of human development. In J. Nadel & G. Butterworth (Eds.), *Imitation in infancy.* Cambridge: Cambridge University Press.

Plutarch. (1965). Coriolanus. In *Makers of Rome: Nine lives by Plutarch* (I. Scott-Kilvert, Trans.). Harmondsworth, UK: Penguin Books.

Post, R. M., Weiss, S. R. B., Li, H., Smith, M. A., Zhang, L. X., Xing, G., Osuch, E. A., & McCann, U. D. (1998). Neural plasticity and emotional memory. *Development and Psychopathology, 10*, 829–855.

Rakic, P. (2000). Setting the stage for cognition: Genesis of the primate cerebral cortex. In M. S. Gazzaniga (Ed.), *The new cognitive neurosciences* (2nd ed., pp. 7–21). Cambridge, MA: MIT Press.

Rizzolatti, G., & Arbib, M. A. (1998). Language within our grasp. *Trends in Neurosciences, 21*, 188–194.

Rizzolatti, G., & Gentilucci, M. (1988). Motor and visual-motor functions of the premotor cortex. In P. Rakic & W. Singer (Eds.), *Neurobiology of neocortex* (pp. 269–284). New York: Wiley.

Rizzolatti, G., Fadiga, L., Matelli, M., Bettinardi, V., Paulesu, E., Perani, D., & Fazio, F. (1996). Localization of grasp representations in humans by PET: I. Observation versus execution. *Exp. Brain Res., 111*, 246–252.

Sanes, D. H., Reh, T. A., & Harris, W. A. (2000). *Development of the nervous system.* San Diego, CA: Academic Press.

Smith, E. E., & Jonides, J. (2000). The cognitive neuroscience of categorization. In M. S. Gazzaniga (Ed.), *The new cognitive neurosciences* (2nd ed., pp. 1013–1022). Cambridge, MA: MIT Press.

Stendhal. (1958). *The charterhouse of Parma.* Harmondsworth, UK: Penguin Books. (Original work published 1839)

Steriade, M. (1999). Coherent oscillations and short-term plasticity in corticothalamic networks. *Trends in Neurosciences, 22,* 337–345.

Wenning, A. (1999). Sensing effectors make sense. *Trends in Neuroscience, 22,* 550–555.

Young, J. G. (in press). The concept of culture. In J. G. Young, P. Ferrari, S. Malhotra, S. Tyano, & E. Caffo (Eds.), *Brain, culture, and development.* New Delhi: Macmillan India.

Young, J. G. (in press). Neural mechanisms mediating etiological influences: The developing brain, evolution, and culture. In J. G. Young, P. Ferrari, S. Malhotra, S. Tyano, & E. Caffo (Eds.), *Brain, culture, and development.* New Delhi: Macmillan India.

16
CHAPTER

J. Gerald Young
João Gomes-Pedro
J. Kevin Nugent
T. Berry Brazelton

The Infant and Family in a New Century: Integrating Clinical and Neuroscience Perspectives

Magallanes, Señor, fué el primer hombre
Que abriendo este camino, le dió nombre.
Magellan, Sir, was the first man
Both to open this route and to give it name.

Alonso de Ercilla, *La Araucana*
Canto I, strophe 8, 1569 (cited in Morison, 1978, p. 614)

As we finish this leg of our journey, we view our exploration as both opening a new route and generating appropriate names for the objects of our exploration. Scientific disciplines assign names with great specificity as new findings emerge, using this precision to organize their conceptual frameworks. At some point, however, the disciplines intersect in their activities and the differing nomenclatures are a barrier. Once again, naming becomes a pivotal element of exploration, as names now become both link and foundation to an integrated conceptual framework. Investigators concerned with the development and care of children are no different—as we understand something with greater clarity, we attempt to give it a name, or change its name, so that the continuing process of interpretation and validation can proceed. This book contains many perspectives, each using its own system of names, its own dictionary. One step in our journey to help children is to persist in our efforts to build a common vocabulary for the varying facets of their development.

☐ From Predictive Signal Mapping to Early Intervention Strategies: Applying Concepts of Brain Development to Infant Care

The essential question remains: Can we apply the emerging understanding of brain development to the clinical care of infants? Or is the distance separating the two domains still too great? Obviously, we do not use brain imaging techniques to guide our advice to parents for the emotional care of a normal infant. Where are the links between laboratory and clinical data? When we encounter a specific infant and family, matters are always more complex than in the neuroscience laboratory, creating a tendency to separate the two activities. A practical place to look for useful, authentic links would be by directly comparing the descriptions of data and theory from laboratory and clinical experts. Having ventured that it is now possible to associate the parallel paths of brain development and emerging skills in the infant, we will attempt this in a review of earlier chapters in our book, looking for evidence of matching processes at cellular and clinical levels of observation. We will ask whether principles emerge from developmental neuroscience research that are sufficiently practical to guide our advice to parents and policymakers—most significantly, whether the clinical theory and advice of experts appear to match our understanding of the dynamic development of the brain in the infant.

In the first chapter, Dr. Gomes-Pedro recalls many of the elements that, on the one hand, clinicians repeatedly identify as the central concerns of families seeking help and, on the other, are the fundamental components of early childhood development that preoccupy clinicians as they organize their observations theoretically. He invites us to join him on a journey, and provides a map indicating sectors of experience that will be explored at different levels in this book: the *unique characteristics* of a child, as evident in individual differences, individual developmental needs, distinctive attachment behaviors, specific competencies, and varying status of self-esteem; *motivation* as a central influence on families, including how it is developed in families and how it is transmitted to children; *social and cultural influences* as manifest in social inheritance, cultural identity and individual identity, cultural memories and cultural traditions, as well as cultural threats to adaptation; *threats to the child's adaptive responses and to development*, as viewed through the lenses of vulnerability and risk factors, responses to vulnerability, sources of resilience, types of stress, changing family structures, and the inevitability of change generally; *the evolution of human adaptive capacities*, including individual adaptative responses, life-span adaptation, attachment behaviors influencing adaptation, and cultural influences on attachment behaviors; and, finally, the conspicuous advantages of *early interventions.*

Well guided by the map provided by Dr. Gomes-Pedro, what will we find along the way? His map uses the language of clinical conceptualization, but we now aspire to fabricate a shared language that fits both clinician and laboratory neuroscientist. The concepts have converged sufficiently that we can use reasonable hypothetical models about underlying events that blend the observations of both clinician and neuroscientist, and be able to generate a preliminary integrated language, as described in the previous chapter. The following provides an initial series of examples indicating how this tentative common language can be used to group the observations from earlier chapters in the book.

☐ Applying Emerging Knowledge Through Public Policy

Initially, however, we must firmly locate our purposes: The ultimate goal in the consulting room or in the laboratory is to provide aid to as many infants and families as possible. To do so requires energetic attention to public policy, which means that we must ensure that knowledgeable experts have access to whatever indispensable forum will make it possible for their voices to influence public policy.

Dr. Brazelton focuses on themes such as cultural identity and risk factors, but he particularly accentuates the neglect of the developmental needs of children. He offers a fundamental challenge: the unforgiving fact is that we already know many of the critical environmental parameters affecting the development of cognition, emotion, and behavior in children, yet we do not apply this knowledge. He uses his own country, the United States, as the unhappy example of the most powerful country in the world persistently and systematically neglecting its own children. He prods us to begin at the national level because national policies affect so many fundamental influences on the lives and development of millions of children.

To choose a simple example from among factors affecting the infant, we consider his need for stability of environment and relationships. Bronfenbrenner's Developmental Principle Five suggests a way in which the detrimental effects of daily instability are mediated. Stability across the settings in which the child and his or her parents live is obligatory for the development of mutual trust, accommodation, communication, and information exchange; when settings become isolated this breaks down. Realization of this simple need becomes remarkably complex in modern cultures because it encompasses not only the child's home and school, but also the locus of child care programs and workplaces for each of the parents. Stress in the father's job is especially crucial, even more so than in the mother's workplace. This means that achieving stability is no longer under the control of the child's parents alone, requiring employer and community cooperation, and the initiation of government policies—all operating at the level of cultural influences. And what is the goal of these cooperative efforts? They are quite specific—to ensure reasonable stability of a setting nurturing the attachment situation so that the mother can provide physiological and behavioral regulation for the infant, and simultaneously be a stable educational platform enabling the infant to form primary memory prototypes, during synaptogenesis and other developmental processes, that will be conducive to his happiness and adaptation now and later in his development.

Bronfenbrenner's Developmental Principle 6 expressly states this amplification: Public policies and practices at all levels of a culture that affect the development of children must be active and effective, if we expect each child to adapt and function well in their lives. Is this extension of Principle 5 repetitious? Possibly, but it could be judged as indispensable because the tension between familial and government control over the lives of children is long-standing and confusing. Principle 6 indicates that it is not sufficient to be aware of infant needs, such as a stable environment, but that a culture must actively and effectively pursue their realization. It is an essential protection for children that their parents have initial and strong rights to determine the nature of the care and education for these children, and government intrusion must be minimized. This must *not* be confused, however, with government abrogation of its responsibility to recognize and implement basic policies and procedures reflecting the principles nourishing optimal development in children. Moreover, we must recognize that economic and philosophical-religious influences weigh heavily at this point, too often undermining the development of very large numbers of children to preserve the wishes and priorities of adults. Neglect of this cultural challenge is perilous for any society.

☐ Experience

While we focus on practical matters related to prevention, parent counseling, and clinical care, we are reminded by Dr. Greene that how we approach these activities is influenced by fundamental theoretical perspectives, which are easily neglected because they are so familiar, concepts as basic as development itself. Moreover, examination of the child by his or her dissection into components, which is necessary for many research studies and for theory building, can lead to the unintentional misunderstanding of his or her development if we neglect to put the child back together again.

Most importantly, Dr. Greene reminds us of the emerging focus on the "normalization" of the child: the fictitious creation of a "normal" child growing up in an "expectable" environment, rather than the rich and endlessly diverse experiences with which individual children are challenged and must cope—not an abstract set of experiences destined to channel their development along predictable, even acceptable, lines. This emerging recognition of the individuality of experience, which is obvious to a clinician listening to many children, demands that each child's reactions be considered in the context of each child's actual experiences. While this consequential recognition of context, meaning, and values in the lives of children is essential to viable child care and theories, it also is true that these same influential factors are those which clinicians caring for children have stressed for decades. Regrettably, these clinicians were insistently criticized for invoking the formative significance of these influences, because they were viewed to be scientifically unsubstantiated and invalid. While the clinicians might not have utilized the necessary research methodologies, they were good observers, and now theoreticians and many investigators are recognizing these discoveries. Those caring for, investigating, and theorizing about children operate at different levels of perspective, vocabulary, and evidence, but all need to be respectful of the work of others. Ultimately, the clinician must cope with the challenges of the most complex of these phenomena, the complete and whole child operating within the fullness of a rich and varied environment. It is not surprising that mustering evidence for clinical observations and theories has been more difficult than monitoring the response of mice in laboratory experiments. Each of the many research methodologies contributes to a more accurate view of the whole child. It is not methodologies that create the misapprehensions that encumber our theories, but our gradual, unintended fidelity to a method or its related theory as we necessarily focus our efforts on one element of investigative work. One powerful tactic for encouraging all investigators to remain attentive to the unique context of each child's development—the repetitive responses from the familial and other environment around each child—is to increasingly emphasize the nature of the infant's necessarily molecular, gradually expanding, learning about the massive stimuli confronting her during the prenatal, neonatal, and infant periods of development. Dr. Greene's focus on the individual context of each child carries us to a focus on how this is mediated: How does the child "internalize" this context so that it becomes the matrix of his or her adaptive responses, and how is it represented in brain functioning? At this point we reset our program, as we return to our design that *experience* is the core of our inquiry in the book, meaning how experience is transformed from environmental stimuli and genetic influences into brain function. The term *experience* connotes that the child, at any moment, is confronted by a massive and unique stimulus array—now identified by many clinical investigators as *context*—and responding to it. How do we examine "experience"? We begin with the brain's utilization of the stimulus array for adaptive purposes, as it identifies motivationally significant signals and slowly sculpts the primary and secondary memory prototypes that will be the foundation of the child's coping strategies.

☐ Predictive Signal Mapping: Candidate Stimuli, Perceptual Discrimination, and Stimulus Significance Detection

We repeat our now familiar discovery, that the child—whether fetus, neonate, or infant—is an active learner, preparing herself for future contingencies. Preparedness is a prominent issue in the first months of life, and the development of the central nervous system makes it possible. Fifer presents data that we expect but commonly neglect as too difficult to verify, which indicates that this preparation for responding adaptively to environmental stimulus arrays begins prior to birth. He has demonstrated that the newborn, within the first day of life, can discriminate his or her mother's voice, and prefers her voice to either silence or an unfamiliar female voice. Moreover, a filtered maternal voice, altered to approximate the intrauterine maternal voice, was preferred over the unaltered maternal voice. Similarly, newborns prefer to listen to the sound of female voices speaking the language that the neonates heard in utero, suggesting their recognition of characteristic language features, such as intonation patterns. This is a highly significant finding, because it indicates that perceptual discrimination, and specifically the type of discrimination of sound regularities and patterns that is an essential initial step preparatory to building primary memory prototypes for spoken language, has already been initiated by the time the infant is delivered. By the time of birth, the neonate is already selecting predictive stimuli from among candidate stimuli, and using stimulus significance detection. Moreover, the response of the fetus is not limited to the very end of pregnancy. Preterm infants (26–34 weeks) also show discrimination of sounds in the environment, as indicated by fetal heart rate changes, suggesting that this type of learning has been progressing for a significant period of time. Aversive stimuli are also beginning to be separated from candidate stimuli, as fetal responses to high intensity (e.g., vibroacoustic) stimulation suggest that the fetus could respond to it as stressful.

Fifer's data document that, not only did the myth of a brain unresponsive to the environment during infancy not withstand scrutiny, but that now its capacity for response can be extended to the fetal period. This recognition consolidates our understanding of brain function, which is ceaselessly receptive to stimuli in the environment, recording them and determining their significance, then to be stored in memory. An active brain is available for participation in the crucial biological functions for each specific developmental period; we know that, during the earliest period of life (even the fetal period), when initial learning takes place, the first fund of memories and knowledge are burgeoning, attachment processes fundamental to the infant's development are active, the first experiences of emotions within oneself and emanating from others have their impact, and adaptive motivations in response to stimuli are being established. We are far from understanding the role of fetal experiences in establishing emotions and adaptive behaviors in the young child, and we do not yet understand parallel changes in neural and molecular functions, but tools for these "impossible" studies are emerging and carry promise for the future. If the fetus is capable of elementary responses to the environment, Fifer reminds us that we must consider that stress effects on the fetus also might be possible, and that emerging fetal indices might be useful for indexing possible disabilities otherwise silent at that time.

Dr. Lipsitt places cultural and clinical data describing the child's development, amassed in the twentieth century, firmly in the context of the neurosciences. His documentation of the infant's progress in developing sensory systems—examining data emerging about specific features of each sensory modality, including specific qualities, intensity thresholds, and preferences—indicates the infant's specific domains of increasing knowledge about the world as she puts together the building blocks of cognition. This description provides examples from decades of clinical research elucidating detailed sensory-perceptual processes in infants, which now can be linked to the more recent neuroscience explication of molecular and cellular events underlying these activities. These are processes selecting predictive stimuli from among candidate stimuli, and using them to develop more complex knowledge.

Dr. Lipsitt reviews data indicating the infant's progress in the development of the basic elements of perceptual skills. This progress increasingly is manifest in the baby's attention to composite elements or species-specific features fundamental to the development of emotions, behavior, motivation, and other basic processes. For example, early behavioral responses indicating the infant's immediate receptivity to human interactions are notable, and suggest elements biasing him toward the pleasurable motivations associated with a preference for being with other humans; these behavioral configurations are probably rooted in the fundamental biology of attachment behaviors. The cry of another newborn is recognizable to a neonate, causing restlessness and crying, and is distinguishable by the neonate from a computer-simulated cry, which does not produce the same behavior (Simner, 1971). At the outset of life, therefore, in addition to the basic sensory elements developing in each modality, the neonate recognizes the human voice and responds by imitation or some mechanism that eventually evolves into an empathic response. Moreover, Dr. Lipsitt tells us that the human female voice elicits cardiac deceleration in the neonate, while the male voice making the same sounds does not evoke similar responses indicating attention or observation. Thus, we recall the high-pitched sounds uttered by men to tiny babies, men who would otherwise not think of making such noises. Experience teaches us what babies like, and we respond accordingly. The attachment situation and genetic programming help guide experientially guided preferences in the learning infant, including the higher pitched voice of the mother, which becomes a predictive stimulus discriminated as highly significant. This matches Dr. Kuhl's findings concerning the infant preference for a high-pitched voice and the use of "motherese" by adults (Kuhl, 2000).

Dr. Lipsitt similarly argues that newborns manifest gradations of pleasure preferences, suggesting that motivational parameters can be defined at the beginning of life. Dr. Lipsitt reviews the work of his group examining patterns of newborn sucking bursts and pauses in response to varying concentrations of sweetness, indicating that the neonate monitors the pleasurable sweetness, with indicator responses both in patterns of sucking and in heart rate changes. They demonstrated that the biasing of behavioral preferences by experience (i.e., memories) is already identifiable in neonates. Using sucking rate as the indicator response, they found that the sucking rate (preference) for water was less in a newborn who had just had a 15% sucrose solution than it was for a newborn receiving only water (Kobre & Lipsitt, 1972). Significance detection and motivation already are consequential influences in neonates, and long-term memory formation makes preference-based choices possible.

☐ Formation of Memory Templates

At what age is there evidence for the presence of memory templates available for comparison with later environmental stimuli? Habituation techniques, indicating the presence of memory function, have been used to demonstrate that an infant is biologically at risk following a perinatal event, such as the presence of the cord around the neck or effects of obstetrical anesthesia on the infant. Dr. Lipsitt comments that habituation to a sound, indexed by the gradual reduction of their suppression of sucking, occurred much more slowly when compared to normal infants. Moreover, classical conditioning occurs in the neonate, as indexed by several methods, again attesting to the presence of active memory processes, including the formation and availability of memory templates.

☐ Formation of Primary Memory Prototypes

If memory templates are formed in the neonatal period, are they soon consolidated sufficiently through developmental processes—especially synaptogenesis—to endure and guide the subsequent adaptive responses of the infant? Very rapidly after birth, differential responses to stimuli can be observed, and begin to reflect experiences—sensory preferences are appearing, and environmental contingencies have begun to shape the responses of the baby. Dr. Lipsitt suggests that data indicating the baby's immediately growing experiential knowledge is validation of the clinician's emphasis on the importance of early life experiences; it is not to say that the outcome of many of them cannot be altered by future experiences differing substantially from the early ones, but that, all things equal, the initial months and years at least have the opportunity to shape the preferred adaptive responses of the infant and toddler. If there are no compelling and continuing experiences counter to this, then it persists. We can describe this as the enduring influence of primary memory prototypes formed during infancy, unless substantially important and continuing environmental changes alter the use of this set of memories for predictive purposes.

Dr. Lipsitt points out the significance of the transitional period, generally from 2 to 4 months of age, when genetically programmed, automatic reflexes are gradually replaced by voluntary responses shaped by experience with the environment. He postulates that an infant, lacking an obvious deficit but having a relative weakness in a significant function, might be more dependent on the results of coping experiences related to this function—because they are replacing the weaker function. This would maximize his success in a compensatory sense, in spite of his original relative deficiency, making him less vulnerable to challenges from the environment during this transitional period toward voluntary responses. As an example, he hypothesizes that the lack of such experiences in a child might contribute to his vulnerability to crib death, which occurs predominantly during this period. Of course, the environment can be helpful, and this is another example of how attachment can be a facilitator of development, as the mother recognizes a vulnerability and is particularly watchful and helpful in supporting the infant. Matters are not so obvious, however, as it is also possible that less ministration to the infant might lead to more experiences in coping herself. Again, the fragile balance of the transition from automaticity and dependence on the mother to increasingly autonomous responses is apparent. The sensible selection of experiences by the mother during this period is a defining determinant of how successfully the emerging cortical pathways supplant the subcortical responses, and how well the resultant primary memory prototypes serve the adaptive needs of the infant.

☐ Motivation

Can we say that infants are motivated to respond to certain stimuli in preference to others? Dr. Brazelton (1993) reminds us that recognition by parents of the need for *motivation* is evident in their emphasis on learning to succeed, rather than learning to fail, and the accentuation of the idea that "the child's success in development becomes experienced as their own success as parents" (p. 9). The biological foundation for motivational driving of behavior is apparent even in the newborn period, according to Dr. Lipsitt. Temporal conditioning of feeding schedules show classical conditioning features and render clear anticipatory phenomena, not only the expected increase in bodily activity, but also in the blood leukocyte count. Tactile, auditory, and visual stimuli have been used successfully in classical conditioning studies with infants.

Operant conditioning research also clearly demarcates the infant's capacities to be motivated by experience, Dr. Lipsitt reminds us, directly using memories of prior responses to determine subsequent behaviors. Examples are elements of the sucking response to influence fluid delivery or different shaped nipples to access the regular commercial nipple for sucking without a fluid. Memories of prior experiences enable the infant to respond to differential incentive conditions. Novelty is a powerful incentive that is used to indicate discrimination in different modalities (visual, auditory, tactile) from the first days of life.

Dr. Macfarlane also furnishes us with considerable wisdom about the motivation of families and children when making decisions about their own health. He makes it clear that abstract information, no matter how instructive and important, is less persuasive than expected unless it is accompanied by specific data (e.g., results of routine blood tests related to the information) about the individual's own health risks in relation to this general information. This immediately makes it difficult for the individual to pretend that this information has little relation to him. Moreover, he cogently points out that true effectiveness of public health presentations in the media is more likely to be achieved if there is individual follow-up by family pediatricians, visiting nurses, or other professionals. These comments indicate a practical and realistic understanding of the primary importance of motivation and its context for an individual.

A similar insight into a child's or adolescent's mind—meaning authentic recognition of the enduring imperative role of motivation in each individual's life—adds an important additional perspective to how we should plan population-based attempts to improve the mental health of children. Dr. Macfarlane reminds us that, from the prepubertal years onward, adolescents view themselves as responsible for their own health, even though parents recognize that it is their continuing responsibility. Therefore, any program which fails to include an intense effort to consider and respond to the perspectives and motivations of adolescents will lack fundamental elements necessary to achieve the motivation of the adolescents necessary to achieve the goals of the concerned clinicians. This includes the need for thinking through strong, essential motivations for teenage mothers when they are requested to follow specific guidelines during their pregnancies.

☐ Emotion and Emotional Memories

Emotion in the infant is not a common topic, but Dr. Lipsitt describes a most instructive illustration of its cardinal effects during the newborn period. Missing from most discussions of the neonatal period is a consideration of anger and aggression on the baby's part. While crying is a very common topic, it is often treated as if it is congenital and mechanistic, rather than reflecting a definite feeling state, one component of which might be anger. The example chosen by Dr. Lipsitt is apt, as it describes a predictable source of frustration bound to elicit a response from the infant: occlusion of the infant's nostrils by the breast or bottle/artificial nipple during feeding, interrupting his ability to breathe and causing him to forcefully turn his head away, move his arms vigorously, object vocally, and appear red in the face. The emotion is clearly recognizable to the mother, and is possibly the initial opportunity for an infant's anger to be misinterpreted. An individual's deep understanding of the causes of anger is an ability that has both useful and deleterious effects. In this instance, many inexperienced mothers would be likely to feel hurt by this angry display by their baby, and might completely misapprehend the actual cause. Mothers often say that breast-feeding was not successful with their infants without understanding why, and this is one common possible reason. Here again, the attachment situation has benefits, because the likelihood of repeated opportunities to observe the unintentional smothering is enhanced. Similarly, this train of events has a meaningful impact on the motivation of the mother to care for the infant, and, too often, an infelicitous grouping of several types of disengagements between infant and mother can initiate a prejudice in the mother that this is a "difficult" baby, or that "I always felt that he didn't like me." Humans fill in reasons where knowledge is lacking, and it is this type of situation that is fertile ground for a lingering misunderstanding. It is hoped that accurate knowledge about the baby's needs and behaviors will be more widespread in the future.

It should also be understood that this is another example of the concept that babies are not simply passive recipients of what the environment brings them, because they not only protest and free themselves from the occlusion, but also learn to position their heads differently in order to avoid the experience. However, this has an associated risk, because a determined mother might misunderstand the baby's purpose and behaviorally demand that the infant attach and hold herself in the same, specific (blocking) manner. In this instance, breast-feeding loses its motivational coloring, and the infant's dissatisfaction registers with the mother and leads to a switch to bottle feeding, and, very possibly, complex emotions (guilt, anger, confusion, regret, etc.) in the mother. Dr. Lipsitt properly emphasizes the pleasure focus of these transactions, because the pleasure of freeing itself from the blockage of breathing is a very strong incentive, just as pleasurable feeding is. Suitable instruction in how to feed the infant without disrupting breathing is a powerful facilitator of the child's pleasure through the mother, and, therefore, of their mutual attachment. Pleasure and, therefore, motivation become the heart of the solutions, and a major element of a felicitous outcome is the deepened motivation of each partner to interact.

When repeated sufficiently, these are not merely unpleasant experiences, but become emotional memories for both infant and mother—but most significantly for the infant, because the emotional memories, if sufficiently reinforced by similar experiences, can become primary memory prototypes that color the infant's emotional appraisal of the mother. This influence should not be exaggerated, because it is one among many, but we can now understand why such occurrences can take on a disproportionate importance while acting among the initial experiences defining each of the partners in the mind of the other—once again, most significantly for the partner in whom synaptogenesis and other developmental processes are occurring. The formation of these multiple primary memory prototypes can cumulatively give a tenor to the mother–infant relationship that affects stimulus discrimination and motivation, but, most importantly, emotional language.

☐ Sensitive Periods

Our repeated mention of the potentially enhanced significance of these events in the first year of life elicits consideration of possible "sensitive periods" in early childhood. The potential benefits of rapid intervention in the first hours and days of life are obvious, and have been validated by research by Dr. Kennell and colleagues showing that mother–child interactions are altered months later. In particular, expected attachment behaviors are less frequent, while interactions related to a perception of vulnerability and illness in the child are increased. Extended contact between the mother and infant in the first days of life may have an even more potent effect than early contact, to the point of reducing the rate of serious mothering disorders, such as infant battering and infant abandonment. Elegantly responsive reciprocal interactions documented between mother and infant in these first days are the playing out of the genetically entrained attachment behaviors, both prompted by and facilitating for neural and neuroendocrine activities that keep these biological processes active. However, while the biological impetus of these attachment behaviors is present, they will not be fully active if environmental obstacles arise. It would seem that little is required, only such likely events as prolonged quiet periods together for the mother and infant; these periods are highly gratifying, so there appears to be little threat to the emergence of attachment behaviors. Nevertheless, threats to the inception of attachment behaviors are too common in hospital settings, in spite of the increasing awareness of their importance. The power of these interactions within the attachment situation is suggested by many observations, including that extended time for interactions with the infant by the father also leads to increased caregiving behaviors by the father weeks later.

Dr. Lipsitt remarks on the mutually satisfying and pleasant interactions that fuel the baby's progress through "increasingly complex manipulations of the environment and other people." He recalls that "some types of learning disability and psychopathological conditions may well have their origins in the interplay between constitutional and experiential factors impinging on the baby from the first days. Our knowledge about these processes remains woefully inadequate today" (p. 70). We have much to learn about the trajectory of the gradual transmutation of genetic influences and environmental stimuli into behaviors heavily biased by experience. This remains a prime goal in our sciences, as we attempt to understand how fixed the potentially sensitive periods in the early months of life might be, if at all, and which behaviors remain mutable indefinitely, available to us for therapeutic aid later.

☐ Imitation Learning

Parents have long known that younger siblings put the knowledge of older brothers or sisters to good use by imitating their behaviors in every possible manner; this is especially vivid when the two are close together in age and tend to be together a lot, and the younger sibling's need to keep up is accentuated. Dr. Lipsitt reminds us of this distinct category of learning, and that it begins very early in life. As early as the second or third week of life an infant has the capacity for imitative behavior, and the model's behaviors can be held in memory for a few minutes or longer. The neural basis for imitative learning is now better known, including the localization of some types of imitation learning, and the role of mirror neurons, as described by several investigators. Moreover, we also recognize that this is another specific form of interaction and learning that is benefitted by attachment processes. It is obvious that more imitative learning can occur and be functionally useful if the partners involved are consistently close and available to one another during the earliest stages of life of the dependent infant. Attachment promotes more rapid and extensive learning through imitation of reliably present, repetitive behaviors by the mother.

☐ Emotional Language

What evidence do we find for the proposed formation of emotional language, with processes parallel to those occurring in conventional spoken language? Papoušek and Papoušek point out that parents unconsciously teach infants about language, and that this intuitive parental teaching is demonstrated by the sequence of behaviors in which a parent seeks visual contact with the infant, the infant consents, and the parent immediately (in 500 ms or less), and without awareness, replies with a "greeting response." This playful guidance by parents utilizes their continual adjustments to the infant's fleeting emotional and behavioral states in addition to their developing communication capacities. These mutually guided interactions have been captured by many clinical investigators on videotape.

> The intuitive character of this guidance guarantees a regular and repetitive delivery of behavioral patterns that facilitates integrative processes in infants—detection of contingency, conceptualization, prediction, expectance, and control of caregiving, anticipatory coping with interactional sequences that concern highly relevant adaptive capabilities, and thus are associated with a strong intrinsic motivation and expressive emotionality both in infants and caregivers. (Papoušek & Papoušek, 1981, 1987)

These coevolving patterns of exchange are fundamental to vocal development, but also to learning and concept formation generally, and they trace the parent's guidance of the infant through procedural communications to the beginning use of words with specific meanings and associations with objects. Words, and increasingly abstract concepts, launch cultural participation and a more rational, conscious use of communication. This traces the trajectory from a biologically based set of attachment behaviors and intuitive parental behaviors to their replacement by attachment tools that are used "at a distance," and are more conceptual and verbal in nature.

Papoušek and Papoušek remind us that attachment and bonding are not an end in themselves, or sufficient for the infant's progress. Rather, attachment is a key process that enables the emergence of other adaptive elements in the infant's developing repertoire. They meticulously describe how this dance to the melody of preverbal communication between mother and infant proceeds, and how it is vulnerable to both biological and environmental variation. As attachment enables and facilitates preverbal communication, so does the latter enable a gradual elaboration of attachment processes at a more complex level, as communication confers additional competencies and a push toward beginning attempts at autonomy in the infant. Moreover, embedded within this spiraling set of competencies and communicative abilities, there is a mounting development of emotional language between the partners.

☐ Attachment Behaviors

Genetic Predisposition and the Development of Stimulus Discrimination through Experience

Do we have evidence that attachment behavior in humans encompasses maternal regulation of infant physiology and behavior, as in studies of laboratory animals? Dr. Lipsitt points out that studies of smell exemplify aspects of the biology of attachment demonstrated in animal studies, such as their capacity to identify relatives hierarchically; infants orient to the odor of their mother preferentially by turning their faces toward their mother's used breast pad in preference to a nonodorous pad or a used breast pad from another woman (Macfarlane, 1975). While animal research suggests strong genetic influences on their discrimination capacity, this study of infants indicated that the capacity was not present in the first few days of life and might be strongly influenced by experience. In either case it shows the preparedness of the brain to register and respond to a caregiving mother immediately following birth, and gives a concrete, understandable example of the types of physiological regulators within the mother that directly affect the biology and behavior of the infant. These regulators operate within the context of attachment biology, reaffirming how important the physical proximity of the baby is in the first days of life. It also demystifies some of the findings reported by Kennell and his group, as it shows one of the physiological elements underlying the bonds. It is, further, a demonstration of the formation of memories that will have a strong effect on future pleasure preferences related to the mother. Dr. Lipsitt also notes that sensory preferences motivating the infant are not limited to the peripheral level, but can involve the cortex, as demonstrated by the neonate not overcoming habituation to a single component of a mixture of odors to which it had earlier habituated.

While evolution has structured attachment behaviors in the mother and neonate so that they are relatively automatic, there are clear benefits for instruction and guidance from the earliest days, as indicated by Lipsett. Tactile responses in the infant can initiate defensive behavior when he experiences possible motoric restraint or respiratory occlusion, and this can occur inadvertently while the mother is feeding the infant. If the mother fails to recognize the source of the infant's turning away and not feeding, her misinterpretation can impair the developing attachment emotions and emotional memories that motivate the mother and interfere with her attachment.

The Development of Motivation within the Context of Attachment Behaviors: Emotion and Emotional Memories

After examining the ecology of human development over many years, Dr. Bronfenbrenner has extracted specific principles that he identifies as the basis for a child's optimal chance to fulfill his genetic potential for adaptive capacities. There are six developmental principles cited by Dr. Bronfenbrenner, and his Developmental Principle 1 is stated as follows:

> In order to develop intellectually, emotionally, socially and morally Baby XXI requires the same thing: progressively more complex, reciprocally contingent interaction with one or more older people with whom he or she develops a strong, mutual, and irrational emotional attachment, and who are committed to her well-being and development, preferably for life. (p. 45)

This principle is itself complex, and contains many elements which themselves might be considered a separate principle. Bronfenbrenner emphasizes that there must be "an irrational emotional attachment," and that this commonly evokes questions about why it should be "irrational." We now know something of the nature of this answer and can provide guidance about why this should be the case. He identifies this irrational emotional attachment as "love," and comments how difficult it is to sustain a progressively more complex, reciprocally contingent interaction—it is hard work and requires motivation and considerable attention. Love fuels this arduous process, and this love must be active, reciprocal, and increasingly complex. Moreover, the interactional process is more fruitful when it is the infant who increases the complexity by introducing something new.

In sum, Dr. Bronfenbrenner specifies fundamental elements, necessary for a child's developmental progress, that are galvanized through reciprocal interactions with one or more persons who are developing mutual attachments with the child. This attachment is with an older person who is committed to her well-being and development, preferably for life, but certainly for the long term, and it is this commitment which provides a stable context. It has an "irrational" emotional element, identified as love, that is pleasurable and motivating and makes it possible to accomplish the hard work entailed: to deploy continuing attention to the child and his circumstances, and to participate in interactions that must be, to induce learning, active, contingent, and progressively more complex, and that are most fruitful when the child injects the novel element.

Influences Affecting the Development of More Complex Processing Units during Predictive Signal Mapping: Stability of the Attachment Situation and Physical Health

Bronfenbrenner's Developmental Principle 3 extends and emphasizes the concept of attachment, because it encompasses a long-term commitment to an older person, stating that the child's development will be facilitated by the reciprocal activity only if this activity occurs regularly over extended periods of the child's life in circumstances that are not repeatedly disrupted or subject to significant strains from the environment. Such circumstances, of course, favor joint attention and response selection, especially important when the adult must be making judgments about optimal responses that will enable the infant to move to a higher level of complexity. When frequent interruptions or significant stresses continue, they slow or stop the child's progress. Progress can be reestablished, but the ease of this process depends on familiar clinical factors, such as the length of time it was interrupted, the nature and intensity of the stress, or whether the child is no longer at the developmental level appropriate to his age. The parent and child *can* recover progress in their reciprocal activities, however; while there are sensitive periods in children, there do not appear to be critical periods that make reorganization impossible for these interactive phenomena. Nevertheless, the longer the delay, the more difficult to reestablish progress, as accumulating experiences and memories bias the child's adaptive preferences and behaviors.

The actual physical and neurological capacities of the infant to perform the attachment behaviors are typically ignored in discussions of attachment, and Montagner alerts us to the peril of overlooking these competencies. The intactness of the requisite systems can be viewed from three perspectives. First, an infant must possess the rudimentary physiological and anatomical equipment to carry out the behaviors; interference by a serious developmental disorder affecting the musculature or the nervous system, for example, could prevent the child from performing one or more of the attachment sequences in response to environmental stimulation. Second, the infant's *memories* associated with the primary attachment figure could be so compelling as to interfere with the full exhibition of the infant's skills: earlier motor responses to the mother, accompanied by intense emotional memories, might preempt the use of some recently acquired skills for a period of time until the child gradually learns the potential use and gratifications associated with the newer skills. Third, *imitation* of the mother's movements and behaviors will gradually lead to learned adaptations. However, as Montagner points out, the differing abilities and skill levels of a mother as compared to an infant— with an infant attempting to imitate aspects of the mother's behavior that he is not developmentally capable of performing—might disguise actual capacities that are visible when the infant is with other age peers, and "under conditions which 'compensate' their tonico-postural immaturity" (which otherwise make them unstable in the sitting position and unable to regulate the position of the head; these investigators used a specially designed seat and jacket to support the infants). In this setting, the two equal (infant) partners use the same equipment and can imitate each other and respond to each other in quite recognizable ways, all within their current developmental capacities (rather than attempting to imitate behaviors of an adult which they cannot manage yet). In the process, the infant demonstrates the possession of capacities that were previously invisible to observers, and that "form the foundation of its emotional, interactive, social, perceptual and cognitive development, especially with regard to maternal influence . . . " (p. 112). What are some of the functional indicators of these capacities? He specifies more gaze toward the face, hands, eyes, or feet of the other child; more gestures in relation to the other child, and of greater diversity; reproduction of the movements and utterances of the other child; and significant modifications of behaviors over the first few sessions, especially in the direction of increased contact with the other infant.

☐ Ensuring Maternal Capacities for Regulating Her Infant's Status and Activities

Bronfenbrenner's Developmental Principle 2 posits that the emotional attachment and reciprocal interaction between the child and her caregiver are dependent to a great degree on another adult who is available and involved through assistance, encouragement, and affection for the caregiver. It is helpful if this individual is of the opposite sex, but not essential. This principle reflects the realities of the hard work of being a parent: motivation is essential, and, while the child himself inspires motivating love, a different kind of love, for another adult, along with shared parental responsibilities, decision making, and planning, make this additional adult a powerful augmentation of the likelihood of developmental success for the child.

Bronfenbrenner reminds us to be attentive to cultural influences on developing children, in this instance the current high prevalence of single-parent families. He reviews cross-cultural studies indicating the risk of children in single-parent families for a great range of detrimental developmental outcomes in later childhood and adolescence. However, the data are complicated by the fact that these families also tend to have a history of problematic relationships and interactions from the early preschool years, which might be a more fundamental cause of the separation of the parents. Not all of these children have a poor developmental outcome, and the primary predictor of a good outcome seems to be the involvement of the father in assisting the mother with responsibilities for the children, even more than direct ministrations to the children themselves, or the presence of other family or friends to aid the mother and children.

Other cultural factors are identified by Bronfenbrenner as even more destructive to the favorable development of children, however (1979). He particularly emphasizes poverty and the instability and inconsistency of modern daily life, which affect all socioeconomic classes. A loving, supportive parent can sustain a child in spite of these forces, although the oppressive environment has increasingly damaging effects the older the child is. A long list of poor outcome descriptors fits these children, with a much greater chance that these cultural factors will have a deleterious effect on the child than the effect of a single-parent family alone. Poverty and daily instability interfere with attachment processes at all ages by occupying the parent's time, energy, and emotions. Opportunities for sustained learning, in a consistent situation that facilitates repetition of the material to be learned, is disrupted each time the mother is pulled away from the young child, interfering with emotion regulation and learning—particularly learning the subtleties of emotional language.

Biological or cultural variation in the infant and in the parent is expected and compensated for, and even useful. Yet in Chapter 8 Papoušek and Papoušek remind us that when either becomes too extreme, especially if it is coincident with a deficit in the other of the pair, then there is the danger that communication will be threatened.

Thus, it is well known that parents must be alert to the possibility of a biological deficit in the child which might curtail his or her capacity for participation in this rhythmic communication. More generally, the intrinsic motivation for these free-flowing, intuitive exchanges between parent and infant is to be found in the associated pleasurable emotions. But such emotions also reflect the ambience of the parent's life, and are vulnerable to disruptions when a parent suffers significant problems and dysphoric responses. These can easily taint and alter the interaction with an infant—for example, the emotional language accompanying conventional spoken language might vary much more than usual, confusing the infant's attempts to learn her emotional language, or the mother might alter her sleep schedule and the infant's state regulation might be disrupted sufficiently so that his attention deteriorates and his capacity for predictive signal mapping might deteriorate. While this type of emotional change in a parent will most often occur because of specific personal problems suffered, more general cultural shifts can also lead to a greater likelihood of parental dissatisfaction in their lives, and more difficulty for a parent when wishing to engage emotionally in a potential communicative situation with the infant. Poverty, neglect of the needs of families and children by government policymakers, and work hours ill-fitting for parents of preschool children are some of the common current cultural challenges to the necessary nurturance of parent–infant interactions. While intuitive parental responses, shaped by genetic inheritance, will remain the foundation of successful caregiving for infants, enhanced scientific knowledge of the needs of infants, and the practical influence of this knowledge on government policy and business decision making can have a markedly beneficial effect on the development of infants.

☐ An Expanded Model for Attachment Functions: Maternal Regulation of Infant Experiential Learning and Primary Memory Prototype Formation During Synaptogenesis and Other Developmental Processes

Maternal–Infant Interactions and Regulated Learning in a Social Context

Human learning is preferentially and specifically oriented toward the social world, which enables enhancement of the those adaptive capacities related to social stimuli, as opposed to other available stimuli in the environment. This reflects the evolutionary molding of the developmental phases characteristic of very young children: There is a prolonged period of dependency, which imparts vulnerability while the child is completely dependent on her parents or other adults—yet, this long period also is suffused with learning, and confers immense adaptive advantages for the child in the future. This tenuous balance between adaptive advantages and vulnerabilities is the focus of parental ministrations, individual habits, cultural customs, and government policies. Several familiar behavioral characteristics of the child bias his or her development toward success, however, including attachment behaviors, a preference for social learning, and the capacity to appraise, select, and seek varying rewards.

The attachment situation is the vehicle providing the base for stable learning. It provides an initial framework which spawns shifts in the types of parental aid provided to promote the child's adaptation to the environment, from parental control of the child's physiology and behavior, through all forms of learning, up to teaching the use of symbols and, eventually, abstract thinking. In a formal sense, it provides a stable base on which shared databases can be enlarged and new categories added. Reciprocal interactions kindle developmental progress within the stable framework provided by attachments to developmentally mature persons (parents or others) committed to her, her well-being, and her development for an indefinitely long period of time.

Human social learning must be active, like any other learning. This implies that there are "results" during the learning, meaning that by acting the child learns something about the environment: Will this action (looking, listening, attending, reaching, thinking while using a new category, trying out something as a possible new symbol, etc.) lead to a result that is, in the general sense, noxious, rewarding, or indifferent and uninteresting? There is also a requirement for reciprocity, which means that there is a selection and presentation of the information by the parent. This is the basis for the significance of the "style" of interaction on the side of the mother. Most important is the need for the mother to be aware of what information might be most useful for the child. This requires that the mother attend meticulously to the actions and communications of the baby, and then insert a pause which ensures that the child has completed her action; therefore, the mother has clearly attended to and absorbed the action, and the child has a second to shift to a receptive mode. The mother then selects a response which, if she is to optimize its utility for the infant, has two primary characteristics: it is contingent (it recognizes the interests and purposes of the child's initiating actions and responds specifically to them, often by repeating as validation of the child's understanding) and it is rewarding (it uses intonation, facial expression, and touching or other activities in a manner known to be gratifying to the baby). The reciprocity permits the learning to move forward because the back and forth gives repeated opportunities for validation and responses to subtle variations on the learning topic. These delicate variations are the initial introduction of increasing complexity, but a bigger jump in novelty can provide substantially more complexity, and it is the parent who must be able to judge whether a new level of complexity is sufficiently recognizable and understandable to the child to be useful, or whether it is confusing, uninteresting, or creates anxiety.

Later on the child learns a powerful new paradigm for learning, which is the use of the negative. In order to test his learning he does something and then awaits the parental response, thus initiating a testing session. This learning strategy is more appreciated by the child than the parents, who greet its full inception with the descriptor "the terrible twos." He is testing not only the predicted result, but related aspects of it, such as its reliability, its level of generalization, possible reasons for its occurrence, and similar matters. The child is now outside the close *physical* framework of the attachment situation (although still within the emotional, cognitive, and increasingly symbol-driven framework of the attachment situation), and his or her standardized reference system is no longer available to ease learning. Thus, a new strategy is needed for active learning and seeking validating responses, which the child supplies by doing things at a greater physical distance, which, nevertheless, gain the attention of the mother. We again emphasize that it is inherent and essential in all of these interactions that they are fueled by motivation, which is chiefly the irrational emotion known as "love," which is pleasurable and rewards the hard work of both partners in the interactions, but particularly the parent. It is detrimental to the development of a child if we fail to recall that rewards guide behavior.

Augmented Predictive Signal Mapping in the Infant: The Elaboration of Increasingly Complex Processing Units and Genesis of Novel Primary Memory Prototypes, Including Symbols

In Chapter 4, Bronfenbrenner's Developmental Principle 4 states: "The establishment of patterns of progressive interpersonal interaction under conditions of strong, mutual attachment enhances the young child's responsiveness to other features of the immediate physical, social and—in due course—symbolic environment that invite exploration, manipulation, elaboration and imagination. Such activities, in turn, also advance and support the child's psychological development" (p. 47). The stability and gratification of the child's interactions with his or her parents create sufficient trust and self-confidence that the child's curiosity and pursuit of gratification begin to shift to other elements in the environment. Bronfenbrenner cites the significance of this principle in relation to the choice of objects for the child's environment, and illustrates potential consequences of these choices by recalling the nature of toys, dolls, and related objects in relation to their effects on adaptive approaches such as activity versus passivity, encouraging imagination versus discouraging imagination, elaboration inducing versus elaboration deterring, mechanized versus not mechanized, exploration inviting versus exploration discouraging, violent versus nonviolent, and other adaptive contrasts. The objects favored by Bronfenbrenner are "whatever induces sustained attention and evolving activity of body and mind. . . . " Many objects in "postmodern societies" are well able to attract attention, but might not sustain attention or might have other deficiencies as indicated above. His guiding, but broad principle of selection of objects, is that they "are appropriate to the child's developing physical and psychological capacities" (p. 48).

This shift of dominant attention away from the parents is a vital step in the child's development, as it indicates that her predictive signal mapping begins a solid focus on the environment outside the attachment figures. As this occurs, she discriminates predictive stimuli in the wider environment with increasing success, and gauges the utility of various stimuli with greater sophistication as her significance detection capacities guide her and her motivation fuels her explorations. She forms primary memory prototypes in relation to all of these stimuli, so that her understanding of her wider environment achieves much greater breadth. She elaborates more processing units characterized by increasing complexity which, in turn, spawn additional primary memory prototypes. Most significantly, she is not only becoming familiar with the concrete features of her toys and objects around her, but is continuing to extend the languages that she is learning within the attachment situation. This enables her to begin to use the toys and other objects in a representational manner, playing out sequences of activities integral to her own needs. Objects can be categorized and relational elements among them established, but, most significantly, their dynamic use as powerful symbols becomes central to her activities, reinforced by her mother's responses.

We again underline that the child's needs and interests are heavily influenced by the attachment experiences that have been the foundation for his or her preferred adaptive strategies; these attachment experiences are the basis for the child's memories, which shape his or her interpretation of the meaning of events, especially for predicting later noxious or rewarding events. How does this transduction of attachment experiences into a child's adaptive preferences occur? Tracing a few of the infant activities affected by attachment activities with his or her mother gives a hint of the mediating events. For example, the child's disposition of attention is an intentional focusing on a stimulus, retaining the capacity to also deploy it over multiple stimuli, as contrasted to purposeless, anxiety-driven distractibility. An anxious, depressed mother, overwhelmed by poverty, will be inattentive to her baby at times, and his own increasing needs and anxiety will disrupt his capacity to focus on a single activity. Moreover, sustained anxiety within the mother—vividly portrayed to the watching baby through her altered facial expressions and gestural language, and her halting, indecisive speech—can have pronounced effects because it is occurring at the time at which face recognition and emotional language capacities are emerging in their respective cortical areas through synaptogenesis and the formation of primary memory prototypes. The specific nature of this predictive signal mapping places the infant himself at risk for protracted periods of anxiety or depression, or other responses to the mother's distress, including speech patterns that mimic his mother's speech or facial expressions or gestural communications that reflect what later would be described as anxiety or depression.

Imagination is an essential capacity for a child, as it enables the use and manipulation of memories, their categorization and elaboration into increasingly complex memory sequences, the recombination of all into novel configurations, and the increasing use and manipulation of symbols. Why is this important? Imaginative play opportunities are necessary for the child to be able to "try out" what he has learned, manipulate possible actions and outcomes, and consolidate his "findings" and preferences into a modified map of the world and how it works, producing modified adaptive strategies. In other words, the child forms, and increasingly consolidates, novel primary memory prototypes by repeated comparisons of these new prototypes (templates) with varied stimuli in the environment. This further stimulates the formation of more complex processing units, as necessary, to capture new category recognition or previously unappreciated relationships. Thus, nurturing outlets for the exploratory needs of the child, and responding to his novelty-seeking wishes, is more than trying to keep him happy—it encourages the development of increasingly complex categorization, relationships, and conceptual capacities generally, with a correspondingly related amplification of his symbolic capacities.

Bronfenbrenner emphasizes the role of these emerging capacities, such as for attention and for active and contingent interactions, which become the containers and are the prerequisites for a child's ability to fully respond to and utilize formal education. Moreover, these easily ignored capacities contain the cognitive ingredients that fuel adaptation in a modern society, such as thinking causally and logically, being attentive to the emotions and behaviors of others, learning respect for the needs and wishes of others in the context of diversity and individuality, organizing oneself in multiple ways, learning the importance of long-term goals and the patience required to reach them, recognizing sustained work and effort as the means toward accomplishing long-term goals, and similar practical concepts easily taken for granted.

In Chapter 9 Montagner specifies "five core skills revealed by our experimental studies on interactions between children 4 to 7 months old and other children of the same age" (p. 113). They are (1) the capacity for sustained visual attention; (2) a "hunger" for interaction; (3) increased affiliative behavior; (4) targeted organization of gestures; and (5) imitative behavior. These core skills of the first year are the foundation for more complex behaviors that arise during the first three years. They also reflect the extension of the infant's interests and capacities beyond those related primarily to the mother, as just described above. Developmentally disabled children, one group with autism and another group with cerebral palsy, were shown to have impairments in the five core skills. Nevertheless, Montagner indicates that they have data indicating that "under specific human and spatial conditions" the performance of these disabled children on the five core skills is significantly improved.

☐ Behavioral and Physiological Alterations Following Early Childhood Stress

In Chapter 5 Dr. Lipsitt makes a sensible plea that we utilize routine and unavoidable aversive, painful hospital experiences for infants (e.g., venipuncture, circumcision) to explore the conditioning that occurs in order to improve our understanding of the effects of stress at the outset of life, both deleterious and salutory (due to its promotion of adaptive strategies), and how behavioral effects might be sustained, especially in their relationships with caregivers. The advantage of such a paradigm is the relative simplicity of the interacting variables when compared to an older infant or child, for whom experience has already made the response to stress a complex matter. For example, is it possible that there would be a beneficial effect of mild aversive stress, until it reaches a threshold at which the painful stimulus begins to have a disorganizing effect? As he comments, the effects of the infant's immediate memory of the concrete event would likely be lost within the next weeks, but its effects on molding a habitual response to stress could be quite significant and continue to have repercussions years later.

☐ Culture and Cultural Identity

Paying Attention to the Stimulus Array Actually Processed by the Child's Brain

Recognition of the central role of cultural identity is evident in Brazelton's admonitions from Chapter 2 that efforts to facilitate the development of children must be embedded within their families and communities, and "respect and attention to diversity" is an essential element of any program. This reflects our understanding of how the child's *actual* experiences guide the development of her brain, and how to use our knowledge of her resulting preferences to optimize our supports for the young child's adaptation.

Cultural Influences on the Maternal Regulation of Infant State and Physiological Escape Phenomena

Dr. Kennell examines the effects of social inheritance at the level of a family's culture—

how cultural traditions, as cultural memories, are forged into a composite cultural identity that has profound effects on the behaviors of individuals when undertaking complex tasks like parental behaviors, especially when caring for infants and very young children. He analyzes how rapid cultural change, characteristic of modern times, can disrupt child-rearing patterns that evolved over centuries, and become a source of vulnerability for a young child. As an example, he portrays a cluster of risk factors related to attachment and bonding.

In Chapter 3 Dr. Kennell describes how advances in care for children in relation to their protection from medical disorders themselves led to procedures that caused secondary problems in mother–infant interactions. For example, the delivery of babies in hospitals instead of at home was a practice designed to combat high infant and maternal mortality rates, but it generated new problems. The increasing incidence of hospital infections in infants and mothers led to restrictions on the contact between the baby and family members, even including the mother, so that more care was given by nurses. While a reasonable solution, a byproduct was that the mother lost family sources of support during this trying period and the infant had reduced contact with its mother, diminishing the bonding between mother and infant in the first few days of life. Additionally, the use of sedation and analgesia altered the responsive capacities of the mother and diminished her abilities to become attached to the infant in the usual manner and to enact the anticipated maternal attachment roles. This led to, effectively, a separation for a few hours after the delivery. The simultaneous changes in family structures in the past decades leave fewer extended family members available for help and support to the mother, and to be advocates for the traditional practices surrounding childbirth, making it easier to intrude on the mother–infant relationship. Of course, the major reason that the relationship was not protected was a lack of knowledge among physicians, who dismissed any maternal complaints or requests as secondary to medical considerations and as unscientific and emotional.

This converging set of factors made it possible to neglect the developmental needs of infants by ignoring the evolution of human adaptive capacities that foster attachment behaviors between the infant and mother. Dr. Kennell points out that the essential adaptive role of attachment behaviors for the infant is undermined by this cultural threat to the infant's adaptation. The lack of recognition of the significance of attachment behaviors subverted an appreciation for the specific ties between culturally prescribed behaviors during delivery and the perinatal period on the one hand, and attachment behaviors on the other. This is a potent example of the relation between attachment behaviors and culture. It is best understood in the context of his group's review of birth practices in 183 societies, demonstrating that in 180 of these societies there is a period of days to weeks in which the mother and infant are together, enjoying the chance to extend their mutual bond, and not enduring the separation enforced by modern hospitalization. Formation of emotional bonds is not automatic and immediate within an hour after birth, as they demonstrate, but requires an opportunity for proximity. This, in turn, favors the action of "expectable" environmental stimuli (mother for the child, child for the mother), which induce the genetically endowed neural and endocrine mechanisms mediating bond formation—thus ensuring proper regulation of the physiological and behavioral systems of the infant. The initiation of these bonds is a fragile process that has been shown to be vulnerable to interfering processes, such as illness, and may alter maternal–child behaviors months or years later (Klaus & Kennell, 1982).

Enhancing Maternal Capacities for Regulating Infant State and Learning

In order to underline the vital role played by culture, we offer another example of the beneficial effects of respectful attention to cultural traditions—cultural memories that act as prescriptions affecting the biology of social interactions. This is the salutory effect for a mother, coping with the strains of labor and delivery, of the presence of a supportive woman, known as a *doula*. The presence of a doula contributes to significant health advantages for the mother and infant, such as a shorter period of labor, and fewer obstetrical interventions, including caesarian sections. Moreover, there are also indirect effects that facilitate the genesis of attachment behaviors between them. Dr. Kennell also cites data suggesting that the larger context of social support for a mother from pregnancy onward—the continuing presence of a male partner and family members—might have a significant effect on obstetrical outcome. Once again, these effects are presumably embedded in the neural and neuroendocrine activities of the caregiving woman during labor, and family members during pregnancy. This indicates the central role of human interactions and relationships throughout the life span, grounded in their biological roots and interacting effects, and suggests the basis for cultural rituals and practices—cultural memories—that enhance social interactions.

"Memes": Shaping Maternal Behavior through Influences from Her Culture and Her Infant

There are many unexpected turns on the road of our journey, as novel research findings guide us in new and sometimes startling directions. Many professionals and parents are surprised, for example, by the meticulous work already accomplished in the study of fetal responses and learning, as described by Dr. Fifer. Similarly remarkable is the potential impact of the challenge advanced by Dr. Nugent in chapter 7 for culturally inclusive research, and even more the challenges to conventional assumptions about the nature of development. This perspective emphasizes "*the primacy of context*," which implies questions about the appropriateness of research design, assessment tools, treatment strategies, and program goals in our clinics and offices.

Dr. Nugent emphasizes that shaping activities move in both directions, from the family and culture to the child, but also from the child to the culture. The child's temperament is one of the determinants of how the family and culture respond to her, with a strong influence on whatever the family or culture judges to be permissible or beneficial. Prescriptions for child-rearing techniques arise not only from cultural traditions, but become cultural traditions because the infants of the culture behave in a manner suggesting that this prescription will be useful and practical. This interaction is also an example of how important it is for a family or culture to respond to the individual child, nurturing and guiding him according to *his* needs, not an abstraction from elsewhere. The child, in turn, awakens in adults the memories of earlier instances of various behaviors, and their accompanying emotional memories, all of which drive the responses of the adults. We recall that these memories are both familial and cultural memories, and, therefore, can be thought of in terms of "memes," the postulated self-replicating units that are hypothesized to be units of cultural transmission (Blackmore, 1999; Dawkins, 1976).

The Influences of Cultural Mutation on Maternal–Infant Interactions in Multicultural Countries: The Advantages of Expanded Adaptive Strategies and the Risks of Dysregulation of Infant State and Learning

Dr. Nugent quotes statistics on the swift migration of populations, breeding multicultural countries across the globe, and corroborating that cultural diversity is becoming the rule and is no longer the exception. The need for an understanding of the effects of culture on infants and young children is greater than ever before, both to help these immigrant families and to learn more about child rearing and child development patterns in different cultures. In addition, the neglect of a child's cultural context brings with it an enormous distortion of our understanding of the development of children, a distortion that we are not even aware of.

Experimental and controlled designs bring with them the confidence that this scientific approach will bring unbiased results. This is true, but in a more restricted domain than we would prefer to think. What is left out of the study can be crucial, and nowhere is this more salient than potential cultural influences. Dr. Nugent vividly makes the point with examples of research producing decidedly counterintuitive results until relevant cultural factors indicate viable explanations. Examples include the stable state organization and low activity levels of Navajo infants, permitting their mothers to carry them on cradle boards; the better outcome at 30 days of infants of heavy marijuana-using mothers in a Jamaican subculture (vs. nonusers), due to more optimal environments; and the excellent mother–child play of Irish unmarried mothers with their one-month-old infants, and their lack of clinical depression, as the cultural response to their unmarried status shifts to an unanticipated favorable response to a mother and her baby. Most interesting was the study of sleep disturbances in Japan, clearly revealing the role of cultural expectations in the choice of responses to an infant's needs. In a culture promoting *amae* in its children—dependence or obedience—infants up to 3 years of age sleep with their parents or other family members, and sleep problems in these children are much less common than in the United States. However, examination of the infants indicated:

> that the behavioral repertoire of the Japanese newborn with his or her capacity for shutting out negative stimuli while asleep, as well as his relatively low tolerance for excessive levels of stimulation, serves as an enabling predisposition that ensures that the baby can deal with negative unpredictable stimuli when asleep but needs parental support when this stimulation becomes excessive, for his system at least. (p. 94)

This is a very different practice than in the American culture, in which infants sleep alone in a separate room. Each has its advantages and disadvantages, and neither can be termed *correct*. Yet, a clinician in a single culture will often emphatically defend a single solution for infant sleeping arrangements, unaware of the profound cultural determinants of adult solutions for a baby's needs. The discrimination of genetic and cultural influences is typically much more difficult than one might imagine, and many of our own culture-bound assumptions are necessarily quite unconscious. Developing a sensitivity to other possibilities is enhanced by an openness to the child-rearing practices of other cultures and makes us more thoughtful about our conventional interventions. The most significant danger, however, is that the restricted focus of much of our research, useful as it is for some purposes, will continue to fool us as we ignore the

immense power of the cultural context of parental behaviors that can have unanticipated beneficial effects on the child. We see ourselves and our culture when we observe and appreciate the nuances of another culture, and how they guide the infant's
adaptive capacities, beginning with the discrimination of predictive stimuli and their
significance, and leading inevitably to the forging of complex primary memory prototypes at a symbolic level—using symbols indigenous to the baby's culture.

For Dr. Nugent, a corollary of these considerations is that it can be risky for the
career of a clinical investigator if he is to put too much emphasis on cultural context at
the present time in the United States, because the current culture of psychiatric research does not emphasize this factor, in spite of admitting its relevance. Culture is
difficult to quantify, and is therefore easily dismissed as a soft, unquantifiable influence. Links between research at the cultural and controlled clinical investigation levels
are needed, and concepts from the developmental neurosciences offer possible connections.

Cultural Influences on the Regulation of Learning Parallel Spoken and Emotional Languages

It is always a surprise when a familiar scene is illuminated and viewed by someone
with a new lens, casting light on details in the picture that were present but not focused on previously. Papoušek and Papoušek examine the relationship of "nature" and
culture through meticulous observations of the initial preverbal communication between mother and infant. A bias in one direction or another leads to an overemphasis
on genetic or cultural influences, so we recognize that these are interacting forces and
both must be considered. They recall that not only are genetic influences handed down
from generation to generation, but that culture is passed from one generation to another through learning—just as precultural phenomena are passed down from generation to generation of animals as special skills that have been learned (they remember
examples such as migratory routes in herds, communication variants in birds, and
food cleaning techniques in primates). The early developmental period is central to
picking up these simple precursors of culture, as, for example, the requirement for
learning and play if primates are to gain the basic skills of tool use; lacking this opportunity, the use of tools remains at a less mature stage. If other animal species share
protocultural transmission of skills, it implies that we be attentive not only to the social
transmission of influences, but also to evolution and the genetic transmission of capacities that enable the cultural development of the specific adeptness of a species of
animals. Papoušek and Papoušek selected the capacity of the newborn to "trigger
speech" in caregivers: upon seeing a baby the caregiver speaks to her, knowing that
she cannot understand or answer. They have documented this preverbal vocal behavior, and examine it as an example of the extensive unconscious, intuitive parenting
behaviors emerging from genetic predisposition and additionally shaped by culture.
They view preverbal vocal behavior as more than an expression of emotion, but a beginning of the mutual entrainment of the parent and infant as they support developing
communication in the infant; in doing so, they utilize unconscious predispositions in
the parent to support preverbal vocal activities in the infant. They emphasize that verbal communication does not arise only as a product of human culture, but emanates
from precursors of speech observed in animal communication. We recall as an example
the research demonstrating vocal learning, using matching or labeling communica-

tion, in bottlenose dolphins, who appear to imitate sounds made by other dolphins; moreover, young dolphins take on a signature whistle pattern, akin to a name, early in life and use such signaling for social communication (Janik, 2000). The unique, newly evolved capacities of the human species, together with the progress of human culture as it aggregated knowledge, led to the unparalleled complexity of human communication. This reflects not only the remarkable evolution of communication capacities, but the intermingling and parallel development of conventional spoken language and emotional language.

☐ Interventions

Enhancing Maternal Capacities for Regulating Infant State

Brazelton developed "a system for reaching out to new parents" (p. 24), based upon "the points at which a change in the system is brought about by the baby's spurt in development"—a system known as "touchpoints" (p. 26). Nodal developmental periods are used as times for scheduled interventions to aid the family and help them prepare for coming changes (Brazelton, 1992). This approach is a model for a scientifically authentic intervention system that is, at the same time, practical and appealing to the parents who will benefit from it.

As our knowledge about the infant's developing organization of behavior and emotions has progressed so dramatically, the communication of this knowledge to those who need it most—parents—has persistently lagged behind. Recognition of this need for structured guidance to parents of infants, and finding a means for organizing it in a manner both developmentally attuned to the needs of the baby and accommodating to the reciprocal challenges emerging for the parents, is now possible, as demonstrated by the Brazelton program and others, notably the one described by Barnard and Sumner in Chapter 10. The content and goals of the latter were mapped onto "a specific progression during the first 12 weeks of the infant's life," and individualized for each family as necessary. The topics are the common features of infancy that are known to parents, yet of universal concern as parents hear different opinions and explanations from family members and friends: sleep–wake-feeding patterns; fussiness and crying; and smiling, eye contact, and other social behaviors. Parents learn to understand what is occurring in the baby and make choices about how to help the infant through the curriculum provided to them; they also are helped to anticipate novel changes in the infant in the coming weeks. The parents are tutored in the practical concepts from several different content areas, including "infant state, infant behaviors, infant nonverbal language, state modulation, and parent–infant interaction."

The type of training organized by Barnard and Sumner helps replace the guidance provided in the past through the parents' culture, religion, and extended family, but which might no longer be available. Yet, this parent guidance goes beyond this, in that it provides a condensation of the most important information drawn from clinical and laboratory sciences about the infant's development and needs, and how a parent can understand the baby's behaviors and can best respond to his or her needs. This is a notable advantage for any parent.

We have hinted at a universe of "small" facts and deeper conceptual understanding that previously was passed to new mothers in the filtered, sometimes factually mistaken, form of "tradition," and which was consoling to young mothers searching for guidance in infant care—but with the dispersion of families and cultures it began to fade. For example, an understanding of sleep–wake states, and knowledge about how to recognize each, is heartening to parents and likely to give them comfort in the first six months of life as they cope with this often worrisome aspect of infant life. More fundamentally, this can be protective of an infant's optimal development. For example, Barnard and Sumner remark that parents "occasionally mistake the active sleep state as a signal that the infant is waking." Similarly, mothers are notoriously concerned about their infants' nutrition, as are interested relatives. In this program mothers have a concrete guide to discern when they might be concerned about food intake: "We are concerned if infants in the first weeks of life have fewer than six feedings in a 24-hour period." Similarly, they break down infant behaviors of interest to parents into recognizable units that underlie interactions of infants and parents and are open windows for the influence of parents on a child (e.g., orientation to voice, habituation, consolability). This spurs a positive response to the infant that is more focused on the now recognizable needs of the baby. Through this understanding gained during the program developed by Barnard and Sumner, parents develop a greater breadth of responses to the array of behaviors and needs in their infant and rely less on a habitual, all-purpose comforting response, such as feeding or rocking. This targeted response enhances state regulation in the infant and optimizes the conditions for his or her attention to predictive signal discrimination, significance detection, and building spoken and emotional languages as precursors to a well-adapted life.

Enhancing Maternal Capacities for Regulating Infant Social Interactions and Learning

Interactive communication is more vivid and intelligible for parents following instruction about engaging and disengaging cues, both "potent" and "subtle," as well as cue clusters signaling states like hunger or satiation. The training program used by Barnard and Sumner provides simple instruction in caregiving techniques for infants, including suggestions for positioning of the baby, which enables the baby to see her mother better, and in itself encourages more interactions with her mother and strengthens the bonds between them. Instruction concerning the abilities of an infant can open a new world to mothers who were unaware of them and begin to engage and observe the infant in a more elaborated manner. Comments about temperament aid the mother's understanding of the individual characteristics of her baby and their normalcy, and encourage individualization of her responses. Such alterations in parental responses affect the quality and duration of interactions, the infant's control and pleasure in the interactions, and the infant's trust and interest in the parents. This is true not only for primiparous mothers, but also for experienced mothers who follow what they know and cannot respond to what they were never taught to understand. Similarly, by urging the parents to fill out a record of prespecified observations between visits, the training program helps parents to refine their observational skills, improve their conceptual understanding of infant development, and highlight areas of confusion. Moreover, enhanced understanding of matters such as infant states, and how to intervene to modulate and stabilize these states, helps parents know how to help regulate the infant's functioning in a natural manner, not only aiding the infant's comfort and development, but, more significantly, thwarting the development of significant problems that impair mother–infant interactions and can alter the image of the infant in the mother's mind, such as persistent sleep problems that cause the family to be persistently tired and irritable. Similarly, it is easy to underemphasize the importance of assisting the infant's motor development, and how the influence of these activities is amplified as they affect other sectors of development, such as maternal–infant interactions and the level of enthusiasm and role of activity in the infant's life. The authors focus on infant massage, infant exercises, and physical games as vehicles for engaging the infant in motor activities. These activities provide new and recurring sensory experiences to be integrated into the baby's growing repertoire of predictive signals to be detected as significant predictors of pleasurable occurrences associated with the mother or other caregiver. As in other interactions with children and families, the perceptiveness with which the clinician makes the intervention, particularly the responsiveness to individual family members, is the fuel that keeps everything moving. Validation of the responses and judgments of family members is essential, and compliments from expert clinicians are highly rewarding.

Understanding what is occurring, even if the parents can do little about it, can reduce tension in the parents, and the pressure to do something and be active, even if mistakenly. Barnard and Sumner make the point that this is particularly true when the parents understand the remarkable rate of brain development occurring, as well as the extraordinary learning that occurs as the infant makes sense of the mass of stimuli reaching him. Reducing parental anxiety can prevent the development of too much frustration and anger, and subsequent mistaken parental responses and the formation of negative mental representations of some qualities of the infant. Moreover, parents are in a receptive mood in the first months of an infant's life—curious, desirous of understanding more, frustrated by the noncommunication and puzzles presented by the infant—and this can be taken advantage of to set parents onto a more knowledgeable and involved path with the baby. Fathers can be especially gratified by their inclusion and their more informed understanding of their infants.

At the center of these instructions in the Barnard and Sumner program is augmentation of the parent's growing capacity for contingent responding to the infant, who learns trust, love, and the efficacy of his responses. This is a fundamental basis for cognitive growth, as the infant begins to form chains of predictable action–response sequences. This is among the mediating factors for the known predictor of better behavioral outcome in middle childhood in relation to the mother's higher educational level. At its most fundamental level, the baby is learning to recognize stimuli in her environment and understand their predictive meaning, and gaining a beginning sense of their significance—in short, engaging in predictive signal mapping.

Maternal Regulation of the Development of More Complex Processing Units and Emerging Skills

In Chapter 9, Montagner proposes the organization of space in the areas in which the child lives, even outside the home, in such a manner as to aid in the full development of these skills, creating "a strong probability of the emergence and development of the core skills that appear to be the foundation for the regulation and the future of emotional, affective, interactive, relational, social and cognitive systems in children" (p. 121). He describes the functioning of two such centers and their impact on the children and families under their care. The central theme emerging from these proposals is that they "show how a mother's view and behavior can change while the child itself changes" (p. 135). They describe "strategies and settings that, by enhancing the emergence of the skills of young children and enabling them to demonstrate them to their mothers and families, modify for the better their behaviors, views and images" (p. 135).

This unusual approach to the study of mother–infant attachment and interactions reawakens our recognition that there is a biological foundation to attachment behaviors. Montagner's research makes a crucial link between brain development enabling the emergence of component functions necessary for the full flowering of attachment and interaction processes, and how each of them must be recognized and nurtured if optimal development of attachment processes is to occur. This research is among the best demonstrating that problems with these component functions will have an impact on the behavior of the mother, following an initial period of her full engagement, as she ascertains that the expected responses of the child are not forthcoming. This is in agreement with clinical observations of clinicians caring for children with developmental disabilities. It is here that professional interventions can aid the mother and child by enhancing the child's capacity to demonstrate his best capacities and providing professional aid to encourage his mother's understanding and continued nurturing activities.

Public Health Applications

The reality of these needs for children, and how difficult they are to accomplish, hits hard when we reflect on Dr. Macfarlane's description. from chapter 11. of the needs for total population pediatrics worldwide in the twenty-first century. The context of multiple competing health problems, and the difficulties encountered when selecting priorities, awaken us to the need for mental health professionals to be highly imaginative if we are to accomplish the goals we set for ourselves. It is also true that pediatrics is awakening to the primacy of child development and mental health problems in outpatient, ambulatory pediatrics, and its pivotal role even within the hospital. Pediatricians are generally lagging in sophistication about the range of etiologies of these problems and the best interventions, and they have a very limited amount of time to respond to these problems. Mental health professionals have a strong mandate from pediatric population data to be advocates for bettering the development of children, effective administrators of viable and practical programs, investigators and monitors of diagnostic and intervention data, and efficacious front-line clinicians.

As we survey our varied strategies to help infants and families, we find ourselves returning to public policy as an essential arena for so many of these challenges, whatever the level of intervention. Dr. Caldwell recognizes that gathering information and recommendations from so many sources about a complex question—like what is best for very young children—generates its own challenges. The information from Chapter 13 reflects differing perspectives on a complex problem, and differing levels of analysis, yet requires integration into a plan of action to help young children. This presents uncommon challenges as these complex factors must be reduced to pragmatic actions that are effective and efficient, as well as acceptable and attractive to experts and the general public. Dr. Caldwell illuminates how easily these efforts can go astray, as well as the types of responses that might lead to success.

We have predicated our care for infants on our increasing understanding of their needs, but we also must consider the needs of adults—clinicians, investigators, administrators, parents—as we make decisions about implementation. This requires having a grasp of their understanding of the multiprong information and of their motivations. Dr. Caldwell reminds us that undertaking an effort to alter the ideas of the public about services for infants requires that the concepts be presented in an understandable manner with simple concepts and familiar language, with the recognition that for most parents the concepts will be unfamiliar; they are not clinicians or developmentalists. At the same time we must be thoughtful about the understanding of professionals, due to the bias contributed by their own professional discipline and training perspective. In this instance the significant element will be that the commentary will include remarks indicating reasons for the chosen strategy, gauged to respectfully help a professional put his or her own perspective into the overall framework of the strategy, rather than assume that an erroneous strategy has been developed.

Educare: An Inclusive Strategy for Public Policy

Most importantly, parents and professionals have varied motivations that must be woven into the structure of all strategies. Professionals working on specific sectors of the overall field bring biased perspectives and the natural competitive need to emphasize the point of view represented by their own field. Dr. Caldwell's approach illustrates the benefit of being inclusive, constructing a broad conception of the intended help to children—"educare"—permitting the various professionals to find their natural competitive domains within this broad area.

Supplementary care for children, especially young children, is required in all socioeconomic strata of society. The discussion of day care for children of poverty should be linked to a consideration of the roles of "nannies" or "babysitters" or day care in the lives of children of middle class or wealthy families. Dr. Caldwell makes a fundamental point too often neglected or misunderstood: to discuss with parents, particularly mothers, and to find supplemental care for their children, not only so that they can work, but also so that they can find time for their own personal needs, whether organizing their personal lives or taking time for pleasurable pursuits of any kind. The need is not questioned, but the forms of fulfilling these needs should be examined in the light of scientific information that will enable us to make the best choices at any given state of knowledge. It is, for example, peculiar that the effects of babysitters on young children receive so little attention from clinical investigators who themselves utilize their services for their own children. It is unquestioned that there are specific principles, spawned by the developmental needs of children at different ages, that must be fulfilled by a caregiving arrangement. These needs, and the available responses from caregivers, are what this book examines. These needs must be included within the boundaries of any integrated, comprehensive program that, nevertheless, remains flexible enough to respond to individual differences. Therefore, beginning with an inclusive conceptualization (e.g., educare) that does not ignore any of these needs for children, is the strategy that is optimal and will allow both parents and professionals to individualize programs according to their own knowledge of individual circumstances and needs.

These needs for families have always been present, but were remarkably amplified in the United States by the sudden entry of women into the workforce. Now most women also work outside the home and consideration of the quality of childcare arrangements cannot be ignored. As Dr. Caldwell points out, words and concepts emerge from earlier words and concepts. Thus, if we use a word or concept describing required care for very young children that neglects (purposely or not) an essential need, then we have handicapped our children and our own efforts at the outset. The inclusion of components that she describes reflects common sense and intelligent planning: health care (including safety recommendations), research (particularly outcome studies), training (far beyond the minimal levels so often observed today), and funding mechanisms. Of course, as in most human endeavors, economic constraints mold most of what is occurring, from unavailability of childcare for so many families who cannot afford it, to the dismal salaries for childcare workers that demean the field, imperil children, and reflect the actual valuation of children by Americans.

The shortsightedness of neglecting needs during early childhood development is astonishing in terms of the subsequent economic costs. Nothing is more important to any nation, but it is continually neglected due to the convenience of not understanding this need for society, and the reality that these are long-term goals whose results are conveniently obscured by time. Nevertheless, enough information is already available to assure us that appropriate strategies protect and nourish very young children sufficiently so that they have improved lives later. Better lives imply reduced economic expenditures. The current crises of terrorism surely warn us of the pitfalls engendered by ignoring sectors of populations whose lives are mired in poverty and hopelessness.

Interventions, Culture, and Public Policy: Models for Success

Most important is that the work of leading investigators demonstrates that there can be practical and successful interventions at the cultural level. Drs. Kennell and Klaus and their colleagues confirm this through their successful attempts to help the American public become aware of the benefits of "bonding" for the infant and mother (Klaus & Kennell, 1982); this is a good example of the utility of public education following upon the analysis of research data. Drs. Brazelton and Nugent and their colleagues have awakened popular knowledge and curiosity about infants through their "touchpoints" paradigm for parents, available through their publications and media education for parents. Communication is now worldwide, and the wisdom of caring and knowledgeable experts guides us in the care for our children wherever we might live, and using the major languages of the world (e.g., Brazelton, 1993). These are dramatic, positive cultural influences that deserve replication in relation to an expanding collection of topics. Our new understanding of any matter of substance is a gift for the next generation, to be valued and presented with the greatest possible clarity, and accepted with the respect that it earns, for it enhances the chances for happiness and productivity in future generations of children.

> Finally, the mother said, "When filial piety is gone, there can be no family. When family is gone, there can be no civilization. When civilization is gone, men are no better than beasts."
>
> Bette Bao Lord
> *Spring Moon* (p. 371)

☐ References

Blackmore, S. (1999). *The meme machine.* Oxford: Oxford University Press.

Brazelton, T. B. (1993). *Niños y padres: Del ano a los tres años.* (Traducción: Constanza Fantín de Bellocq). Buenos Aires, Argentina: Emecé Editores.

Bronfenbrenner, U. (1979). *The ecology of human development: Experiments by nature and design.* Cambridge, MA: Harvard University Press.

Dawkins, R. (1976). *The selfish gene.* Oxford: Oxford University Press.

Janik, V. M. (2000). Whistle matching in wild bottlenose dolphins (*Tursiops truncatis*). *Science, 289*(5483), 1355–1357.

Klaus, M. H., & Kennell, J. H. (1982). *Parent–infant bonding* (2nd ed.). St. Louis, MO: C. V. Mosby.

Kobre, K. R., & Lipsitt, L. P. (1972). A negative contrast effect in newborns. *Journal of Experimental Child Psychology, 14*(1), 81–91.

Kuhl, P. K. (2000). Language, mind, and brain: Experience alters perception. In M. S. Gazzaniga (Ed.), *The new cognitive neurosciences* (2nd ed., pp. 99–115). Cambridge, MA: MIT Press.

Lord, B. B. (1981). *Spring moon.* New York: Avon Books.

Macfarlane, A. (1975). Olfaction in the development of social preferences in the human neonate. In *Parent–Infant Interaction.* CIBA Foundation Symposium, 33, 103–117.

Morison, S. E. (1978). *The great explorers: The European discovery of America.* New York: Oxford University Press.

Papousek, H., & Papousek, M. (1987). Intuitive parenting: A dialectic counterpart to the infant's integrative competence. In J. D. Osofsky (Ed.), *Handbook of infant development* (2nd ed., pp. 669–720). New York: Wiley.

Papousek, M., & Papousek, H. (1981). Musical elements in the infant's vocalizations: Their significance for communication, cognition and creativity. In L. P. Lipsitt (Ed.), *Advances in infancy research,* vol. 1 (pp. 163–224). Norwood, NJ: Ablex.

Simner, M. L. (1971). Newborn's response to the cry of another infant. *Developmental Psychology, 5,* 136–150.

AUTHOR INDEX

SUBJECT INDEX

Acts of Meaning (Bruner), 180
adaptation, 14–19, 203–205, 243–244
  abuse and, 269–270
  attachment and, 214, 244–245
  attunement and, 250–252
  context and, 270–271
  hospital birth and, 319
  maternal regulation of physiological/
    behavioral systems, 245–249
  memory and, 219
  predicting behavior and, 213–214
  success of, 260–261
adolescents, 12, 16, 49, 227
affect matching, 252
affiliative behavior, 116–117, 123
aggression, 223
amae (dependence), 94
ambulatory care services, 165
American Academy of Pediatrics, 194
American Public Health Association, 194
amygdala, 237–243. *see also* brain
anger, in newborn, 70–73
anticipatory guidance, 7, 139–141, 155–156.
    see also behavior; parent-child interac-
    tion; touchpoints
  Nursing Child Assessment Satellite
    Training records for, 141, 147–151
  physical activities for parents, 151–155
arealization, 207
attachment, 17–19, 40–42, 106, 126, 304–
    305. *see also* childbirth; core skills;
    separation
  adaptation and, 214
  attunement and, 250–252
  changing family structure and, 11–13
  genetics and, 310–313
  health issues and, 312–313
  language learning and, 280–289

  later adaptive choices and, 249–250
  love and, 32–33, 46, 294–296, 311
  maternal employment and, 11–12, 194–
    195, 294
  mother-infant interaction and, 32–35,
    244–249, 252–255
  proximity maintenance and, 244–247
  as reference for learning, 290–293
  regulating infant state and, 289–290, 314–
    318
  Strange Situation test and, 195
  study of, 109, 112
  success of breast-feeding and, 9–10, 307–
    308
attentional development, 293
attunement, 250–252
audition
  classical conditioning and, 66
  deafness, 59, 66
  operant conditioning and, 69
  sensory mapping and, 212–213
  speech recognition, 79–84, 228–229, 232–
    234, 303
auditory cortex, 240
autism, 119–121
avoidance behavior, 70–73, 109, 116, 119–121

Babkin reflex, 62, 65
Baby and Child (Leach), 183
*Baby XXI-Child and Family: Changing Patterns
    at the Turn of the Century* conference, 3
Bagnols-sur-Cèze Maternity Hospital, 128–130
barn owls, 212–213
behavior, 142–144, 182–183. *see also* feeding
    schedule; infants; parents; sleep-wake
    cycle
  activities to encourage infant develop-
    ment, 151–155

335